STUDY GUIDE
TO ACCOMPANY DELMAR'S

COMPREHENSIVE MEDICAL ASSISTING

Administrative and Clinical Competencies

Fifth Edition

Barbara M. Dahl, CMA (AAMA), CPC
Program Director, Retired
Whatcom Community College
Bellingham, WA

Julie A. Morris, RN, BSN, CBCS, CCMA, CMAA
Director of Career Services
Medtech College
Atlanta, GA

Angela P. Rein, RMA (AMT), AS, BSHM, CPC, MAHS, CPC-H
Medical Program Director
Vatterott College–Online Division
St. Louis, MO

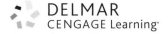

DELMAR
CENGAGE Learning®

Australia • Brazil • Japan • Korea • Mexico • Singapore • Spain • United Kingdom • United States

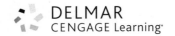

Study Guide to Accompany Delmar's Comprehensive Medical Assisting: Administrative and Clinical Competencies, Fifth Edition
Barbara M. Dahl, Julie A. Morris, Angela P. Rein

Vice President, Careers & Computing: Dave Garza

Publisher: Stephen Helba

Executive Editor: Rhonda Dearborn

Director, Development–Career and Computing: Marah Bellegarde

Product Development Manager: Juliet Steiner

Product Manager: Lauren Whalen

Editorial Assistant: Courtney Cozzy

Executive Brand Manager: Wendy Mapstone

Senior Market Development Manager: Nancy Bradshaw

Senior Production Director: Wendy Troeger

Production Manager: Andrew Crouth

Content Project Manager: Brooke Greenhouse

Senior Art Director: Jack Pendleton

Technology Project Manager: Brian Davis

Media Editor: William Overocker

Cover image(s): www.Shutterstock.com

For product information and technology assistance, contact us at
Cengage Learning Customer & Sales Support, 1-800-354-9706
For permission to use material from this text or product,
submit all requests online at **www.cengage.com/permissions.**
Further permissions questions can be e-mailed to
permissionrequest@cengage.com

Library of Congress Control Number: 2013933619

ISBN-13: 978-1-133-60301-6

Delmar
5 Maxwell Drive
Clifton Park, NY 12065-2919
USA

Cengage Learning is a leading provider of customized learning solutions with office locations around the globe, including Singapore, the United Kingdom, Australia, Mexico, Brazil, and Japan. Locate your local office at: **www.cengage.com/global**

Cengage Learning products are represented in Canada by Nelson Education, Ltd.

To learn more about Cengage Learning, visit **www.cengage.com**

Purchase any of our products at your local college store or at our preferred online store **www.cengagebrain.com**

Notice to the Reader
Publisher does not warrant or guarantee any of the products described herein or perform any independent analysis in connection with any of the product information contained herein. Publisher does not assume, and expressly disclaims, any obligation to obtain and include information other than that provided to it by the manufacturer. The reader is expressly warned to consider and adopt all safety precautions that might be indicated by the activities described herein and to avoid all potential hazards. By following the instructions contained herein, the reader willingly assumes all risks in connection with such instructions. The publisher makes no representations or warranties of any kind, including but not limited to, the warranties of fitness for particular purpose or merchantability, nor are any such representations implied with respect to the material set forth herein, and the publisher takes no responsibility with respect to such material. The publisher shall not be liable for any special, consequential, or exemplary damages resulting, in whole or part, from the readers' use of, or reliance upon, this material.

Printed in the United States of America
2 3 4 5 6 7 16 15 14

CONTENTS

This Study Guide is part of a dynamic learning system that will help reinforce the essential competencies you need to enter the field of medical assisting and become a successful, multiskilled medical assistant. It has been completely revised to challenge you to apply the chapter knowledge from *Delmar's Comprehensive Medical Assisting: Administrative and Clinical Competencies*, Fifth Edition, to develop basic competencies, use critical thinking skills, and integrate your knowledge effectively.

STUDY GUIDE ORGANIZATION

The Chapter Assignment Sheets are divided into the following sections: Chapter Pre-Test, Vocabulary Builder, Learning Review, Certification Review, Learning Application, Chapter Post-Test, and Self-Assessment. The content of the Study Guide has been designed to give you a creative and interpretive forum to apply the knowledge you have learned, not simply to repeat information to answer questions. Realistic simulations appear throughout the Study Guide that reference the characters in the textbook. This gives the material a real-world feel that comes as close as possible to your future experiences in an ambulatory setting. Clinical principles, such as infection control or communication and patient education, are repeatedly reinforced through simulation exercises that require the ability to use your knowledge effectively and readily.

COMPREHENSIVE EXAMINATION

Feel certain that each procedure and concept you master is an important step toward preparing your skills and knowledge for the workplace. A final comprehensive examination is presented at the conclusion of the Study Guide, covering all the essential topic areas that medical assisting graduates must master. This examination has 200 questions and provides excellent practice for national certification examinations.

FINAL THOUGHTS

The textbook, Study Guide, Competency Manual, and Premium Website have all been coordinated to meet the core objectives. Review the Learning Outcomes at the beginning of each chapter in the textbook before you begin to study; they are a road map that will take you to your goals.

Remember that you are the learner, so you can take credit for your success. The instructor is an important guide on this journey, and the text, Study Guide, Competency Manual, and practicums are tools—but whether or not you use the tools wisely is ultimately up to you.

Evaluate yourself and your study habits. Take positive steps toward improving yourself, and avoid habits that could limit your success. Do family responsibilities and social opportunities interfere with your study? If so, sit down with your family and plan a schedule for study that they will support and to which you will adhere. Find a special place to study that is free from distraction.

Because regulations vary from state to state regarding which procedures can be performed by a medical assistant, it will be important to check specific regulations in your state. A medical assistant should never perform any procedure without being aware of legal responsibilities, correct procedure, and proper authorization.

As you pursue a wonderful career in medical assisting, make the most of your education and training.

Chapter Assignment Sheets

CHAPTER **1**

The Medical Assisting Profession

CHAPTER PRE-TEST

Perform this test without looking at your book.

1. Certification demonstrates that a medical assistant has the body of knowledge associated with the profession. Which of the following describes certification?
   a. It is governed by state agencies.
   b. One must sit for and pass a national exam.
   c. It is mandatory.
   d. None of the above.

2. Once the CMA certification exam is passed and the credentials are awarded, what must be done to maintain that certification?
   a. Obtain continuing education credits that are sanctioned by the credentialing body.
   b. Retake the certification exam.
   c. Have continuous employment in the field.
   d. a or b

3. In 1978, which governmental agency recognized the profession of medical assisting?
   a. American Association of Medical Assistants
   b. Office of the Inspector General
   c. Department of Education
   d. National Healthcareers

4. In order to sit for the Certified Medical Assistant certification exam, one must:
   a. Have completed an accredited medical assistant program.
   b. Have a clean legal record.
   c. Be licensed in the state where they work.
   d. a and b

5. American Medical Technologists offers which certifications?
   a. RMA
   b. CCMA
   c. AAMA
   d. None of the above

6. Which professional organization defined the role of the professional medical assistant as "a multi-skilled member of the health care team who performs administrative and clinical procedures under the supervision of licensed health care providers"?
   a. CCMA
   b. NCCT
   c. NHA
   d. AAMA

7. National Healthcareer Association offers which of the following certification(s):
   a. Registered Medical Assistant
   b. Certified Clinical Medical Assistant
   c. Certified Medical Assistant
   d. b and c

8. Scope of practice is defined as:
   a. The limits placed on a professional's activities in the provision of patient care
   b. The granting of professional privileges
   c. A part of the accrediting process for medical assisting programs
   d. None of the above

9. Select the accrediting body that grants approval for the standards and guidelines for medical assistant programs.
   a. The Accrediting Bureau of Health Education Schools (ABHES)
   b. The Department of Education (DOE)
   c. The Commission on Accreditation for Allied Health Education Programs (CAAHEP)
   d. a and c

VOCABULARY BUILDER

Misspelled Words

Find the words below that are misspelled; underline them, and then correctly spell them in the space provided. Then insert the correct vocabulary terms from the list that best fit the statements below.

ambulatorie care settings	bachelor's degree	lisense
asociate's degree	competancy	professionalism
attributes	compliance	

_____   _____

_____   _____

1. _____ with standards and guidelines as stated by CAAHEP allows a medical assisting program to obtain programmatic certification.

2. Demonstrating _____ is a key to being a successful medical assistant.

3. Medical assistants find employment most often in _____.

4. Degrees available in medical assisting include _____ and _____ degrees.

5. Medical assistants are certified, but they do not hold a _____.

6. Successfully obtaining certification demonstrates _____ as a medical assistant.

7. An externship, or _____, is an opportunity for the student to apply classroom knowledge and skills in a real-world medical setting.

8. Integrity, responsibility, and compassion are _____ that are necessary for a medical assistant.

LEARNING REVIEW

Short Answer

1. Define ethics.

   _____

2. What are the benefits of certification?

   _____

3. Describe continuing education activities.

   _____

   _____

4. List five attributes of professionalism.

   _____

   _____

5. Describe the role of a Certified Medical Administrative Specialist.

   _____

   _____

6. Describe the history of the organization known as the American Association of Medical Assistants.

   _____

   _____

   _____

7. The U.S. Department of Labor, Bureau of Statistics, lists medical assisting as the fastest-growing allied health profession. Name eight settings where medical assistants are usually employed.

   _____

   _____

   _____

8. What is the purpose of the CARE bill?

   _____

   _____

   _____

9. State the benefits of graduating from a program accredited by either CAAHEP or ABHES.

_____

_____

10. What are some of the benefits that medical clinics receive as a result of being a practicum site?

_____

_____

_____

_____

Matching

A medical assisting curriculum should provide a variety of clinical, administrative, and general skills courses. Write a C next to each clinical course, an A next to each administrative course, and a G next to each general course.

_____ 1. Medical Records

_____ 2. Medical Law and Ethics

_____ 3. Urine and Blood Testing in the Laboratory

_____ 4. Insurance, Billing, and Coding

_____ 5. Pharmacology

_____ 6. Medical Terminology

_____ 7. Word Processing

_____ 8. Anatomy and Physiology

_____ 9. Appointments and Scheduling

_____ 10. Electronic Medical Records

_____ 11. Patient Education

_____ 12. Infection Control

_____ 13. Temperature, Pulse, Respirations, and Blood Pressure

_____ 14. Drawing Blood Samples

CERTIFICATION REVIEW

These questions are designed to mimic the certification examination. Select the best response.

1. Which of the following statement(s) best describe(s) the professional medical assistant?
   a. Has good written and oral communication skills.
   b. Looks and acts professional at all times.
   c. Is aware of the scope of practice and stays within the legal boundaries.
   d. Assists the provider in all areas of the ambulatory care setting.
   e. All of the above.

2. Medical assistants display their professional attitude by:
   a. discussing their personal lives at work because it is therapeutic for them
   b. talking with their coworkers to help them with their problems

    c. reminding their providers that they work only 7.5 hours per day

    d. helping patients in a friendly and empathetic manner

    e. doing a basic workload

3. To become involved with their professional organization, medical assistants could:

    a. attend local chapter or state meetings

    b. attend a national conference or state convention

    c. join their national organization

    d. offer to serve on a local, state, or national committee

    e. all of the above

4. A system of values that each individual has that determines perceptions of right and wrong is called:

    a. laws

    b. ethics

    c. attributes

    d. attitudes

5. Stepping into a patient's place, discovering what the patient is experiencing, and then recognizing and identifying with those feelings is:

    a. sympathy

    b. association

    c. flexibility

    d. empathy

6. Which of the following contribute(s) to a professional appearance?

    a. Good nutrition and exercise

    b. Healthy looking skin, teeth, and nails

    c. Daily showering and use of deodorant

    d. All of these answers

7. Courses in a professional medical assisting program include a complement of general knowledge classes such as anatomy and physiology and:

    a. assisting with minor surgery

    b. CPR

    c. medical terminology

    d. all of the above

8. The type of regulation for health care providers that is legislated by each state and is mandatory in order to practice is:

    a. licensure

    b. registration

    c. certification

    d. a and c

9. The period in which a student is able to apply their newly acquired skills as a medical assistant prior to graduation is known as:

    a. practicum

    b. residency

    c. orientation

    d. none of the above

LEARNING APPLICATION

Critical Thinking

1. Describe two benefits for medical assistants who join their professional organizations.

   _____

   _____

2. Explain what opportunities are available for medical assistants to improve their skills while on practicum (externship).

   _____

   _____

   _____

   _____

3. Many employers require credentialed medical assistants. Give two specific reasons why this is the case.

   _____

   _____

4. Explain two ways in which a certified or registered medical assistant can remain current with changes in health care and technology.

   _____

   _____

   _____

   _____

5. Research which of the credentials is most widely accepted in your geographic area. How would pursuing a different professional credential affect your ability to find employment?

   _____

   _____

   _____

   _____

   _____

Case Studies

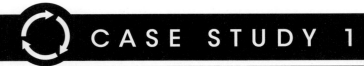

CASE STUDY 1

During your course of studies to become a medical assistant, you have an opportunity to volunteer to help out at a multiprovider urgent care center downtown in a large city to gain some firsthand experience in a professional setting.

CASE STUDY REVIEW QUESTIONS

1. Would this opportunity be interesting to you? Would you want to volunteer in this professional setting?

   _____

2. Even though you are a volunteer, why is it important to look and behave like a professional?

_____

_____

_____

_____

_____

CASE STUDY 2

Linda Ludamann is preparing for her practicum. Linda is an excellent student, detail oriented, responsible, and professional in her dress and attitude. Linda is eager to experience her practicum with a large general practice or clinic with open hours built into the schedule for emergency patients, such as Inner City Health Care. Linda is intrigued by the idea of working with a group of providers and a diverse patient population where she can really work on improving her screening skills. Linda, however, is shy and quiet; she has difficulty meeting new people and relies on a core group of friends.

CASE STUDY REVIEW QUESTIONS

1. Is Linda really suited to practicum at Inner City Health Care? What are the potential advantages or disadvantages of this practicum placement?

_____

_____

_____

_____

_____

2. What would be some ways in which Linda could overcome the difficulty she experiences when meeting new people?

_____

_____

3. Being able to work with diverse populations is just a small part of being a health care professional. What suggestions would you offer Linda in reaching her goal of professional growth?

_____

_____

4. Consider your own short- and long-range goals. How important is it to challenge yourself, personally and professionally, with experiences that contribute to your growth and knowledge? How can you use your practicum placement to work toward fulfilling your goals?

_____

Role-Play

Assign the role of provider, office manager, and medical assistant to a group of students in your class. Role-play a roundtable discussion regarding the benefits of certification and the merits of each certification that is offered.

Web Activities

1. Visit the American Medical Technologists (AMT) Web site at http://amt1.com to discover the answers to the following questions:
   a. Which allied health professionals, other than medical assistants and medical laboratory technicians, are credentialed by AMT?
   b. Does AMT have a code of ethics for the medical assistant?
   c. What are the eligibility requirements for individuals to sit for the RMA examination?

2. Visit the American Association of Medical Assistants Web site at http://aama-natl.org to discover the answers to the following questions:
   a. What allied health professions does the AAMA sponsor?
   b. What are the eligibility requirements for individuals to take the CMA (AAMA) examination?
   c. What resources are available on the Web for medical assistants that are interested in continuing education?

3. Visit the National Healthcareer Association Web site at http://nhanow.com to discover the answers to the following questions:
   a. What are the five functions of the organization?
   b. What is the NHA's goal?
   c. What is NHA's continuing education program?

CHAPTER POST-TEST

1. Which of the followings settings are appropriate for a professional medical assistant's practice?
   a. Medical laboratory
   b. Surgery center
   c. EKG department
   d. All of the above

2. Examples of licensed professionals are:
   a. physicians
   b. medical assistants
   c. nurses
   d. all of the above

3. The transitional experience for the medical assistant between education and employment is referred to as:
   a. practicum
   b. externship
   c. internship
   d. all of the above

4. Formal education of the medical assistant takes place in which of the following settings:
   a. community or junior colleges
   b. on the job
   c. proprietary schools
   d. a and c

5. Which accrediting bodies are responsible for evaluating medical assisting programs?
   a. CCMA
   b. ABHES
   c. CAAHEP
   d. b and c

6. What is the best definition of "attributes"?
   a. Characteristics or personal qualities.
   b. Morals and ethics.
   c. Certifications.
   d. None of the above.

SELF-ASSESSMENT

1. As you begin your education as a medical assistant, you may not be sure whether you want to work in the administrative and clerical area or in the clinical and laboratory areas. What are some ways for you to explore the various options?

   _____

   _____

   _____

2. For each of the attributes listed in your textbook to describe a professional, identify individuals from your family, circle of friends, work, or community who possess one or more of those traits. Explain why you chose them.

   _____

   _____

3. Imagine your first day in your practicum. What will you wear? How will you prepare the night before? How will you look? Would you change your hairstyle? Makeup? Jewelry?

   _____

   _____

   _____

   _____

   _____

   _____

   _____

   _____

   _____

   _____

CHAPTER **2**

Health Care Settings and the Health Care Team

CHAPTER PRE-TEST

Perform this test without looking at your book.

1. A branch of the healing arts that gives special attention to the physiological and biochemical aspects of the body's structure and includes procedures for the adjustment and manipulation of the articulations and adjacent tissues of the human body:
   a. Integrative medicine
   b. Osteopathy
   c. Chiropractic
   d. Osteopathic manipulative treatment

2. Provides comprehensive care of the eye and its structures and other vision services:
   a. Neurology
   b. Ophthalmology
   c. Immunology
   d. Otolaryngology

3. The most familiar managed care operation is a(n):
   a. Health Maintenance Organization (HMO)
   b. Independent Provider Association (IPA)
   c. Preferred Provider Organization (PPO)
   d. Ambulatory care setting

4. This type of medical professional will physically and chemically analyze, as well as culture, urine, blood, and other body fluids and tissues.
   a. Health unit coordinator
   b. Medical laboratory technologist
   c. Medical assistant
   d. Surgical technologist

5. _____ facilitates communication between the right and left sides of the brain with the patient in a state of focused relaxation when the subconscious mind is open to suggestions.
   a. Aromatherapy
   b. Acupuncture
   c. Biofeedback
   d. Hypnotherapy

6. Develops activity plans for each individual that integrate a complete approach to fitness and wellness through exercise, strength training, and proper diet:
   a. Occupational therapist
   b. Registered dietician
   c. Athletic trainer
   d. Personal fitness trainer

VOCABULARY BUILDER

Misspelled Words

Find the words below that are misspelled; circle them, and correctly spell them in the spaces provided. Then insert the correct vocabulary terms from the list that best fit the descriptions below.

accupuncture

ambulatory care settings

concerge

health maintainance
   organizations (HMOs)

homeopathy

independent provider
   association (IPA)

intagrative medicine

managed care operation

preferred provider
   organization (PPO)

screening

urgant care

_____   _____   _____

_____   _____   _____

1. _____ Organizations designed to provide a full range of health care services under one roof or, more recently, through a network of participating providers within a defined geographic area

2. _____ An independent organization of providers, whose members agree to treat patients for an agreed-upon fee

3. _____ Treatment using highly diluted doses of certain substances derived from plants, animals, or minerals that are manufactured by pharmaceutical companies under strict guidelines

4. _____ Medical setting that provides services on an outpatient basis

5. _____ A form of medicine where sterile fine needles are inserted in specified sites of the body

6. _____ Organizations in which providers network to offer discounts to employers and other purchasers of health care

7. _____ Alternative forms of health care increasingly perceived as complements to traditional health care

8. _____ A for-profit center that provides services for primary care, routine illnesses, and injury, as well as minor surgery

9. _____ Another avenue of health care that provides exclusive services for fees ranging from $2,000 to $6,000 per year.

10. _____ Assessment of patient needs to determine the priority of medical action

11. _____ A standard of patient care that seeks to provide quality care while containing costs

LEARNING REVIEW

Short Answer

1. How has managed care changed medical settings as the health care profession works to offer high-quality, cost-effective care to patients? What is the medical assistant's role in contributing to the efforts of the health care team in an era of managed care?

_____

_____

_____

_____

_____

_____

_____

2. Since medical assistants are often patients' first contact with the facility and the provider, what attributes must medical assistants possess?

_____

_____

3. Name six administrative duties of the medical assistant as a member of the health care team.

_____

_____

4. Name five clinical duties of the medical assistant as a member of the health care team.

_____

_____

_____

5. In the medical field, the abbreviation "Dr." is used, and the title *Doctor* is used to address the person qualified by education, training, and licensure to practice medicine. List the medical degree associated with each of the following credentials, and define each specialty.

MD	
DPM	
DC	

ND	
DO	
OD	
DDS	

6. Using a medical dictionary to help you, define the following seven medical and surgical specialists. (Refer to Chapter 2 of your textbook for a complete listing of medical and surgical specialties.)

Radiologist	
Obstetrician/ gynecologist (OB/GYN)	
Pediatrician	
Allergist and Immunologist	
Dermatologist	
Cardiologist	

7. Medical assistants are only one of many allied health and other health care professionals who form the health care team. Although medical assistants may not work directly with each professional, they are likely to come into contact with many of them through telephone, written, or electronic communication. List six of those types of professionals.

_____

_____

_____

8. In an effort to offer and receive alternative therapies, many health care providers and patients are pursuing integrative medicine as a complement to traditional health care. Name eight alternative forms of health care that may be currently perceived to supplement and complement traditional health care.

_____

_____

9. List at least five services that a so-called "boutique" or "concierge" medical practice offers.

_____

_____

_____

10. What is the role of the physician assistant? How does a physician assistant relate to a medical assistant?

_____

_____

_____

_____

Medical Settings Activity

For each of the three forms of medical practice management, list appropriate medical settings. Describe the patient's experience with care under each form of medical practice management. Note how patient experiences may differ and why this is possible.

1. Sole Proprietorships

   Medical settings: _____

   Patient experience: _____

   _____

2. Partnerships

   Medical settings: _____

   Patient experience: _____

   _____

   _____

   _____

3. Corporations

   Medical settings: _____

   Patient experience: _____

   _____

   _____

CERTIFICATION REVIEW

These questions are designed to mimic the certification examination. Select the best response.

1. The form of medical practice management under which personal property cannot be attached in litigation is a:
   a. partnership
   b. sole proprietorship
   c. corporation
   d. group practice

2. The minimum amount of time it takes to become an MD without specialization is:
   a. 6 years
   b. 8 years
   c. 12 years
   d. 4 years

3. In the ambulatory care setting, the medical assistant may prefer which of the following tasks?
   a. Educating patients
   b. Administration such as coding and billing
   c. Performing various laboratory tests
   d. All of the above

4. The American Society of Clinical Pathology is the professional organization that oversees credentialing and education in what allied health area?
   a. Nurses
   b. Medical laboratory
   c. Registered dietician
   d. Physical therapy

5. The specialty that is based on the belief that the cause of disease is violation of nature's laws is called:

   a. chiropractic

   b. osteopathy

   c. podiatry

   d. naturopathy

6. HMOs are organizations designed to:

   a. provide a full range of health care services under one roof

   b. employ providers who network to offer discounts to employers and other purchasers of health care

   c. include environments such as a medical clinic and a primary care center

   d. serve as an emergency room

7. In order to practice medicine, a physician must:

   a. go to college

   b. pay a fee

   c. take online courses

   d. obtain a license to practice from a state or jurisdiction of the United States

8. Another name of the organization where providers network to offer discounts to employees and other purchasers of health insurance is:

   a. IPA

   b. HMO

   c. PPO

   d. group practice

9. Another term for assessing the patient's needs is:

   a. screening

   b. prescribing

   c. taking vital signs

   d. monitoring

LEARNING APPLICATION

Critical Thinking

1. Evaluate the different health care settings and discuss the pros and cons of working in each setting.

   _____

   _____

   _____

   _____

   _____

2. From a patient's point of view, which health care setting do you think offers the most benefits? Why?

   _____

   _____

   _____

   _____

3. Review the three forms of medical management models. Which is probably the most advantageous from the provider's point of view? Justify your responses.

_____

_____

_____

_____

_____

_____

_____

_____

4. Recall a few types of allied health professionals and, working in small groups, create scenarios in which the medical assistant needs to coordinate patient care with two or three allied professionals.

_____

_____

_____

5. Identify as many reasons as you can for why patients might be seeking alternative approaches to traditional medicine. Explain your choices.

_____

_____

_____

_____

6. Compare doctors of osteopathy and chiropractic. When and why might one be selected over the other?

_____

_____

_____

_____

_____

_____

7. Discuss the validity of licensure or national certification for health care practitioners.

_____

_____

_____

Case Studies

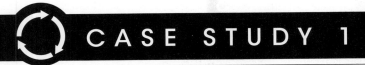

Abigail Johnson is an older woman in her 70s with adult-onset diabetes. She is having trouble managing her diet. She lives alone but craves social contact and seems to enjoy her visits to the family provider's clinic. She has an appointment today for dietary counseling.

CASE STUDY REVIEW QUESTIONS

1. How can Mrs. Johnson be encouraged to consider herself part of the health care team?

   _____

   _____

2. What is the role of the medical assistant?

   _____

   _____

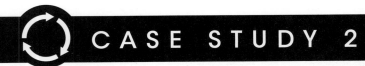

Herb Fowler is an African American man in his early 50s. Herb is a heavy smoker, is significantly overweight, and has a chronic cough. He believes the cough is caused by bronchitis and stubbornly insists on being prescribed antibiotics. Today, Herb is at the medical clinic for a preventive medicine appointment.

CASE STUDY REVIEW QUESTIONS

1. How can Mr. Fowler be encouraged to consider himself part of the health care team?

   _____

   _____

   _____

2. What is the role of the medical assistant?

   _____

CASE STUDY 3

Juanita Hansen is a single mother in her mid-20s with one son, Henry. Juanita arrives at the urgent care clinic for the fourth time in a month. Henry has fallen down the stairs twice, suffered a burn on the hand, and is now refusing to eat. There are bruises on various parts of Henry's body, as well.

CASE STUDY REVIEW QUESTIONS

1. How can the mother be encouraged to consider herself part of the health care team?

_____

2. What is the role of the medical assistant?

_____

_____

Web Activities

1. Use the American Board of Medical Specialties Web site (http://www.abms.org) to review details of the specialties. What does "board certified" mean? Identify those specialists for whom you would most enjoy working and give your reasons.

2. If you have doubts about alternative medicine, you might want to view the following Web site: http://www.quackwatch.org. Click on "What's new?" It is helpful to research as many thoughts on a subject as possible. Examine the validity of the Web site and whether any biases are evident.

CHAPTER POST-TEST

Perform this test without looking at your book.

1. A _____ performs nonclinical patient care tasks for the nursing unit of a hospital.
   a. registered health information technician
   b. health unit coordinator
   c. medical administrative assistant
   d. practice administrator

2. _____ are licensed by each state to prepare and dispense all types of medications as well as medical supplies related to medication administration.
   a. Nurse practitioners
   b. Medical illustrators
   c. Pharmacists
   d. Clinical laboratory technicians

3. For licensure, all states require physician assistants to complete an accredited, formal education program and to pass the Physician Assistant National Certifying Examination, which is administered by the:
   a. NCCPA
   b. NCLEX
   c. ABHES
   d. ARNP

4. Uses images or symbols to train the mind to create a definitive physiological or psychological effect:

   a. Medical illustrator

   b. Hypnotherapist

   c. Occupational therapist

   d. Guided imagery

5. Evaluates and treats medical conditions that result from trauma or sudden illness:

   a. Primary care physician

   b. Emergency medical doctor

   c. General practitioner

   d. Family practitioner

CHAPTER **3**

History of Medicine

CHAPTER PRE-TEST

Perform this test without looking at your book.

1. The first electrocardiogram machine was invented in:
   a. 1923
   b. 1903
   c. 1912
   d. 1910

2. _____ is the physician most frequently recalled from the Greek culture who created an oath that established guidelines for the practice of medicine.
   a. Jonas Salk
   b. Louis Pasteur
   c. Hippocrates
   d. Frederick Banting

3. _____ started the American Red Cross in 1881.
   a. Robert Koch
   b. Edward Jenner
   c. Clara Barton
   d. Ian Wilmut

4. In the year _____, a combination vaccine for measles, mumps, rubella and varicella became available.
   a. 2005
   b. 2006
   c. 2007
   d. 2008

5. In the United States, the first female physician was:

a. Clara Barton

b. Margaret Sanger

c. Elizabeth Blackwell

d. Florence Nightingale

VOCABULARY BUILDER

Misspelled Words

Find the words below that are misspelled; circle them, and correctly spell them in the spaces provided. Then insert the correct vocabulary terms from the list that best fit the descriptions below.

acepsis	pharmacopoies	typhis
alopathic	pluralistic	yellow fever
bubonic plague	septacemia	
malaria	trephination	

_____   _____   _____

_____   _____

1. In our _____ society, we rely on several philosophies of medicine that serve an individual's needs by respecting ethnic, cultural, and religious traditions while providing the best standard of care to patients and their families.

2. That bacteria can enter the bloodstream to cause infection, or _____, was observed in the nineteenth century by Hungarian physician and obstetrician Ignaz Philipp Semmelweiss.

3. Since the beginning of the twentieth century, the discovery of antibiotics, the development of vaccines, and the institution of proper health and sanitation measures have largely contributed to the containment of many infectious diseases, including _____, _____, and _____.

4. _____ physicians treat illness and disease with medical and surgical interventions intended to alleviate the condition or effect a cure.

5. A _____ is a book that describes drugs and their preparation and details plant, animal, and mineral substances as essential ingredients in effecting cures.

6. In the nineteenth century, _____, the process of sterilizing surgical environments to discourage the growth of bacteria, and anesthesia, the process of alleviating pain during surgery, revolutionized surgical practices throughout the world.

LEARNING REVIEW

Short Answer

1. Religion, magic, and science all play a vital part in the history of medicine. Describe each.

    Religion: _____

    Magic: _____

    _____

    Science: _____

    _____

2. Individual cultures and people throughout history have conferred different, and often changing, statuses upon women in medicine. For each of the five cultures below, describe the status of women in medicine.

    (1) Primitive societies: _____

    _____

    _____

    (2) Chinese: _____

    _____

    (3) Muslim: _____

    _____

    (4) Italian: _____

    (5) American: _____

    _____

3. Trace the progression of medical education by listing the important advances, discoveries, or medical philosophies for each period or century listed. What do you expect for the twenty-first century?

    (1) Prehistoric times: _____

    _____

    (2) Ancient times: _____

    _____

    _____

    _____

    (3) Seventh century: _____

    _____

    _____

    (4) Ninth century: _____

    _____

    (5) Renaissance: _____

    _____

    _____

(6) Nineteenth century: _____

_____

_____

(7) Twentieth century: _____

_____

_____

_____

_____

(8) Twenty-first century: _____

_____

4. Name 15 infectious or epidemic diseases that have been controlled in the twentieth century through medical advances and discoveries such as antibiotics, vaccines, asepsis, and insulin.

_____

_____

5. The Hippocratic Oath, which originated in ancient Greece, embodies within it many ethical standards of treatment and care that providers espouse to this day. In contemporary layperson's language, name the five basic standards contained in the oath.

_____

_____

_____

_____

_____

6. Fill in the blanks below with the three epidemics discussed in the chapter, along with descriptions of each and treatment options.

Epidemic	Description, Causes, Treatment

Matching I

For each of the following, write an R if the statement describes a belief in religion, an M if the statement describes a belief in magic, or an S if the statement describes a belief in science.

_____ 1. A recent research study involved two groups of patients with AIDS: One group received daily prayers from an anonymous prayer group hundreds of miles away, and the other received no prayers. The group receiving the prayers responded better to treatment.

_____ 2. Trephination was used by prehistoric cultures to release evil spirits responsible for illness.

_____ 3. Chinese acupuncture techniques are used to control pain or treat drug dependency.

_____ 4. Botanicals are effective in treating certain conditions. The Chinese pharmacopoeia is rich in the use of herbs.

_____ 5. Some Native Americans believe that someone recovering from a serious illness might hold extraordinary powers.

_____ 6. Some practitioners throughout history have held to the belief that healing involves not just medical treatment, but attention to the purity of the patient's soul and to the faith of the individual as well.

Matching II

Match the individuals listed below with each of their contributions to the history of medicine.

_____ 1. Andreas Vesalius

_____ 2. Sir Alexander Fleming

_____ 3. W. T. G. Morton

_____ 4. Moses

_____ 5. Edward Jenner

_____ 6. Clara Barton

_____ 7. Louis Pasteur

_____ 8. Elizabeth Blackwell

_____ 9. Hippocrates

_____ 10. René Laënnec

_____ 11. Robert Koch

_____ 12. Florence Nightingale

_____ 13. Anton van Leeuwenhoek

_____ 14. Wilhelm von Roentgen

_____ 15. John Hunter

_____ 16. Elizabeth G. Anderson

_____ 17. Leonardo da Vinci

_____ 18. Joseph Lister

_____ 19. Jonas Salk

_____ 20. Frederick G. Banting

A. Developed a vaccine for poliomyelitis

B. "Father of medicine"

C. Developed smallpox vaccine

D. Discovered penicillin

E. "Father of bacteriology"

F. Advocate of health rules in Hebrew religion

G. Invented the stethoscope

H. First female physician in the United States

I. Rendered accurate anatomical drawings of body systems

J. Wrote first anatomical studies

K. Laid the groundwork for asepsis

L. Started the American Red Cross

M. Founder of modern nursing

N. Introduced ether as an anesthetic

O. Discovered lens magnification

P. Discovered X-rays

Q. Founder of scientific surgery

R. Developed culture-plate method

S. Discovered insulin

T. First female physician in Great Britain

CERTIFICATION REVIEW

These questions are designed to mimic the certification examination. Select the best response.

1. Who of the following was not a scientist who contributed to the study of bacteriology?
   a. Louis Pasteur
   b. Robert Koch
   c. Joseph Lister
   d. John Hunter

2. The first female physician in the United States was:
   a. Clara Barton
   b. Elizabeth Blackwell
   c. Florence Nightingale
   d. Joan of Arc

3. The Oath of Hippocrates:
   a. establishes guidelines for all health care providers
   b. establishes guidelines for the practice of medicine
   c. is a well-known document about the ethics of ancient medicine
   d. was the first scientific journal of significance

4. The ancient culture that believed that illness was a punishment by the gods for violations of moral codes was the:
   a. Chinese
   b. Egyptian
   c. Mesopotamian
   d. Indian

5. Ancient healing priests performed many functions that involved the welfare of the entire community or village and were referred to as:
   a. shamans
   b. chi
   c. lipuria
   d. polypenia

6. Medical education in established universities began in what century?
   a. Second
   b. Fifteenth
   c. Eighteenth
   d. Ninth

7. In 1922, insulin was established as a treatment for diabetes by:
   a. Lister
   b. Pasteur
   c. Salk and Sabin
   d. Banting and Best

LEARNING APPLICATION

Critical Thinking

1. With a group of peers, identify the effects of culture on today's medicine.

   _____

   _____

   _____

   _____

2. How does the role of a medical specialist today compare to the role of a medical specialist in the past? Consider both similarities and dissimilarities.

   _____

   _____

   _____

   _____

3. You are the medical assistant. Your practitioner-employer has just prescribed opiates for a young Asian woman suffering from migraine headaches. You overhear the young woman arguing with her mother, who thinks that she should take non-addictive Chinese herbs. What, if anything, would you do?

   _____

   _____

   _____

   _____

4. Discuss with a peer the role of women in medicine today. What difficulties, if any, might a female practitioner face today? Compare today's difficulties with those of female health care practitioners 100 years ago.

   _____

   _____

   _____

   _____

5. Using the example of aromatherapy in the Frontiers in Medicine section, identify any new frontiers using integrative medicine that you know about or have seen used in patient treatment.

   _____

   _____

   _____

Case Studies

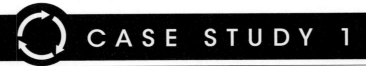

CASE STUDY 1

When 52-year-old Margaret Thomas, Martin Gordon's younger sister, begins to experience mild hand tremors and balance problems, Martin suggests that Margaret go see Dr. Winston Lewis. Dr. Lewis is Martin's primary care provider and had provided treatment for Martin's prostate cancer. Feeling more comfortable with a female physician, Margaret chooses to make an appointment with Dr. Lewis's associate in the group practice, Dr. Elizabeth King. On the day of the examination, she brings her 25-year-old daughter with her to the clinic.

After taking a detailed patient history and undertaking a thorough physical examination of Margaret, Dr. King makes note of signs and symptoms, including a resting tremor, shuffling gait, muscle rigidity, and difficulty in swallowing and speaking. Margaret also complains of a "hot feeling" and odd, uncharacteristic moments of defective judgment when "she just can't keep things straight." Dr. King suspects Parkinson's disease and tells Margaret and her daughter that she would like to refer Margaret to a neurologist for a more specific examination and medical tests. Dr. King explains that there are effective drug therapies for controlling the disease, although it has no known cure, and that the neurologist will outline Margaret's treatment options if a diagnosis of Parkinson's is made. Margaret seems to be shaken but takes Dr. King's words in stride.

Dr. King leaves Margaret and her daughter in the examination room with Audrey Jones, CMA (AAMA), who has assisted Dr. King throughout the examination and asks Audrey to be sure to give Margaret the referral to the neurologist. Margaret's daughter asks Audrey if Parkinson's is the disease that has shown promise in fetal tissue research and if her mother might be a candidate. Before Audrey can answer, Margaret becomes visibly distressed. "We're a good Catholic family, I could never consider that. Me—a grandmother." Looking to Audrey, she adds, "Please tell me I won't be involved with such a thing."

CASE STUDY REVIEW QUESTIONS

1. What part does the role of women in medicine and in society play in this situation?

_____

_____

_____

_____

_____

_____

_____

_____

2. How should Audrey, the medical assistant, reply to Margaret and her daughter? What course of action, if any, should she take?

_____

_____

_____

_____

3. How do religious beliefs make an impact on the attitude toward illness held by the patient? How might these beliefs affect a treatment plan?

_____

_____

4. Discuss the issues that arise when a potential medical breakthrough involves controversial or radical ideas that challenge long-held cultural viewpoints and beliefs.

_____

_____

_____

_____

_____

Web Activities

1. Do an Internet search using the keywords "penicillin discovered" to find some interesting sites. Determine the reasons it took so long to put penicillin into production. What kind of hurdles do new medications face today before they are available on the market to consumers and patients?

2. Search the Internet for "Women in Medicine: An AMA Timeline 1800s." This publication compiled by the American Medical Association provides valuable and interesting information about women in medicine. What surprises you the most? Are female applicants to medical school increasing or decreasing? By what percent?

CHAPTER POST-TEST

Perform this test without looking at your book.

1. In a technique known as _____, we can perform a whole-body trauma scan in less than ten seconds.
   a. magnetic resonance imaging
   b. volume computed tomography
   c. aromatherapy
   d. electromyography

2. This medication was discovered in 1943 and was designated to be the cure for tuberculosis:
   a. Penicillin
   b. Azithromycin
   c. Streptomycin
   d. Augmentin

3. What significant medical event occurred in 1978?
   a. The first heart pacemaker was created.
   b. Ether was introduced as an anesthetic.
   c. The vaccine for adult shingles was approved.
   d. The first baby created by in vitro fertilization was born.

4. What American president was diagnosed with polio in 1921?
   a. Theodore Roosevelt
   b. Lyndon Johnson
   c. Franklin Roosevelt
   d. Herbert Hoover

5. What medical procedure did Dr. Christian Barnard perform in the year 1967?
   a. Heart transplant
   b. In vitro fertilization
   c. Open heart surgery
   d. Lumbar puncture

SELF-ASSESSMENT

1. Make a list of the various ethnic, religious, and cultural groups you and your family members participate in or are descended from.

2. Interview family members to determine how their ethnic, religious, or cultural beliefs make an impact on the kind of medical care and treatment they expect to receive and how attitudes may have changed or evolved from generation to generation. Write a brief summary of your family's beliefs.

3. Write down any folk or home remedies used by your parents or grandparents that may or may not still be used by your family today. Why might these remedies have been more widely relied on by previous generations? Is there a scientific basis for each remedy?

4. An experimental treatment may be the only alternative available for your patient. How would this particular situation affect you, the medical assistant, if it is against your cultural or religious beliefs?

CHAPTER **4**

Coping Skills for the Medical Assistant

CHAPTER PRE-TEST

Perform this test without looking at your book.

1. _____ let events, other people, or environmental factors dictate their behavior.
   a. Outer-directed people
   b. Inner-directed people
   c. Micromanagers
   d. Role conflicts

2. _____ are achievements that may take three to five years to accomplish.
   a. Short-range goals
   b. Long-range goals
   c. Goal setting
   d. Goal focusing

3. The result of stress and frustration, principally brought about by unrealistic expectations, is known as:
   a. Goals
   b. Self-actualization
   c. Burnout
   d. Depression

4. Which of the following is *not* one of the four stages of burnout?
   a. Role conflict
   b. Dissatisfaction
   c. Sad state
   d. Reality

5. The body's response to mental and physical change is known as:
   a. Fight or flight response
   b. Frustration
   c. Management style
   d. Stress

VOCABULARY BUILDER

Misspelled Words

Find the words below that are misspelled; circle them, and correctly spell them in the spaces provided. Then insert the vocabulary terms from the list next to their definitions below.

burnout	outer-directed people	stress
goal	parasympathetic nervous system	stressers
inter-directed peepel	self-actualzation	sympathetic nervous system
long-range goal	short-range goal	

_____   _____   _____

1. _____ Achievements that may take several years to accomplish

2. _____ Fatigue and exhaustion that results from stress and frustration

3. _____ The body's response to change, which may be manifested in a variety of ways, such as increased blood pressure, increased heart rate, or headache

4. _____ People who decide what to do based on events, environmental factors, or other people

5. _____ Demands to change that cause stress

6. _____ People who decide for themselves what they want to do

7. _____ Achievement toward which effort has been directed

8. _____ Interim goal that helps to achieve a larger goal over a longer period of time

9. _____ Developing your full potential and experiencing fulfillment

LEARNING REVIEW

Short Answer

1. List and describe the four stages of burnout.

_____

_____

_____

_____

_____

_____

_____

_____

_____

_____

2. Han Selye's General Adaptation Syndrome (GAS) theory proposes that adaptation to stress occurs in four stages. Identify each stage in the order in which it is manifested and describe the physiologic changes that occur during each stage.

_____

_____

_____

_____

_____

_____

_____

_____

3. Identify six changes in your approach to your work environment and lifestyle that will help you to avoid burnout.

_____

_____

_____

_____

_____

4. List and define the five considerations important in determining a goal.

_____

_____

_____

5. Stressors are divided into three categories. List and describe them.

_____

_____

_____

Matching

Burnout is stress-related energy depletion that takes place in the working world. Burnout occurs gradually over a period of continued stress. Place a P next to those items that promote burnout and an R next to those that reduce the risk for burnout

_____ 1. Keep work separate from your home life.

_____ 2. Have regular physical examinations.

_____ 3. Work harder than anyone else in the clinic.

_____ 4. Feel a greater need than others to do a job well for its own sake.

_____ 5. Prioritize tasks and perform the most difficult ones first.

_____ 6. Prefer to tackle projects yourself rather than consult a supervisor.

_____ 7. Never stop until you achieve your goals, regardless of the personal cost to yourself or loved ones.

_____ 8. Postpone vacation time.

_____ 9. Give up unrealistic goals and expectations.

_____ 10. Maintain a positive self-image and your self-esteem.

_____ 11. Develop interests outside your profession.

_____ 12. Procrastinate.

_____ 13. Wear loose-fitting, comfortable clothes and shoes.

_____ 14. Stretch or change positions. Walk around and deliver charts or laboratory specimens.

_____ 15. Know your limits and be aware of your body's needs.

CERTIFICATION REVIEW

These questions are designed to mimic the certification examination. Select the best response.

1. The body's response to mental or physical change is called:
   a. stress
   b. adaptation
   c. denial
   d. burnout

2. Which of the following is not part of Hans Selye's general adaptation syndrome?
   a. Exhaustion
   b. Alarm
   c. Fear
   d. Fight or flight
   e. Return to normal

3. The four parts of the process leading to burnout are the honeymoon stage, the reality stage, the dissatisfaction stage, and the:
   a. sad stage
   b. angry stage
   c. retaliation stage
   d. giving up stage

4. In order for the body to survive, the sympathetic nervous system prepares the body for:
   a. fight or flight
   b. sleep
   c. developing a good appetite
   d. exercises

5. Time segments for short-range goals may be:
   a. monthly
   b. quarterly
   c. yearly
   d. all of the above

6. The result of long duration stress could be:
   a. making quick judgments
   b. job related
   c. immune system disorders
   d. an adrenaline rush

7. Stressors can be divided into which category(ies)?
   a. Frustration
   b. Conflicts
   c. Pressure
   d. All of the above

8. Needlessly worrying is an example of which type of stress?
   a. Short-term stress
   b. Episodic stress
   c. Long-term stress
   d. Intermediate stress

9. A common cause of stress in an organization would be:
   a. too much time spent on the telephone
   b. lack of motivation
   c. poor time management skills
   d. no smoke breaks

10. Discipline, perseverance, determination, and hard work are necessary in accomplishing:
    a. short-range goals
    b. long-range goals
    c. self-actualization
    d. prevention of burnout

11. The "wear and tear" our bodies experience as we continually adjust to a changing environment is called:
    a. adaptation
    b. stress
    c. prioritizing
    d. conditioning

12. The fight-or-flight response includes all but which one of the following reactions?
    a. Respirations and heart rate increase.
    b. Digestion is activated.
    c. Hormones are released into the bloodstream.
    d. Blood supply is increased to the muscles.

13. When individuals with a high need to achieve do not reach their goals, they are apt to feel:
    a. angry and frustrated
    b. tired and lonely
    c. distrustful and leery
    d. motivated and enthusiastic

14. The best way to treat burnout is to:
    a. cover it up
    b. get a prescription to help you cope
    c. prevent it
    d. encourage it

LEARNING APPLICATION

Critical Thinking

1. You have just graduated from a two-year medical assisting program and have been hired by a pediatric practice as an administrative medical assistant. The practice is busy with many telephone calls daily and many new patients who need charts created and information entered into the database. While in school you learned that you enjoyed the laboratory and clinical work much more than the front-office procedures. How do you think this position will impact your short- and long-duration stress?

_____

_____

_____

_____

_____

_____

2. Identify two long-range goals you personally would like to attain within the next five years. How will you achieve these goals?

_____

3. After you have been on the job for five years, you begin to recognize signs of burnout. How will you manage these symptoms?

_____

_____

_____

_____

_____

_____

Case Studies

CASE STUDY 1

Dr. Angie Esposito is a provider at Inner City Health Care. It was her dream, even as a child, to become a physician and work in an environment where she could help people and benefit the community as well. Proud of her accomplishments, she is the first woman in her family to attend college, and she got herself through medical school with scholarships and student loans. Dr. Esposito works hard, often pulling double shifts. Liz Corbin, CMA (AAMA), has a similar dream and is working to save money to attend medical school to become a pediatrician. Dr. Esposito does her best to encourage Liz's ambitions and has taken Liz under her wing.

Late one night, Liz assists Dr. Esposito in treating three difficult emergency patients in a row. "That's it," Dr. Esposito says. "We're taking a fifteen-minute break. Ask Dr. Woo if he can cover for a short time." When Liz catches up with Dr. Esposito in the employee lounge, she finds her frustrated and in tears. "These double shifts," she says. "I'm so tired. And the patients just keep coming. I want to help them all," she sighs, and her voice trails off, "I just can't help them all. . . ."

CASE STUDY REVIEW QUESTIONS

1. Dr. Angie Esposito is experiencing burnout. What personality traits are promoting her burnout? Identify the stressors in her life.

_____

_____

_____

_____

2. Liz Corbin sees her mentor breaking down under stress. Should Liz reevaluate her own long-range goals?

_____

_____

_____

_____

3. Discuss the importance of keeping goals in perspective.

_____

_____

_____

_____

4. What would be Liz's best therapeutic response to Dr. Esposito?

_____

_____

_____

Web Activities

Search the Internet for additional information about different relaxation and meditation techniques useful in reducing stress. Choose the technique that interests you the most and research it completely. Compile your information into a report for your instructor. Be sure to include a bibliography identifying your Web sources.

CHAPTER POST-TEST

Perform this test without looking at your book.

1. Which of the following is not one of the four characteristics of burnout?
   a. Role conflict
   b. Role overload
   c. Dissatisfaction
   d. Role value

2. Which of the following is a common cause of stress in an organization?
   a. Overspecialization
   b. Burnout
   c. Traumatic events
   d. Failure to satisfy needs

3. Which of the following is not one of the three categories of stressors?
   a. Prioritization
   b. Pressure
   c. Conflicts
   d. Frustrations

4. _____ decide for themselves what to do with their lives.
   a. Outer-directed people
   b. Micromanagers
   c. Inner-directed people
   d. Goal-oriented employees

5. The result or achievement toward which effort is directed is known as:
   a. stressor
   b. aspiration
   c. self-actualization
   d. goal

SELF-ASSESSMENT

Determining how well you now handle stress will help you to identify personal strengths and weaknesses and point you toward the skills you will need to develop to be successful on the job as a medical assistant. Complete the following stress self-test.

How Stressed Are You????

Answer each question with a 0, 1, 2, 3, or 4.

0 = never; 1 = rarely; 2 = sometimes; 3 = often; 4 = very often/always

Instructions for scoring follow the questions.

_____   1) My sleep is poor—delayed onset, wake early, or not restful

_____   2) I have headaches regularly (tension or migraine)

_____   3) I feel tense and anxious

_____   4) I rarely have enough time to complete tasks

_____   5) I experience frustration when trying to get things accomplished

_____   6) I feel like escaping, I wish I were somewhere else

_____   7) I feel like my schedule is controlled by outside factors or other people

_____   8) I feel angry even for no reason

_____   9) I feel overwhelmed by things that shouldn't be that hard

_____ 10) I eat more sugar and junk food than I want

_____ 11) I am not happy with the way I look

_____ 12) I have digestive difficulties (gas, cramping, irregularity)

_____ 13) I feel like I want to cry, I am tearful more often than normal

_____ 14) I can't concentrate

_____ 15) I have constant colds/flu/infections

_____ 16) I feel isolated even when around others

_____ 17) I am forgetful, even important things slip my mind

_____ 18) I have pain in more than one place in my body

_____ 19) I feel irritable

_____ 20) I am unorganized and lose things

_____ 21) I have cold hands and or feet

_____ 22) I am late for appointments or meetings

_____ 23) I have moist or sweaty hands

_____ 24) I talk rapidly

_____ 25) My heart pounds in my chest

Scoring

Add all your points together. You can have a total of 100 points.
The higher the score, the greater your stress response.
Keep in mind that your symptoms may not be just stress related—it is important to see your doctor if you are not feeling well!

0–25 — low

26–36 — low-moderate

37–50 — moderate-high

50–65 — high

+65 — VERY HIGH

(Courtesy of T. M. Geil, PhD. *How Stressed Are You????* PowerPoint presentation retrieved from www.wwu.edu/vpsa/nakama/documents/toi_Geil_TalkNakamaWeb.PDF)

C H A P T E R **5**

Therapeutic Communication Skills

CHAPTER PRE-TEST

Perform this test without looking at your book.

1. _____ involves being aware of what the patient is not saying, or picking up on hints to the real message by observing body language.
   a. Therapeutic communication
   b. Decoding
   c. Active listening
   d. Encoding

2. Which of the following is not one of the five Cs of communication?
   a. Clarity
   b. Cohesive
   c. Complete
   d. Concise

3. The study of body language is known as:
   a. Kinesthetics
   b. Kinesics
   c. Personal space
   d. Position

4. An opinion or judgment that is formed before all the facts are known:
   a. Bias
   b. Roadblock
   c. Prejudice
   d. Personal belief

5. The conscious awareness of one's own feelings and the feelings of others:
   a. Congruency
   b. Bias
   c. Self-esteem
   d. Perception

VOCABULARY BUILDER

Misspelled Words

Find the words below that are misspelled; circle them, and correctly spell them in the spaces provided. Then, insert the correct vocabulary terms from the list that best fits the descriptions below.

active listening	denial	open-ended questions
biases	displacement	prejidices
body language	encode	projektion
closed questions	hierarcky of needs	rationalization
cluster	high-context communication	regression
compinsation	indirect statements	repression
congruancy	interview technikes	roadblocks
cultural brokering	kinesics	therapuetic communication
decode	low-context communication	time focus
defense mechanisms	masking	undoing

_____   _____   _____

_____   _____   _____

_____   _____   _____

1. _____ Allows patients to feel comfortable, even when receiving difficult or unpleasant information, achieved through use of specific and well-defined professional communication skills

2. _____ The person seems to experience temporary amnesia; forgetting or wiping things out of the conscious memory

3. _____ Knowing how to encourage the best communication between the health care provider and the patient

4. _____ Human needs grouped into five levels, each level being satisfied first before moving on to the next

5. _____ Types of questions that require only a "yes" or "no" answer

6. _____ Verbal or nonverbal messages that prevent patients from expressing themselves

7. _____ The study of nonverbal communication, which includes unconscious body movements, gestures, and facial expressions

8. _____ Statements that turn a question into a topic of interest that allows the patient to speak without feeling directly questioned

9. _____ Being aware of what the patient is not saying or the ability to pick up on hints by the patient's body language regarding the real message

10. _____ Personal preferences slanting toward a particular belief

11. _____ An opinion or judgment that is formed before all the facts are known

12. _____ Nonverbal communication that conveys expression or feelings

13. _____ Types of questions that require more than a "yes" or "no" answer, the patient being required to verbalize more information

14. _____ An attempt to conceal or repress one's true feelings or real message

15. _____ Nonverbal messages grouped together to form a statement or conclusion

16. _____ When a person's nonverbal message agrees with that person's verbal message

17. _____ Interpreting the meaning of the message to understand it

18. _____ Creation of a carefully crafted message by a sender to match the receiver's ability to receive and interpret it properly

19. _____ Substituting a strength for a weakness

20. _____ The mind's way of making unacceptable behavior or events acceptable by devising a rational reason for it

21. _____ Refusal to accept painful information that is apparent to others

22. _____ Attempt to withdraw from an unpleasant circumstance by retreating to a more secure state of life

23. _____ Act of bridging, linking, or mediating between groups or persons through the process of reducing conflict or producing change

24. _____ Statements eliciting a response from the patient without the patient's feeling questioned

25. _____ Unconscious behavior used to protect the ego from guilt, anxiety, or loss of esteem

LEARNING REVIEW

Short Answer

1. List the three listening goals of the health care professional.

   _____

   _____

2. The four modes of communication most pertinent in our everyday exchange are:

   _____

   _____

3. Circle the five correct responses. The five Cs of communication are:

               coherent
    constant   curious
    credible   comment
    curt   cooperative

4. Understanding Maslow's hierarchy will help medical assistants assess patients' needs and facilitate therapeutic communication. For each level, list a minimum of three needs that meet it.

    _____

    _____

    _____

5. Identify eight significant roadblocks to communication.

    _____

    _____

6. In order for any type of communication to take place, the patient must trust the health care provider. List the necessary steps in building the patient's trust.

    _____

    _____

    _____

    _____

7. How does therapeutic communication differ from normal communication?

    _____

8. List and explain the four basic elements included in the communication cycle.

    _____

    _____

    _____

    _____

    _____

9. Edith Leonard arrives at the clinic for a routine six-month follow-up examination. At her last visit, she had been referred to an ophthalmologist for removal of a cataract in her right eye. Compose (1) a closed question, (2) an open-ended question, and (3) an indirect statement regarding Ms. Leonard's condition.

    Closed question: _____

    Open-ended question: _____

    Indirect statement: _____

Matching I

Identify each of the following as high-context communication (H) or low-context communication (L).

_____ 1. African American, Western culture

_____ 2. Relies on highly detailed language to communicate ideas

_____ 3. Asian culture

_____ 4. Native American

_____ 5. Relies on relevant phraseology to communicate ideas

_____ 6. Caucasian, Western culture

_____ 7. Hispanic and Latino cultures

_____ 8. Islam

_____ 9. Relies on body language to communicate ideas

Matching II

Biases and prejudices common in today's society have the potential to create hostility. Match each difficult situation below to the corresponding bias or prejudice that motivates it. Put a letter in the space provided.

A. A preference for Western-style medicine

B. The tendency to choose female rather than male providers

C. Prejudice related to a person's sexual preference

D. Discrimination based on race or religion

E. Hostile attitudes toward persons with a value system opposite to your own

F. A belief that persons who cannot afford health care should receive less care than those who can pay for full services

_____ 1. Mr. Gordon refuses to accept a referral to an acupuncturist to help alleviate the chronic pain of advancing prostate cancer.

_____ 2. Medical assistant Bruce Goldman mistakenly assumes that patient Bill Schwartz has AIDS when he arrives at the clinic with a gentleman friend, seeking attention for a recurring black mole on his calf.

_____ 3. Rhoda and Lee Au fear they will not receive adequate medical care because they use Chinese as their first language and speak only broken English.

_____ 4. Corey Boyer resists his gym teacher's efforts to get him to the clinic to check out a recurring rash on his arm because his family has no health insurance.

_____ 5. Mary O'Keefe is relieved to find that the practice's OB/GYN is a female physician, Dr. Elizabeth King.

_____ 6. Edith Leonard, a widow in her 70s, counsels medical assistant Liz Corbin that she should settle down and get married instead of pursuing a dream to attend medical school and become a pediatrician.

CERTIFICATION REVIEW

These questions are designed to mimic the certification examination. Select the best response.

1. Which of the following is not part of communication?
   a. Speech
   b. Facial expression
   c. Gestures
   d. Attitude
   e. Body positioning

2. Which is the most basic need in Maslow's hierarchy?
   a. Food
   b. Safety
   c. Status and self-esteem
   d. Need for knowledge
   e. Self-actualization

3. Your patient refuses to accept a diagnosis, claiming the doctor "must be mistaken." Assuming the doctor is correct, which self-defense mechanism is the patient using?
   a. Repression
   b. Denial
   c. Projection
   d. Compensation
   e. Rationalization

4. Congruency in communication can be described as when:
   a. the verbal message matches the body language
   b. the verbal message does not match the gestures
   c. the verbal message can be interpreted in two or more different ways
   d. two different messages are interpreted as the same

5. The conscious awareness of one's own feelings and the feelings of others is:
   a. congruency
   b. perception
   c. bias
   d. masking

6. The founder of humanistic psychology is:
   a. Jacobi
   b. Freud
   c. Erikson
   d. Maslow

7. The grouping of nonverbal messages into statements or conclusions is known as:
   a. assimilating
   b. feedback
   c. clustering
   d. introjection

8. The goal of therapeutic communication at the point of care is:
   a. to collect a blood specimen
   b. to determine the reason for the visit
   c. to explain the treatment plan for the patient
   d. all of the above

LEARNING APPLICATION

Critical Thinking

1. A 15-year-old girl awaiting a sports physical examination says that she is overweight and has pimples. How will you respond therapeutically?

   _____

   _____

2. Bill, who is 28 years old, comes for his annual checkup. When reviewing his social data sheet, you discover he is now living in an apartment and has a new phone number. He mumbles to you that his wife left him and won't let him see the kids. How will you respond therapeutically?

   _____

   _____

3. You try to be gentle and gracious with Edith. She is fragile and difficult to please. While positioning her for a radiograph, she sneers and says, "You are about the roughest person who ever cared for me." How will you respond therapeutically, and how will you control your body language?

   _____

   _____

   _____

   _____

4. When you report to Herb that his cholesterol is quite high and that the doctor wants to discuss medication and diet, he responds, "That is impossible; you must have made some mistake." Which defense mechanism is Herb using? How will you respond therapeutically?

   _____

   _____

5. How might the unequal relationship between provider and client/patient impact therapeutic communication?

   _____

   _____

   _____

   _____

   _____

   _____

   _____

Case Studies

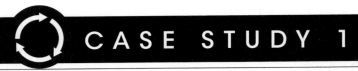

CASE STUDY 1

Wayne Elder arrives at the clinic for an examination to check on a recurrent ear infection that has been treated with antibiotics. Wayne, who is slightly retarded and lives in a group home, is still reporting dizziness and pain in his right ear. He has come to the clinic by himself, taking a bus from his job as a part-time dishwasher. Wayne's boss asked him to return to the clinic because Wayne could not concentrate at work.

Wanda Slawson, RMA (AMT), who is the medical assistant at the clinic, discovers from Wayne that he has not been taking his medication properly; he stopped taking his pills once his ear began to feel better. She must politely ask Wayne to repeat himself several times before she can clearly understand his slurred speech, and she has difficulty holding his attention or maintaining eye contact.

Wanda conveys Wayne's situation to Dr. Ray Reynolds, who examines Wayne and gives him a new prescription for antibiotics, gently explaining the need to finish the entire prescription to get well. After Dr. Reynolds leaves the examination room, however, it is clear to Wanda that Wayne is still confused about why he must take the medication even after he begins to feel better. Wanda carefully explains to Wayne that the infection will continue to heal even though he no longer feels sick. To be sure he understands, Wanda asks Wayne to repeat to her what he must do and why; she then asks Dr. Reynolds to step in briefly to remind Wayne once more to complete the prescription.

CASE STUDY REVIEW QUESTIONS

1. How does the unequal relationship that exists between patients and health care professionals have an impact on the therapeutic communication between provider, medical assistant, and patient?

_____

_____

_____

_____

_____

2. How must medical assistant Wanda Slawson tailor her verbal and nonverbal messages to meet the abilities of her receivers: the provider and the patient?

_____

_____

_____

_____

_____

3. How does Wanda use active listening? Which interview techniques are the most effective in facilitating therapeutic communication? Does nonverbal communication play a role?

_____

_____

_____

_____

_____

4. Using Maslow's hierarchy of needs, discuss how the health care team meets Wayne's special needs resulting from his disability.

_____

_____

_____

_____

_____

_____

5. Do you think the medical assistant acted appropriately? What else could she have done? What should she not do in this situation?

_____

_____

_____

_____

Role-Play Exercises

Active listening is an important element of therapeutic communication. To practice active listening skills, role-play as a patient and a medical assistant. Have the "patient" say each of the phrases below. The "medical assistant" should then rephrase each of the messages listed for verification from the sender and also include a therapeutic response. When you are finished role-playing, write what you have said in response to each statement below.

1. "I don't know what to do. My father takes so many pills he can't remember which is the right one, so he ends up refusing to take any of them."

_____

_____

_____

_____

2. "I can't give you my insurance card because I lost it and I can't remember the name of the company, either. You've always taken care of this before."

_____

_____

3. "I can't help being worried. The doctor just suggested a referral for treatment at that hospital where somebody had their wrong foot operated on. What do you think?"

_____

_____

_____

4. "I feel dizzy just thinking about having my blood taken. Do you really need to do it?"

_____

_____

Web Activities

Select three cultures of particular interest to you personally and search the Internet for information regarding these cultures and their communication traditions. How might this new information be applied to the provider whose clientele is primarily made up of these cultures? How might this new knowledge benefit a medical assistant employed in this type of setting?

CHAPTER POST-TEST

Perform this test without looking at your book.

1. _____ is attributing unacceptable desires, impulses, and thoughts falsely to others to avoid acknowledging they are actually the person's own experiences.
   a. Displacement
   b. Projection
   c. Regression
   d. Repression

2. Behavior that is used to protect the ego from guilt, anxiety, or loss of esteem:
   a. low-context communication
   b. rationalization
   c. defense mechanisms
   d. sublimation

3. _____ is a pattern of many concepts, beliefs, values, habits, skills, instruments, and art of a given group of people in a given period.
   a. Culture
   b. Lifestyle
   c. Ideals
   d. Compensation

4. What religion not only does not allow eating pork but also requires kosher food?
   a. Hinduism
   b. Judaism
   c. Buddhism
   d. Islam

5. _____ relates to whether the patient's attitude toward life is future, present, or past.
   a. Hierarchy of needs
   b. Caregiving expectations
   c. Cultural brokering
   d. Time focus

SELF-ASSESSMENT

Think about your own facial expressions and body language. Are you always portraying the message you want to send? List two situations in which you have been misinterpreted through your nonverbal communication, or situations in which you have misinterpreted someone else's message. Then think of what would have been a verbal message to help make the situation more accurate. That is, explain what you could have said to the person to determine if he or she was really hearing the message you meant to send.

C H A P T E R **6**

The Therapeutic Approach to the Patient with a Life-Threatening Illness

CHAPTER PRE-TEST

Perform this test without looking at your book.

1. The slowing of physical and mental responses, decreased alertness, apathy, withdrawal, and diminished interest in work:
   a. Depression
   b. Psychomotor retardation
   c. Mental retardation
   d. Terminal illness

2. A _____ allows an individual to make decisions related to health care when the patient is no longer able to do so.
   a. living will
   b. durable power of attorney for health care
   c. health care directive
   d. DNR order

3. When patients cannot believe they are dying, this is known as:
   a. Denial
   b. Depression
   c. Bargaining
   d. Acceptance

4. Patients who reach this stage of grief are sad and sometimes quiet and withdrawn:
   a. Denial
   b. Depression
   c. Bargaining
   d. Acceptance

5. This document will inform loved ones of the patient's decision related to whether or not they wish their life to be prolonged:
   a. Health care directive
   b. Medical power of attorney
   c. DNR order
   d. Durable power of attorney for health care

VOCABULARY BUILDER

Misspelled Words

Find the words below that are misspelled; circle them, and correctly spell them in the space provided. Then insert the correct vocabulary terms from the list that best fit the descriptions below.

durible power of attorney for health care   health care directive palyative   living will sychomotor retardation

_____   _____   _____

1. A _____ allows the surrogate to make decisions related to health care when the patient is no longer able to do so.

2. A _____ allows patients to make decisions (before becoming incapacitated) of whether life-prolonging medical or surgical procedures are to continue or be withheld.

3. _____ is the slowing of mental responses, decreased alertness, and apathy.

4. A _____ is a legal document that allows a person to make choices related to treatment in a life-threatening illness.

5. _____ measures are taken to relieve symptoms of disease.

LEARNING REVIEW

Short Answer

1. List five issues that are appropriate to discuss with a patient facing a life-threatening illness.

   _____

   _____

2. The federal government passed the Patient Self-Determination Act in _____, giving all patients receiving care in institutions that receive payments from Medicare and Medicaid written information about their right to accept or refuse medical or surgical treatment.

3. Explain what each of the letters in the acronym "TEAR" means as it relates to the grieving process.

   T = _____

   E = _____

   A = _____

   R = _____

4. What is the best therapeutic response to the patient with a life-threatening disease?

_____

_____

_____

CERTIFICATION REVIEW

These questions are designed to mimic the certification examination. Select the best response.

1. Your patient's culture influences:
   a. his or her views about illness
   b. his or her views about treatment
   c. his or her views about death
   d. all of the above

2. Your patient has just been diagnosed with a life-threatening illness. She tells you that she would much rather die quickly than to suffer through this disease. She asks you not to say anything about her comment to the doctor. What is your best response?
   a. You have had quite a shock. I believe Dr. King would like to talk to you about those feelings. May I go get him for you?
   b. You, above anyone else, know what is best for your life.
   c. I know what you mean; I would feel the same way.
   d. Don't worry about that right now. Dr. King will give you medication to help with the pain.

3. The health care directive and power of attorney for health care documents are legal in how many states?
   a. 10
   b. 25
   c. 5
   d. 50

4. The slowing of physical and mental responses, decreased alertness, withdrawal, apathy, and diminished interest in work are referred to as:
   a. passive-aggressive behavior
   b. fight or flight
   c. psychomotor retardation
   d. mood swings

5. The strongest influence in managing the life-threatening illness of a patient is the:
   a. health care team
   b. family and those closest to the patient
   c. social worker
   d. hospice

6. The range of psychological suffering a patient may experience can lead to:
   a. tachycardia
   b. anorexia
   c. agitation
   d. all of the above

7. What patients fear more than anything else when facing a life-threatening illness is:
   a. pain and loss of independence
   b. dementia
   c. financial issues
   d. becoming addicted to some medications

8. In caring for individuals with life-threatening illnesses, it can be helpful to remember:
   a. that family members have the strongest influence on patients
   b. that pain must be considered within a cultural perspective
   c. that choices and decisions regarding treatment belong to the patient
   d. all of the above

9. One of the most common emotions that a patient with a life-threatening illness may exhibit is:
   a. displacement
   b. denial
   c. depression
   d. assimilation

10. Referrals to community-based agencies or service groups may include:
    a. health departments
    b. social workers
    c. hospices
    d. all of the above

LEARNING APPLICATION

Critical Thinking

1. Discuss with a friend what cultural influences might affect each of you if you were facing a life-threatening illness. What choices would each of you make?

   _____

   _____

   _____

2. Discuss with a classmate your concerns in dealing with patients with a life-threatening illness. Would you choose to work where you seldom lost a patient to a life-threatening illness? If so, what are your reasons?

   _____

   _____

   _____

   _____

3. A danger in having a fair amount of knowledge about life-threatening illnesses and the grief that accompanies them can be that we hope to be able to "fix" everything. With a friend, discuss the following statement made by Dr. Kübler-Ross: "Listen to the dying. They will tell you everything you need to know about when they are dying. And it is easy to miss." What does she mean? Why is it easy to miss?

   _____

   _____

   _____

   _____

Case Studies

CASE STUDY

Jaime Carrera, a Hispanic man in his late 20s, is brought to Inner City Health Care, an urgent care center, by coworkers when he injures his head in an accident at a construction site where he is working. His head is bleeding profusely. As Jaime's coworkers watch the health care team implement Standard Precautions for infection control, one of them, his own shirt and hands covered with Jaime's blood, pulls the medical assistant aside and whispers frantically, "What are you doing? Does he have AIDS?"

CASE STUDY REVIEW QUESTIONS

1. What is the best therapeutic response of the medical assistant?

_____

_____

_____

_____

_____

_____

2. On what criteria do you base this response as the best therapeutic approach?

_____

_____

_____

_____

Role-Playing Exercises

With another student, role-play the following scenarios as medical assistant and patient. What is the medical assistant's appropriate therapeutic response or action?

1. The patient's wife has just found out that her husband has end-stage renal disease. She tells the medical assistant that under no circumstances should her husband be informed about the prognosis.

_____

_____

_____

2. The patient has been diagnosed with HIV. The medical assistant knows the patient is estranged from his or her family.

_____

_____

_____

Web Activities

1. Using your favorite search engine, key in "American Cancer Society" and look for statistics for the current year. Pay particular attention to the area reporting how long patients survive after diagnosis. What are the major changes in the last two years?

2. Search the Internet for sites on grieving or grief. Pay particular attention to sites that have resources for grieving children or teens. What particular help do you find? Do children and teens grieve differently than adults? If so, explain.

CHAPTER POST-TEST

1. The best therapeutic response to the patient with a life-threatening illness will build on the:
   a. person's own culture and coping abilities
   b. capitalize on strengths and maintain hope
   c. show continued human care and concern.
   d. all of the above

2. What does the letter "R" in the acronym TEAR stand for?
   a. Reconstruct a new reality
   b. Reinvent a new reality
   c. Reinvest in a new reality
   d. Readjust to a new reality

3. The most common signs and symptoms of advanced cancer are:
   a. loss of appetite
   b. shortness of breath
   c. confusion
   d. all of the above
   e. a and c only

4. Which of the following is not one of the stages of grief?
   a. Anger
   b. Self-pity
   c. Bargaining
   d. Acceptance

5. Instead of the term "life-threatening," some people prefer to use the term:
   a. terminally ill
   b. life-ending
   c. life-limiting
   d. incapacitated

SELF-ASSESSMENT

If you were faced with a life-threatening illness, would you choose to sustain your life regardless of the probable outcome? How far would you go with treatments? What four factors would enter into your decision? Have you discussed these issues with your family and provider?

C H A P T E R   **7**

Legal Considerations

CHAPTER PRE-TEST

Perform this test without looking at your book.

1. This document allows a patient to name another person as the official spokesperson for the patient should the patient be unable to make health care decisions:
   a. Living will
   b. Advance directive
   c. Durable power of attorney for health care
   d. Do not resuscitate order (DNR)

2. Oral testimony taken with a court reporter present in a location agreed on by both parties:
   a. Mediation
   b. Deposition
   c. Interrogatory
   d. Arbitration

3. Younger than 18 years who are free of parental care and are financially responsible, married, become parents, or join the armed forces:
   a. Mature minor
   b. Designated adult
   c. Minor
   d. Emancipated minor

4. Legal _____ means that a patient is found by a court to be insane, inadequate, or to not be an adult.
   a. Incompetence
   b. Immaturity
   c. Emancipation
   d. Consent

5. The failure to exercise the standard of care that a reasonable person would exercise in similar circumstances:
   a. Libel
   b. Slander
   c. Negligence
   d. Malpractice

VOCABULARY BUILDER

Misspelled Words

Find the words below that are misspelled; circle them, and correctly spell them in the spaces provided. Then insert the correct vocabulary terms from the list that best fit the descriptions below.

administer	despense	litigation
administrative law	docktrines	malfeasance
ajents	durable power of attorney for health care	malpractice
alternative dispute resolution	emanciated minor	miner
arbetrasion	expert witness	neglegance
civil law	expressed contract	noncompliant
common law	feliny	plaintiffs
constitutional law	implied consent	risk management
contract law	incompetent	slander
criminil law	invation of privacy	statutes
deposition	lible	subpena
discovery		tort

_____   _____   _____

_____   _____   _____

_____   _____   _____

_____   _____   _____

1. _____ Establishes agencies that are given power to enact regulations having the force of law

2. _____ Law that includes 27 amendments, 10 of which are the Bill of Rights

3. _____ A 17-year-old person serving in the U.S. armed forces

4. _____ Medical practice acts, or laws, that regulate the practice of medicine, such as licensure and standards of care

5. _____ A patient who refuses needed care, such as a cancer patient who will not complete a series of chemotherapy treatments

6. _____ A provider or health care professional who testifies in court to establish a reasonable and expected standard of care with respect to a specific medical situation so that jurors can understand the nature of medical information

7. _____ The failure to exercise the standard of care that a reasonable person would exercise in similar circumstances

8. _____ Persons who bring charges in a civil case

9. _____ Medical assistants are _____ of their employers.

10. _____ A patient tilts her head back and opens her eyes wide for instillation of medicated eye drops from a medical assistant without any verbal instructions to do so.

11. _____ Professional negligence

12. _____ Court order

13. _____ Persons against whom charges are brought

14. _____ A medical assistant writes in the patient's record, "Jim Marshall is a ruthless, rude man who is very full of himself. Be careful around him."

15. _____ A patient says loudly in the reception area of Inner City Health Care, filled to capacity with waiting patients, "Dr. Reynolds should retire. I know he's not up on the latest medical techniques."

16. _____ A 17-year-old student who lives with his or her parents

17. _____ Actions that make the medical assistant and the employer less vulnerable to litigation

18. _____ Lawsuit

19. _____ Written or verbal contract that describes exactly what each party in the contract will do

LEARNING REVIEW

Identifying Civil and Criminal Law

Identify whether the following actions fall under the domain of civil law (CV) or criminal law (CM).

_____ A. A provider is siphoning off narcotics from an urgent care center's locked drug cabinet and continuing to treat patients while under the influence of the drugs.

_____ B. A woman in the advanced stages of breast cancer sues her insurer when it refuses to provide benefits for a bone marrow transplant.

_____ C. An office manager steals, or embezzles, funds from the medical practice.

Short Answer

1. List and define the four Ds of negligence.

_____

_____

2. Before any invasive or surgical procedure is performed, patients are asked to sign consent forms, which become a permanent part of the medical record. What four things must the patient know to give informed consent?

_____

_____

_____

3. The unauthorized touching of one person by another is called _____.

4. The federal government established laws in 1968 to allow people to make a gift of all or part of their body; it is known as the _____.

5. The law mandates that the proper authorities be informed of certain harms and injuries, such as *(circle all that apply)*:

    A. rape

    B. gunshot and knife wounds

    C. child abuse

    D. elder abuse

6. What term is used now in place of "domestic violence" and what does it mean? Why was this change made?

_____

_____

_____

_____

7. What is the difference between an advance directive and a POLST form?

_____

_____

_____

_____

8. In the case of Good Samaritan Laws, does the medical assistant have any liability if an injury occurs after performing first aid skills?

_____

_____

_____

CERTIFICATION REVIEW

These questions are designed to mimic the certification examination. Select the best response.

1. The Patient Self-Determination Act, which includes health care directives, ensures that patients are able to:

    a. choose their own providers

    b. control their own health care decisions

    c. have guaranteed confidentiality

    d. have health care benefits

2. Which of the following covers the relationship between providers and their patients?
   a. Informed consent
   b. Locum tenens
   c. Medical ethics
   d. Criminal law

3. *Res ipsa loquitur* means:
   a. the thing speaks for itself
   b. the provider is ultimately responsible
   c. the record must be opened in court
   d. patients have a right to their records

4. The 4 Ds of negligence are:
   a. duty, derelict, danger, damage
   b. danger, duty, direct cause, disaster
   c. duty, derelict, direct cause, damage
   d. disaster, damage, direct cause, danger

5. A 17-year-old individual who is in the Navy is considered to be:
   a. *respondeat superior*
   b. an emancipated minor
   c. privileged
   d. a naval dependent

6. *Respondeat superior* is the Latin word that means:
   a. providers are responsible for their employees' actions
   b. the thing speaks for itself
   c. obey your superior
   d. breach of duty of care

7. What must the inventory of controlled substances include?
   a. List of the name, address, and DEA registration number of the provider
   b. Date and time of inventory
   c. Signature of the individual taking inventory
   d. All of the above

8. A provider is legally bound to treat a patient until the patient:
   a. breaks an appointment
   b. does not have health insurance
   c. cannot get a referral
   d. no longer needs treatment

9. If suspicion of child abuse is aroused, the health care provider should:
   a. send the patient home
   b. treat the child's injuries
   c. inform the parents of the child's diagnosis and that it will be reported to the police and social services agency
   d. b and c

10. When a patient is asked to walk across the hall to the treatment room while wearing only a patient gown and is in full view of other patients, this is considered:

    a. a HIPAA violation

    b. implied consent

    c. invasion of privacy

    d. defamation of character

11. Protection of health care professionals who may provide medical care in emergencies without fear of being sued comes under:

    a. Good Samaritan laws

    b. provider's directives

    c. durable power of attorney for health care

    d. litigation

12. An order for a physician to appear in court with a medical record is:

    a. *res ipsa loquitur*

    b. *subpoena duces tecum*

    c. *respondeat superior*

    d. an interrogatory

13. When a patient reports a sore throat and the provider takes a swab for a throat culture to diagnose and treat the ailment, this act is considered:

    a. an expressed contract

    b. implied consent

    c. informed consent

    d. an implied contract

LEARNING APPLICATION

Critical Thinking

1. Do you have a living will or advance directive? Why or why not? Identify to a family member or loved one what your wishes might be if you were seriously injured in an accident and were still in what appears to be an irreversible coma after 10 months.

   _____

   _____

   _____

   _____

2. Discuss the medical assistant's obligations in regard to public duties.

   _____

   _____

3. What is the Good Samaritan Law? What must a medical assistant and any other health care professional remember when giving first aid at the scene of an accident?

   _____

   _____

4. Describe three types of abuse. Tell what your role as a medical assistant is when Juanita brings her 3-year-old son Henry to the clinic. Henry has bruises on his face and chest and appears quite frightened when you approach him. While you prepare Henry for the pediatrician's examination, Juanita's answers to your questions seem evasive.

Case Studies

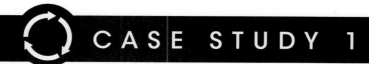

CASE STUDY 1

On a busy afternoon at Inner City Health Care, the reception area is filled with walk-in patients, and the staff struggles to keep up with the patient load. Administrative medical assistant Liz Corbin, CMA (AAMA), gives the patient file for Edith Leonard to clinical medical assistant Bruce Goldman, CMA (AAMA). "Dr. Reynolds wants a CBC done stat on the older adult woman in exam room 1," she tells Bruce, handing him the file. Bruce proceeds to examination room 1. Without identifying the patient, he performs a venipuncture on Cele Little, who has come to the clinic for a hearing problem. Cele asks Bruce why the procedure needs to be performed and states that she does not want to have it. Bruce insists that Dr. Reynolds has ordered the procedure and performs the venipuncture anyway. The procedure frightens Cele, and she begins to fear that her hearing loss is indicative of a more serious illness.

CASE STUDY REVIEW QUESTIONS

1. What errors were made that could leave the medical assistants and provider vulnerable to litigation?

2. How might the errors leave the health care professionals open to potential lawsuits?

3. How could the errors have been avoided through effective risk management techniques?

CASE STUDY 2

Dr. Elizabeth King has just completed a routine physical examination of Abigail Johnson. Elizabeth asks Anna Preciado, RMA, to administer a flu shot to Abigail before the patient leaves the clinic. Abigail, an older African American woman, is accompanied by her daughter. When Anna attempts to administer the flu vaccine, Abigail says, "Is that a flu shot? They make me sick; I don't want it." Abigail's daughter says, "Yes, she does want it. Go ahead and give it to her." Abigail begins to laugh. "Okay," Anna says, "may I give you the vaccinations?" Abigail says nothing, but she rolls up her sleeve. As Anna administers the parenteral injection, the older woman looks up at her seriously and says, "I didn't want any flu shot. My daughter makes me get it every year." However, Abigail does not withdraw physically.

CASE STUDY REVIEW QUESTIONS

1. What errors were made that could leave the medical assistant and provider vulnerable to litigation?

_____

2. How might the errors leave the health care professionals open to potential lawsuits?

_____

_____

3. How could the errors have been avoided through effective risk management techniques?

_____

_____

_____

_____

_____

_____

_____

CASE STUDY 3

Dr. Elizabeth King is going over the daily list of scheduled patients with Ellen Armstrong, CMAS (AAMA). They are standing at the front desk close to the reception area, and several patients are waiting for the first appointments of the day. Dr. King's eyes move down the list and stops over the name Mary O'Keefe. "Mary O'Keefe," she mutters, "she's so neurotic and pestering. It's a small wonder her husband hasn't left her yet; just wait till they have that third child . . . I don't think I have the patience for Mary today."

CASE STUDY REVIEW QUESTIONS

1. What errors were made that could leave the medical assistant and provider vulnerable to litigation?

_____

_____

_____

2. How might the errors leave the health care professionals open to potential lawsuits?

_____

_____

3. How could the errors have been avoided through effective risk management techniques?

_____

_____

_____

_____

_____

CASE STUDY 4

Lydia Renzi, a deaf woman with some residual hearing, comes to Inner City Health Care and has waived her right to a certified sign language interpreter as provided under ADA. She is at the clinic today with a recurrent vaginal discharge. Lydia is diagnosed by Dr. Angie Esposito with candidiasis, a yeast infection caused by the fungus *Candida albicans*. Angie prescribes a vaginal suppository and asks Wanda Slawson, CMA (AAMA), to give Lydia instructions for using the prescription. Lydia wears a hearing aid and has trouble understanding Wanda, who is soft spoken. Wanda is also standing against a brightly lit window, and Lydia has trouble seeing her face. Lydia writes on a pad she has brought with her, "Is this a sexually transmitted illness?" In frustration, Wanda begins shouting, "You just have a yeast infection; it's not like you have herpes or anything." At that moment, another medical assistant, Bruce Goldman, CMA (AAMA), is escorting a male patient past the open door of the examination room. Both men turn their heads away, though it is clear that they have overheard.

CASE STUDY REVIEW QUESTIONS

1. What errors were made that could leave the medical assistant and provider vulnerable to litigation?

_____

_____

2. How might the errors leave the health care professionals open to potential lawsuits?

_____

_____

3. How could the errors have been avoided through effective risk management techniques?

_____

_____

_____

_____

_____

CASE STUDY 5

Construction workers Jaime Carrera and Ralph Samson are required to take a reemployment drug screening test before they can be hired to work on a new site to which they have applied. Jaime and Ralph come to Inner City Health Care, where urine specimens are collected for examination. The test comes back positive for Jaime, and his potential employer does not give him the job. Ralph tests negative. Two weeks later, Ralph returns to Inner City Health Care for a routine physical examination. "Whatever happened to Jaime Carrera?" Ralph asks Bruce Goldman, CMA (AAMA). "I haven't seen him around the site." "Oh," Bruce replies, "He tested positive for chemical substance abuse, and now he's in a rehab program that Dr. Whitney suggested."

CASE STUDY REVIEW QUESTIONS

1. What errors were made that could leave the medical assistant and provider vulnerable to litigation?

_____

2. How might the errors leave the health care professionals open to potential lawsuits?

_____

_____

_____

3. How could the errors have been avoided through effective risk management techniques?

_____

_____

_____

_____

Web Activities

1. Using the Internet, determine whether or when a medical clinic might be required to follow the federal guidelines of the Family and Medical Leave Act (FMLA). Identify reasons to follow the FMLA guidelines.

2. Using your favorite search engine, key in the words "Medical Malpractice Awards." A number of sites will appear. Has a national limit been set on practice awards? What makes this topic a political one? Identify those who favor malpractice award limits and also those who oppose these limits.

3. Research the Internet for the statute of limitations related to claims injuries. What is the time span in your state?

CHAPTER POST-TEST

Perform this test without looking at your book.

1. As long as you do not say the patient's name, you may discuss the patient's illnesses and treatments with:
   a. the physician
   b. the medical assistant
   c. anyone in the clinic
   d. no one at all

2. The patient-provider contract begins when the patient:
   a. makes the appointment
   b. arrives for the appointment and the provider agrees to treat them
   c. makes their first copayment
   d. b and c only

3. If the patient's condition should be treated, is the provider obligated to care for the patient?
   a. YES: unless a formal discharge has occurred, the provider is obligated to treat the patient.
   b. YES: the provider is obligated to treat anyone who walks through the door according to the Hippocratic Oath.
   c. YES: as long as the patient carries an insurance plan where the provider is a contracted participant.
   d. NO: the provider is permitted to select whom he wants and does not want to treat.

4. A medical assistant greets a patient and indicates he/she needs to check the patient's blood pressure. The patient rolls up their sleeve and extends their arm. The patient's action is a form of:
   a. informed consent
   b. implied consent
   c. ethical behavior
   d. standard practice

5. The acronym POLST stands for:
   a. Provider Orders for Life-Sustaining Treatment
   b. Provider Objectives for Life-Sustaining Tasks
   c. Physician Orders for Life-Sustaining Treatment
   d. Physician Orders for Life-Suspecting Treatment

SELF-ASSESSMENT

1. Have you ever been in a situation in which you were asked to disclose information about another person that might have been considered confidential? Or have you ever been told confidential information? If this has happened (or if it happens in the future), what should you have done or said? What will you do/say in the future?

_____

_____

_____

_____

C H A P T E R **8**

Ethical Considerations

CHAPTER PRE-TEST

Perform this test without looking at your book.

1. All providers are reminded to strive to provide the same quality of care to all their patients regardless of race, or _____.
   a. gender
   b. ethnicity
   c. sexual orientation
   d. financial status

2. Issues of bioethics common to every medical clinic are:
   a. Allocation of scarce resources
   b. Dying and death
   c. Women's reproductive issues
   d. Genetic engineering
   e. All of the above

3. Decisions made by Congress, health systems agencies, and insurance companies are termed _____ of scarce medical resources.
   a. macroallocation
   b. microallocation
   c. bioethical dilemmas
   d. exploitation

4. In _____, the ovum is fertilized in a culture dish, allowed to grow, and then implanted inside the uterus.
   a. surrogacy
   b. genetic engineering
   c. artificial insemination
   d. in vitro fertilization (IVF)

5. According to the AAMA Code of Ethics, which of the following is a question that medical assistants should ask themselves in order to uphold the honor and high principles of the profession and its disciplines?

    a. Will I give my full attention to acknowledging the needs of every patient?

    b. Will I refrain from needless comments to a colleague regarding a patient's problem?

    c. Will I encourage others to enter the profession and always speak honorably of medical assistants?

    d. Will I honor each patient's request for information and explain unfamiliar procedures?

VOCABULARY BUILDER

Misspelled Words

Find the words below that are misspelled; circle them, and correctly spell them in the spaces provided. Then insert correct vocabulary terms from the list that best fit into the descriptions below.

bioethics	genetic enginering	microallocation
code of ethics	in vetro fertlzation	serrogate
criopreservation	intimate partner violence	
female genital mutilation	macroallocation	

_____ _____

_____ _____

1. _____ Someone who substitutes for another

2. _____ Biotechnology dealing with sophisticated medical research regarding the prevention of genetic disorders

3. _____ Medical decisions made by Congress, health systems, agencies, and insurance companies

4. _____ Set of principles and guidelines usually found in professional organizations

5. _____ Medical decisions made individually by providers and the health care team at the local level

6. _____ Ethical issues dealing with life

7. _____ An ovum is fertilized in a culture dish, allowed to grow, and then implanted into the uterus.

LEARNING REVIEW

Code of Ethics Matching

The AAMA Code of Ethics presents five basic principles that medical assistants must pledge to honor as members of the medical assisting profession. For each situation presented, identify the AAMA ethical principle that applies.

    A. Render service with full respect for the dignity of humanity

    B. Respect confidential information

    C. Uphold the honor and integrity of the profession

D. Pursue continuing education activities and improve knowledge and skills

E. Participate in community service and education

_____ 1. Marilyn Johnson, CMA (AAMA), in conversation with co–office manager Shirley Brooks, CMA (AAMA), refuses to speculate about whether a diagnosis of AIDS will be confirmed for patient Maria Jover.

_____ 2. Administrative medical assistant Karen Ritter joins a study group to prepare for the CMA (AAMA) certification examination as a method of securing her certification credentials, which must be updated every 5 years.

_____ 3. Clinical medical assistant Anna Preciado, RMA (AMT), agrees to speak to a group of high school students who are interested in pursuing a career in the medical assisting profession.

_____ 4. Liz Corbin, CMA (AAMA), politely reminds older adult patient Edith Leonard that she is a certified medical assistant, not a nurse, but assures Edith that she is qualified to perform the instillation of medicated eye drops ordered by Dr. Susan Rice.

_____ 5. When patient Dottie Tate makes an appointment at Inner City Health Care for follow-up treatment of chronic back pain and a recent history of frequent falls, Bruce Goldman, CMA (AAMA), arranges for a wheelchair to accommodate Dottie's office visit.

_____ 6. Karen Ritter volunteers at the local community office of Planned Parenthood on weekends.

_____ 7. Jane O'Hara gently and kindly guides patient Wayne Elder, whose mild retardation often causes him to become confused in unfamiliar settings, back to the proper examination room after she finds him wandering down the hallway in search of Dr. Ray Reynolds.

_____ 8. When filing a group of recent laboratory reports into the correct patient files, Ellen Armstrong, CMA (AAMA), takes care to complete the task quickly and efficiently. She performs the task at a private office station away from the general reception area and does not leave the charts open or unattended as she works.

_____ 9. Audrey Jones approaches office manager Shirley Brooks, CMA (AAMA), about opportunities for obtaining advanced training to become qualified to perform a wider array of clinical procedures in the ambulatory care setting.

_____ 10. Clinical medical assistant Wanda Slawson assists Dr. Mark Woo in the treatment of patient Rhoda Au, who is diagnosed with lupus erythematosus. Wanda believes the patient is foolhardy when she rejects Dr. Woo's treatment plan of Western drug therapy in favor of an approach that integrates traditional Chinese medicine. However, she respects the patient's heritage and right to choose her own health care.

Short Answer

1. According to the *Current Opinions of the Council on Ethical and Judicial Affairs of the AMA,* advertising by health care providers is considered ethical if the ad follows certain requirements. Which of the following are appropriate types of advertisements? Circle the correct responses.

   A. Testimonials from patients cured of serious illnesses or whose conditions were reversed or controlled under the care and treatment of the provider

   B. Providers' credentials and their hospital or community affiliations

   C. A description of the practice, facility hours of operation, and the types of services available to health care consumers

   D. Guarantees of cure promised within a specific time frame

2. Patient medical records are confidential legal documents. Name three instances, however, in which health professionals are allowed or required to reveal confidential patient information by law.

    _____

    _____

    _____

    _____

3. Issues of bioethics common to every medical clinic are *(circle all that apply)*:

    a. allocation of scarce medical resources

    b. genetic engineering or manipulation

    c. many choices surrounding life and death

4. Individuals who are truly aware of their ethical power are able to *(circle all that apply)*:

    a. not compromise any procedure or technique

    b. not put the patient at risk

    c. hide the truth regarding a possible error

5. Allocation of scarce resources may refer to *(circle all that apply)*:

    a. rationing of health care

    b. denied services

    c. advertising by health care professionals

6. In the case of suspected child abuse, the medical professional should *(circle all that apply)*:

    a. report the case

    b. protect and care for the abused

    c. treat the abuser, if known, as a victim also

7. List the five Ps of ethical power.

    _____

8. List the eight questions adapted from Stephen Covey's book that can be used as guidelines for making ethical decisions.

    _____

    _____

    _____

9. List three factors that constitute intimate partner violence.

    _____

    _____

    _____

    _____

CERTIFICATION REVIEW

These questions are designed to mimic the certification examination. Select the best response.

1. The AAMA Code of Ethics includes all but which one of the following?
   a. We should render service with respect for the dignity of our patients.
   b. We should be paid an equitable salary/wage.
   c. We should respect confidential information.
   d. We should accept the disciplines of the profession.
   e. We should seek to improve our knowledge and skills.

2. Providers may choose who to treat but may not refuse treatment based on certain criteria. Which of the following is untrue?
   a. Providers may not refuse to treat patients based on race, color, religion, or national origin.
   b. It is unethical for a provider to refuse to treat a patient who is HIV-positive.
   c. Providers must inform a patient's family of a patient's death and not delegate that responsibility to others.
   d. Providers who know they are HIV-positive should tell their patients.
   e. Providers should report unethical behaviors committed by other providers.

3. Medical records and information in them are the property of the:
   a. patient
   b. patient and family
   c. provider and patient
   d. provider

4. Once a provider takes a case, the patient cannot be neglected or refused treatment unless:
   a. she did not pay for her last visit
   b. official notice is given from the provider to withdraw from the case
   c. the patient was a no-show
   d. the patient did not keep the last appointment

5. If a provider suspects that an HIV-seropositive patient is infecting an unsuspecting individual:
   a. every attempt should be made to protect the individual at risk
   b. the case should be reported to the CDC
   c. the patient should be dismissed from the practice
   d. the provider should notify the Department of Health

6. When a breach of ethics is about to occur, the health care provider should:
   a. rationalize his or her actions
   b. disregard the outcome
   c. be encouraged to step back and review his or her actions and their likely consequences
   d. not ask for help

7. Providers who know they are HIV-positive should:
   a. refrain from any activity that would risk transmission of the virus to others
   b. wear a mask
   c. inform the patients
   d. retire

8. Revealing information about patients without consent unless otherwise required to do so by law is:

   a. a breach of confidentiality

   b. bioethics

   c. a conflict of interest

   d. genetic manipulation

9. *Roe v. Wade* refers to guidelines for:

   a. artificial insemination

   b. surrogacy

   c. abortion

   d. fetal tissue transplant

LEARNING APPLICATION

Critical Thinking

1. A provider observes another provider put a patient at risk while under the influence of alcohol and does nothing about it. What would constitute ethical behavior?

_____

_____

_____

_____

2. A provider refuses to accept any more Medicaid patients for medical care. Is this the provider's right? Is it ethical? Why or why not?

_____

_____

_____

_____

3. A clinical medical assistant whispers to the administrative medical assistant, "There goes the guy with AIDS." How should the administrative medical assistant view this behavior?

_____

_____

_____

_____

4. The services reported on the insurance claim are more complex than those actually rendered. Is this ethical or unethical? Legal or illegal? State your reasons.

_____

_____

_____

_____

5. A provider performs artificial insemination for a lesbian couple; however, the medical assistant refuses to participate or assist the provider. What are the ramifications of the medical assistant's behavior? Do you believe the medical assistant has a right to refuse?

_____

_____

_____

_____

Case Studies

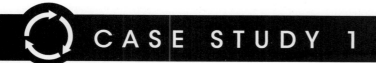

CASE STUDY 1

Lourdes Austen arrives at the offices of Drs. Lewis and King for her annual physical examination. It has been 1 year since Lourdes had surgery to remove a tumor in her breast by lumpectomy with axillary lymph node dissection, followed by a course of radiation. Lourdes's 1-year mammogram and follow-up examination with her surgeon and radiologist find no evidence of a recurrence of the cancer. Lourdes is a single woman in her late 30s. As Dr. King begins the routine physical examination, assisted by Anna Preciado, RMA (AMT), Lourdes begins to cry. "I'm so happy to be alive," Lourdes says. "And so afraid of the cancer coming back. But I want to celebrate life. I've talked to my boyfriend about it and we want to get pregnant. What should I do?" Dr. King takes Lourdes's hand. "I know that living with cancer is hard. You are doing well. There are many things to consider. . . ."

CASE STUDY REVIEW QUESTIONS

1. What bioethical dilemma exists in Lourdes's situation? In your opinion, is Lourdes's choice to become pregnant an ethical one?

_____

_____

_____

_____

2. How do deeply held beliefs and attitudes about parenthood and the role of women in our society have an impact on the patient's decision? How could these beliefs have an impact on the health care team's response to Lourdes?

_____

_____

_____

_____

_____

_____

_____

_____

_____

3. What is Dr. King's best therapeutic response to Lourdes? What medical issues should the health care team consider if Lourdes becomes pregnant?

_____

_____

_____

_____

_____

_____

_____

_____

Web Activities

1. Using the Internet, print the latest issue of the AMA Principles of Medical Ethics. Compare that code with the AAMA Code of Ethics. Do you find this comparison helpful in more clearly understanding ethics, responsibility, and professionalism? Give your reasons.

2. Using your favorite Internet search engine, key in two or three of the bioethical issues and do a small-scale review of items listed. From your research, identify at least three ethical/bioethical questions for your class to discuss.

CHAPTER POST-TEST

Perform this test without looking at your book.

1. Sexual activity between family members is known as:
   a. intimate partner violence
   b. incest
   c. physical abuse
   d. sexual abuse

2. Sometimes ethics is referred to as:
   a. choices
   b. beliefs
   c. morals
   d. standards

3. The majority of states have enacted legislation regarding the abuse of elder adults _____ or older.
   a. 60
   b. 65
   c. 70
   d. 75

4. Failure to provide basic food, shelter, and care of a child is known as:

   a. incompetence

   b. neglect

   c. ignorance

   d. displacement

5. _____ is the term used to describe either a place of residence for those who are dying or an organization whose medical professionals and volunteers are in attendance of someone whose death is imminent.

   a. Home health

   b. Rehabilitation

   c. Skilled nursing facility

   d. Hospice

SELF ASSESSMENT

1. Identify how you are able to demonstrate the five Ps of ethical power in your own life.

   _____

   _____

2. There are eight questions adapted from Stephen Covey's book that can be used as guidelines for making ethical decisions. Identify how your life fits into these guidelines and where/if you are striving to do better.

   _____

   _____

   _____

   _____

CHAPTER **9**

Emergency Procedures and First Aid

CHAPTER PRE-TEST

Perform this test without looking at your book.

1. Of the following, which is the most important in an emergency?
   a. Whether the patient has medical insurance
   b. Whether the patient is HIV-positive
   c. Whether the patient is taking any medication
   d. Whether the patient is breathing

2. The abbreviation BAC stands for:
   a. Biodynamics, airway, circulation
   b. Bleeding, airway, circulation
   c. Breathing, airway, circulation
   d. Bleeding, airway, cardiac

3. Important aspects of preparing for an emergency are:
   a. Developing a policy and procedure manual
   b. Maintaining a crash cart
   c. Maintaining updated CPR certification for staff
   d. All of the above

4. Which of the following describes a second-degree burn?
   a. Superficial, involving only the top layer of the skin
   b. The first layer of the skin is burned through and the dermis is involved
   c. All layers of tissue are destroyed
   d. None of the above

5. The cardiac muscle being unable to contract and provide blood to the body describes which kind of shock?
   a. Hypovolemic
   b. Cardiogenic
   c. Neurogenic
   d. Septic

6. Treatment for frostbite includes:
   a. Warming the area by exposing it to an open flame
   b. Slow warming the area by wrapping in a blanket or clothing
   c. Immersing the affected area in hot water
   d. None of the above

7. A cerebral vascular incident can be described as:
   a. A ruptured blood vessel in the brain
   b. A heart attack
   c. An occlusion of a blood vessel
   d. a and c

8. An example of an open wound is a(n):
   a. Abrasion
   b. Incision
   c. Hematoma
   d. a and b

9. Tearing of ligaments is diagnosed as a:
   a. Sprain
   b. Strain
   c. Fracture
   d. None of the above

10. Cool, clammy skin and a weak thready pulse are symptoms of:
    a. CVA
    b. MI
    c. Shock
    d. Syncope

VOCABULARY BUILDER

Misspelled Words

Find the key vocabulary words below that are misspelled; circle them, and correctly spell them in the spaces provided. Then insert one of the correct vocabulary terms into the sentences below. Not all vocabulary terms will be used.

anaphalaxis	crepitation	sprane
avultion	explicit	syncopy
cardiopulmonary resuscitation	hypothermea	treeage

_____   _____   _____

_____   _____   _____

1. After administering the antibiotic, the patient exhibited symptoms of _____.

2. When a bone is fractured, there is often _____ at the site.

3. A _____ is an injury to a joint.

4. When the body temperature drops to a dangerous level, it is called _____.

5. Fainting is also known as _____.

6. _____ is abbreviated as CPR.

Matching I

Identify each of the following terms as an emergency condition (EC), an emergency or first aid procedure performed by health care professionals (EP), emergency equipment (EQ), or an emergency service provided to assist in emergency situations (ES).

_____ A. First aid

_____ B. Screening

_____ C. Syncope

_____ D. Shock

_____ E. Wounds

_____ F. Crash cart

_____ G. Occlusion

_____ H. Universal emergency medical identification symbol and card

_____ I. Hypothermia

_____ J. Chest compressions

_____ K. CPR

_____ L. Sprain

_____ M. Emergency medical service (EMS)

_____ N. Fracture

_____ O. Splints

_____ P. Strain

_____ Q. Rescue breathing

Matching II

Match each of the terms in Matching I with its definition below.

_____ 1. A break in a bone; there are several types, but all are classified as open or closed

_____ 2. A tray or portable cart that contains medications and supplies needed for emergency and first aid procedures

_____ 3. An injury to the soft tissue between joints that involves the tearing of muscles or tendons and occurs often in the neck, back, or thigh muscles

_____ 4. A break in the skin or underlying tissues, categorized as open or closed

_____ 5. Closure of a passage

_____ 6. An injury to a joint, often an ankle, knee, or wrist, that involves a tearing of the ligaments; most are minor and heal quickly; others are more severe, include swelling, and may not heal properly if the patient continues to put stress on the affected joint

_____ 7. A local network of police, fire, and medical personnel trained to respond to emergency situations; in most communities, the system is activated by calling 911

_____ 8. Identification sometimes carried by individuals to alert to any health problems they might have

_____ 9. Any device used to immobilize a body part; often used by EMS personnel

_____ 10. An extremely dangerous cold-related condition that can result in death if the individual does not receive care and if the progression of the condition is not reversed; symptoms include shivering, cold skin, and confusion

_____ 11. Fainting

_____ 12. The immediate care provided to persons who are suddenly ill or injured, typically followed by more comprehensive care and treatment

_____ 13. A condition in which the circulatory system is not providing enough blood to all parts of the body, causing the body's organs to fail to function properly

_____ 14. The combination of rescue breathing and chest compressions performed by a trained individual on a patient experiencing cardiac arrest

_____ 15. To assess patients' conditions and prioritize the need for care

_____ 16. Performed on individuals in respiratory arrest, this is a mouth-to-mouth (using appropriate protective equipment) or mouth-to-nose procedure that provides oxygen to the patient until emergency personnel arrive

_____ 17. The combination of rescue breathing and chest compressions; known as CPR

LEARNING REVIEW

Short Answer

1. While awaiting the arrival of EMS, what aspects of the patient's condition should the medical assistant continuously monitor?

_____

_____

2. What five infection control measures can health care professionals follow to greatly reduce the risk for transmitting infectious disease when providing emergency care?

_____

_____

_____

3. For each of the patient symptoms or conditions below, identify the type of shock that is most likely:

Patient Symptom/Condition	Type of Shock
Patient suffers heart attack	_____
Patient experiences severe infection after colon surgery	_____
Patient experiences reaction to food allergy	_____
Diabetic patient lapses into a coma	_____
Patient has serious head trauma	_____
Accident victim experiences extreme loss of blood	_____

4. A common procedure for treating closed wounds is to RICE them. What do the letters of this acronym stand for?

_____

Chapter 9 • *Emergency Procedures and First Aid* **83**

5. Match each type of open wound (incision, puncture, laceration, avulsion, abrasion) to its defining characteristics.

Characteristics   **Type of Open Wound**

A wound that pierces and penetrates the skin. This wound may appear
insignificant, but actually can go quite deep.   _____

These wounds commonly occur at exposed body parts such as the fingers,
toes, and nose. Tissue is torn off and wounds may bleed profusely.   _____

A wound that results from a sharp object such as a scalpel blade.   _____

A painful wound. The epidermal layer of the skin is scraped away.   _____

A wound that results in a jagged tear of body tissues and may contain
debris.   _____

6. For each type of wound, describe proper emergency concerns, care, and treatment.

_____

_____

_____

_____

_____

_____

_____

_____

_____

_____

7. Name three sources, other than heat, that can cause burns. For each, describe the proper emergency concerns, care, and treatment.

_____

_____

_____

_____

_____

_____

_____

_____

8. Musculoskeletal injuries, or injuries to muscles, bones, and joints, can be difficult to assess, especially for closed fractures. List five assessment techniques that health care professionals can use to determine the seriousness of musculoskeletal injuries.

_____

_____

_____

9. Identify the method of entry into the body for each of the following poisons:

_____ 1. Carbon monoxide

_____ 2. Insect stingers

_____ 3. Chemical pesticides used in the garden

_____ 4. Spoiled food

_____ 5. Poison oak

_____ 6. Cleaning fluid fumes

CERTIFICATION REVIEW

These questions are designed to mimic the certification examination. Select the best response.

1. Which of the following is not an appropriate treatment for hypothermia?
   a. Give the victim warm liquids to drink.
   b. Remove any wet clothing.
   c. Rub the victim's skin vigorously to increase circulation.
   d. Use warm water to warm the person if possible.

2. In anaphylactic shock, the patient may:
   a. feel a constriction in the throat and chest
   b. have difficulty breathing
   c. have swelling and tingling of the lips and tongue
   d. all of the above

3. While waiting for EMS to arrive, what should be checked?
   a. Degree of responsiveness
   b. Airway, breathing
   c. Heartbeat (rate and rhythm)
   d. All of the above

4. Closed wounds that are painful and swollen require that a cold compress be applied:
   a. until the victim feels tingling
   b. for 10 minutes, then off for 40 minutes
   c. for 20 minutes, then off for 20 minutes
   d. for at least 1 hour, then off for 2 hours

5. To control nosebleeds, the patient should be seated, the patient's head elevated, and nostrils pinched for:
   a. 10 minutes
   b. 20 minutes
   c. 30 minutes
   d. 40 minutes

6. When a patient calls regarding a poisoning or suspicion of poisoning, the advice to give is to:
   a. call the poison control center
   b. give the patient charcoal
   c. tell the patient to drink milk
   d. flush the mouth with water

7. The best treatment for patients who are experiencing a seizure is to:
   a. restrain them
   b. stick a tongue depressor in their mouth
   c. protect from injury and care for them with understanding
   d. stop the seizure

8. Shock that occurs as a result of overwhelming emotional factors such as fear, anger, or grief is called:
   a. neurogenic
   b. psychogenic
   c. anaphylactic
   d. septic

9. The type of burn that may occur resulting in an entrance and exit burn wound area is:

    a. chemical

    b. electrical

    c. solar radiation

    d. explosion

10. In burn depth classifications, third-degree burns are also called:

    a. superficial

    b. full thickness

    c. partial thickness

    d. sunburns

11. The type of fracture often caused by falling on an outstretched hand that involves the distal end of the radius is called:

    a. greenstick

    b. spiral

    c. Colles

    d. implicated

12. Jaw and left shoulder pain; a rapid, weak pulse; excessive perspiration; and cold, clammy skin may be symptomatic of:

    a. seizure

    b. heart attack

    c. stroke

    d. sepsis

LEARNING APPLICATION

Critical Thinking

1. A teenaged patient, Myles Parris, has been recently diagnosed with epilepsy. When he arrives at the office for today's appointment, he states that he feels "odd." He then begins to seize. The front desk staff notified the medical assistant who was responsible for triage in the clinic and she responded immediately.

    a. What actions should the medical assistant take initially?

    _____

    _____

    b. List several underlying diseases besides epilepsy that can cause seizures.

    _____

2. Ms. Cosper, a 52-year-old woman, came into the clinic for a routine follow-up appointment for her diabetes. She suddenly lost consciousness and slumped over in her chair in the waiting room. What immediate steps should be taken by the medical assistant?

    _____

3. Describe the purpose of a crash cart and list five medications and five supplies that should be found there.

    _____

    _____

_____

_____

_____

_____

_____

_____

4. Recall three types of bandages and give examples of their use.

_____

_____

_____

_____

5. Describe the difference between first-, second-, and third-degree burns.

_____

_____

_____

_____

6. Recall and describe the four routes of entry for poisons entering the human body.

_____

_____

_____

_____

_____

_____

_____

7. Explain when, why, and the technique for utilizing abdominal thrusts and back blows in an emergency situation.

_____

_____

_____

_____

_____

Case Studies

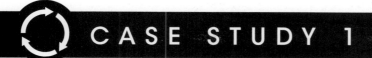

CASE STUDY 1

Mary O'Keefe calls Dr. King's office in a panic. Gwen Carr, CMA (AAMA), answers the telephone.

Mary: "Oh my God, help me. I need Dr. King."

Gwen: "This is Ellen Armstrong. Who is this calling? What is the situation?"

Mary: "It's my baby, oh God, get Dr. King."

Gwen: "Dr. King is unavailable, but we can help you. Now, tell me your name."

Mary: "It's Mary O'Keefe. Help me, I think my baby is dead."

Gwen: "Are you at home?"

Mary: "Yes."

Gwen: "Ok. Try to calm down. Speak slowly and tell me what's happened."

Mary: "My son Chris pried the plug off an outlet and he's electrocuted himself!" Mary cries. "He's just lying there. I'm so scared, if I touch him, will I electrocute myself? Oh my God, my baby, my baby. What should I do?"

Gwen, who has been writing down the details on a piece of paper, motions to Sam Tyler, another CMA (AAMA) in the office, and hands him her notes. Sam immediately accesses the O'Keefe address from the patient database and uses another telephone to call EMS with the nature of the emergency situation and directions to the O'Keefe residence. Meanwhile, Gwen remains on the line with Mary. Dr. King is on rounds at the hospital this morning and will not be in the office for at least another hour. Gwen tells Mary, "Mary, we are calling EMS, and they will be there as soon as possible. In the meantime, I'm going to need you to focus and answer my questions, okay?"

CASE STUDY REVIEW QUESTIONS

1. What steps did the medical assistant take to screen the emergency situation?

_____

_____

_____

2. What questions should Gwen ask Mary regarding the emergency situation?

_____

_____

_____

_____

3. What should the medical assistant do after EMS arrives and takes over emergency care? What follow-up procedures are necessary?

_____

_____

_____

_____

_____

_____

_____

_____

_____

_____

⟳ CASE STUDY 2

Lenore McDonell, a wheelchair-bound woman in her early 30s, experiences a serious laceration to the right arm sustained from a fall while performing an independent transfer from the examination table to her wheelchair. Sam Tyler, CMA (AAMA), assists Dr. Winston Lewis in administering emergency care.

CASE STUDY REVIEW QUESTIONS

1. What Standard Precautions must the health care professionals follow before administering emergency treatment?

_____

2. Sam and Dr. Lewis attempt to control Lenore's bleeding by applying a dressing and pressing firmly. When the bleeding does not stop, what two actions should the health care professionals perform?

_____

3. In the unlikely event that bleeding continues, what piece of medical equipment will the health care team use in substitution for a tourniquet? Why is this alternative equipment effective and widely used today?

_____

_____

_____

4. The bleeding stops, and Sam applies a pressure bandage over the dressing. The patient is prone to fractures, and a radiograph will need to be taken. What is the next emergency procedure Dr. Lewis will perform? Why is this procedure necessary, and what equipment will the provider and medical assistant require?

_____

_____

_____

5. Before applying a sling, what do the health care professionals check to be sure that the medical equipment used has not been too tightly applied?

_____

_____

6. What Standard Precautions will the health care team follow after the emergency treatment of the patient is successfully completed?

_____

_____

_____

7. What information will the health care team include in documenting the procedure for the patient's medical record?

_____

_____

_____

Screening Activity

In an urgent care setting, two or more patients may present with emergency symptoms. The order in which emergency patients will receive care depends on the health care professionals' abilities to screen patients' symptoms to determine who needs care most urgently. The following five patients present simultaneously on New Year's Eve at Inner City Health Care, an urgent care center. Office manager Lynn Garrett, CMA (AAMA), is working the evening shift with Dr. Mark Woo. In what order will Lynn and Dr. Woo screen the priority of treatment? Number the patients 1 (most urgent) through 5 to correspond to the urgency of their conditions.

Patient	Urgency
Patient A presents with a gunshot wound to the leg that is bleeding severely. The patient is conscious but his pupils are dilated and he is unable to answer simple questions put to him by Lynn and Dr. Woo. He cradles his right arm and will not let anyone touch it, although there is no immediate evidence of an open wound to the arm.	__
Patient B, an elderly man, is brought in by his grandson. He describes debilitating chest pains, difficulty breathing, and nausea after eating a large family dinner. The patient's medical record indicates that he has a hiatal hernia, intervertebral disc disease, high blood pressure, and mild angina. The man is walking and speaking with moderate distress and is extremely anxious.	__
Patient C, a young woman, presents with her boyfriend. She appears to have multiple abrasions on her right palm and knee, with damage to the right knee and ankle joints sustained after a fall while on in-line skates. Both joints are swollen and painful.	__

Patient D, a man in his mid-30s, presents with the cotton tip of a swab stuck in his ear canal. Although the man feels a dull consistent pain in the ear, he says he has no trouble hearing. The outside of the ear appears normal, there is no bleeding evident, and the man appears annoyed but not distressed.	_
Patient E, a young woman, presents with a group of friends, all college students, with an eye injury sustained by a champagne cork. The cork, which had a metal covering over its tip, hit the patient's eye. The young woman's eye is red and tearing and she is experiencing severe pain in the eye.	_

Web Activities

1. Search the Internet for sites and resources with information on Emergency Medical Services (EMS). Research the EMS service in your county.

2. Visit the American Association of Poison Control Centers website at http://www.aapcc.org/. Research prevention as it relates to health care providers.

CHAPTER POST-TEST

Perform this test without looking at your book.

1. A traumatic tear in the body tissues that can be contaminated with debris is called a(n):
   a. abrasion
   b. fracture
   c. laceration
   d. sprain

2. If a patient sustains a closed injury to the soft tissues, the best method of treatment is:
   a. sutures
   b. application of a cold compress
   c. cleaning with soap and water
   d. all of the above

3. Shock that results from exposure to substances that elicit an allergic response is called _____ shock.
   a. anaphylactic
   b. neurogenic
   c. cardiogenic
   d. hypovolemic

4. When rescue breathing is required in an ambulatory care setting, it is best practice to use:
   a. direct mouth-to-mouth technique
   b. an Ambu bag
   c. a resuscitation mouthpiece
   d. all of the above

5. Risk management techniques to respond to an emergency situation can include:
    a. CPR-certified staff
    b. policy and procedure for common emergencies
    c. a well-stocked and maintained crash cart
    d. all of the above

6. Submerging the affected area in cool saline or water is the treatment for which burn?
    a. First-degree
    b. Second-degree
    c. Third-degree
    d. Electrical

7. Rendering immediate and temporary emergency care to persons who are injured or disabled prior to the arrival of trained health care personnel is called:
    a. CPR
    b. rescue breathing
    c. first aid
    d. none of the above

8. A painful separation of the bone from its usual position is called:
    a. fracture
    b. sprain
    c. strain
    d. dislocation

9. The treatment for a period of cardiac fibrillation is:
    a. cardioversion
    b. rescue breathing
    c. abdominal thrusts
    d. all of the above

10. To hold a dressing in place on the lateral aspect of the ankle, which of the following bandages would be utilized?
    a. Spiral
    b. Figure-eight
    c. Tubular gauze
    d. Sling

SELF-ASSESSMENT

1. A. On a scale of 1 to 5, rate your personal comfort in regard to the following emergency situations that medical assistants may find themselves involved with in an ambulatory or urgent care setting.

    1 = extremely uncomfortable

    2 = uncomfortable

    3 = somewhat comfortable

    4 = comfortable

    5 = very comfortable

___ Assisting in treatment of patients with injuries clearly sustained by an act of violence or abuse

___ Administering back blows and thrusts to a conscious infant

___ Performing rescue breathing on someone who has poor personal hygiene

___ Bandaging the open wound of an HIV-infected person

___ Caring for a person experiencing a seizure

___ Administering care to a patient who faints after venipuncture

___ Administering care to a patient in extreme pain

___ Administering care to a patient who is verbally abusive or uncooperative

2. On a scale of 1 to 5, rate your level of agreement with the statements that follow.

1 = never

2 = occasionally

3 = sometimes

4 = most of the time

5 = all of the time

___ Life-threatening emergencies frighten me.

___ I respond well under pressure.

___ I am bothered by the sight of blood.

___ I lose my temper easily, becoming openly frustrated and angry.

___ I become frustrated and overwhelmed by feelings of helplessness in emergency situations.

___ I remain calm and clear-headed in emergency situations.

___ I forget about myself completely and focus on the emergency victim.

___ I am concerned about administering care in emergency situations in which danger to myself may exist when giving such care.

___ I am comfortable speaking to the family or friends of emergency victims.

C H A P T E R **10**

Creating the Facility Environment

CHAPTER PRE-TEST

Perform this test without looking at your book.

1. A reception area should:
   a. Be comfortable and inviting
   b. Be clean and uncluttered
   c. Contain current reading materials for all ages
   d. All of the above

2. Patients who are very ill, injured, or upset should not have to wait in the reception area, but rather should be:
   a. Asked to reschedule for the end of the clinic day
   b. Shown to an examination room away from other patients
   c. Immediately referred to the emergency room at the hospital
   d. Told to calm down immediately or the provider cannot examine them

3. Keeping the reception area clean is a responsibility of:
   a. The administrative medical assistant
   b. The bookkeeper
   c. The laboratory technician
   d. The office manager
   e. All of the above

4. A poorly illuminated reception room may suggest to patients that it looks like it has:
   a. Soiled carpets
   b. Faded draperies
   c. Poor housekeeping
   d. All of the above

5. Discussions with elderly adults regarding their health care should involve:

    a. Making certain they know what circumstances to report back to their primary provider for follow up

    b. Providing clear and concise written instructions in easy-to-read print

    c. Making certain they understand their prescription instructions

    d. All of the above

VOCABULARY BUILDER

Misspelled Words

Find the words below that are misspelled; circle them, and correctly spell them in the spaces provided. Then insert vocabulary terms from the list that best fit into the descriptive sentences below.

accessibility   Americans with Disibilities Act   characteristic
accountibility   cataract   enviroment

_____   _____   _____

1. _____   The physical space of the reception area

2. _____   A typical or distinguishing quality

3. _____   Being ultimately responsible

4. _____   Being readily reachable

5. _____   Mandates that facilities and equipment be available to all users

LEARNING REVIEW

Short Answer

1. What is the purpose of the ADA?

    _____

    _____

2. When creating the facility environment, why is accessibility a major consideration?

    _____

    _____

    _____

3. Why are some medical clinics experimenting with the use of water, such as aquariums and water walls, and music in their facilities?

    _____

    _____

4. Name four ways an ambulatory care setting can accommodate the physically challenged.

   _____

   _____

5. Identify at least four things to be done in the reception area to accommodate children.

   _____

   _____

6. What is the medical assistant's role in preparing for a natural disaster or emergency?

   _____

   _____

   _____

   _____

   _____

7. List the evacuation procedures that must be considered in the medical clinic.

   _____

   _____

   _____

   _____

8. Create a checklist of five activities to perform on opening a medical facility for the day.

   _____

   _____

9. Create a checklist of five activities to perform on closing a medical facility for the day.

   _____

   _____

   _____

10. Any drugs identified in the Controlled Substances Act list of narcotics and non-narcotics must be *(circle all that apply):*

    a. logged

    b. in a locked and secured cabinet

    c. checked when leaving the clinic

    d. counted

11. In each of the following situations, health care professionals should strive to empower the patient with as much control and dignity as possible.

    Case 1. Bill Schwartz is referred to a dermatologist by Dr. Ray Reynolds for examination of a suspicious mole on his calf. The dermatologist tells Bill that a full-body inspection will need to be done to ensure that no other areas of the skin are affected. Bill must appear disrobed in front of the dermatologist and medical assistant, who are both female.

    What strategies can health care professionals use to respect the patient's dignity and lessen the sense of disproportion between health care providers and the patient?

    _____

    _____

    _____

    _____

Case 2. Ellen Armstrong, CMA (AAMA), places a Holter monitor on patient Charles Williams. After the Holter monitor is in place, Charles has several questions about the patient activity diary that he would prefer to discuss with Dr. Winston Lewis.

What strategies can health care professionals use to respect the patient's dignity and lessen the sense of disproportion between health care providers and the patient?

_____

_____

_____

_____

_____

_____

Physical Office Environment Review

The physical clinic environment can contribute to the patient's sense of confidence and comfort, or it can be viewed by the patient as intimidating or anxiety producing. For each clinic area below, describe why the area could be perceived by patients as a frightening place. What can be done to make each area a more comforting and welcoming environment for patients?

A. Reception area:

_____

_____

_____

_____

B. Corridors:

_____

_____

_____

_____

C. Examination rooms:

_____

_____

_____

_____

_____

Fill in the Blanks

Fill in the blanks in the sentences below, which discuss the future environment for ambulatory care.

1. The number of primary care providers willing to take new patients who are 65 years or older must

   _____.

2. _____ requires providers to have patients sign a release so the family members can be kept informed.

3. The greatest frustration of elderly patients regarding their health care experiences is the _____ given by all health professionals.

4. It is important to provide clear and concise _____ instructions whenever possible in easy-to-read print.

5. The medical environment should enable all patients to _____ from one department to another with ease.

CERTIFICATION REVIEW

These questions are designed to mimic the certification examination. Select the best response.

1. HIPAA has changed the way we organize our entrance and reception areas in the following way:
   a. Patients must be able to see the receptionist at all times
   b. Patients must have adequate parking
   c. Patients must not be able to see or hear confidential information about other patients
   d. The magazines must be current

2. ADA states that:
   a. patients must not know the names and diagnoses of other patients
   b. handicapped patients must have access to all patient areas with reasonable accommodations
   c. visually impaired patients must have adequate lighting and contrast for better viewing
   d. an interpreter must be present with any non–English-speaking patient

3. Patient safety within the reception area is accomplished by:
   a. providing chairs that are sturdy and in good repair
   b. containing wires and cords and keeping them out of reach
   c. attaching rugs to the flooring without loose edges
   d. containing toys within a designated play area
   e. All of the above

4. The reception area should accommodate:
   a. at least one hour's patients per provider plus a friend or relative who may accompany each patient
   b. only adult patients
   c. 2.5 seats for each examination room
   d. a and c

5. Before entering the exam room, health care professionals should:
   a. turn their cell phones off
   b. knock before entering
   c. wash their hands
   d. put on lab coats

6. According to the ADA, there must be one accessible entrance that should:
   a. have a padlock
   b. state that it is an exit
   c. have a doorbell
   d. be protected from the weather by a canopy or overhanging roof

7. The administrative medical assistant should be able to:
   a. perform telephone screening
   b. remember that the patient's comfort is of primary concern
   c. log data into the computer
   d. All of the above

8. A good way to check a room's readiness is to:
   a. lie on the examining table and look around
   b. place yourself in the room as a patient
   c. ask yourself how you feel about being there and what mood the surroundings create for you
   d. b and c only

9. When closing the facility for the day, it is most important to:
   a. contact the answering service to notify them that the clinic is closed and who can be reached in an emergency
   b. clean all rooms
   c. lock the doors
   d. turn off the lights

10. Making facilities and equipment available to all users is called:
    a. maintenance
    b. accessibility
    c. promotion
    d. standardization

11. HIPAA requires that clinic facilities:
    a. have adequate corridors and bathrooms to accommodate wheelchair patients
    b. place an administrative medical assistant in an area seen and heard by all patients
    c. protect the confidentiality of patients checking in at the reception desk
    d. provide space for children in the clinic

12. The primary goal of maintaining a comfortable environment in which patient care is given is to:
    a. feed anxiety
    b. aggravate illness
    c. promote health
    d. stimulate the senses

13. Space planners suggest:
    a. that the reception area accommodate at least two hours' patients per provider
    b. that the reception area accommodate a friend or relative who might accompany each patient
    c. that there be 2.5 seats in the reception area for each examination room
    d. b and c only

14. Any drugs kept in the clinic that are identified as controlled substances must always be kept:
    a. in the refrigerator
    b. in a locked, secure cabinet
    c. in the provider's desk drawer
    d. in the administrative medical assistant's desk drawer

LEARNING APPLICATION

Critical Thinking

1. What can an interior designer or space planner suggest to create a pleasant atmosphere for patients in a medical facility? If there is an interior design program in your school, consult with their students on planning a medical office environment.

_____

_____

_____

_____

_____

_____

_____

_____

_____

2. Describe the most pleasant clinic you have ever seen. What made it special? What were your first impressions?

_____

_____

_____

3. Recall your provider's clinic. Is it accessible to all patients? If not, what would you do to make it accessible to all patients?

_____

_____

_____

4. As the administrative medical assistant employed in a busy ambulatory setting, how will you keep your manner pleasant, warm, and genuinely friendly and caring even on days when you are having your own personal difficulties?

_____

_____

_____

_____

_____

_____

5. Describe what you might do to monitor children aged 4 and 6 years while their parent is in the examination room.

_____

_____

6. If you believed the facility in which you are employed could benefit from the services of an interior designer either for minor adjustments or a major remodel, what suggestions would you make to your employer to convince him or her of the benefits of such a suggestion?

_____

_____

_____

Case Studies

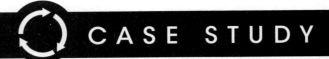

CASE STUDY

Lydia Renzi, a near-deaf woman with some residual hearing, is a patient of Dr. Angie Esposito at Inner City Health Care. Lydia is fluent in American Sign Language (ASL) and usually wears a hearing aid when she is away from home. Lydia calls to make her appointment at Inner City Health Care using a telecommunications device for the deaf (TDD) and the services of a government-funded relay operator. Although Lydia often chooses not to be accompanied by an interpreter, Inner City Health Care, in compliance with the ADA, always provides the option to supply the services of a qualified professional sign language interpreter. When Lydia arrives at Inner City Health Care with a high fever and a suspected case of the flu, the staff accommodates Lydia's special needs in several simple ways. Remembering that people who are hearing impaired rely on visual images to receive and to convey messages, Liz Corbin, CMA (AAMA), always faces Lydia directly so that the patient can see her facial expressions and lip movements. Liz holds eye contact with Lydia and does not break it until she is sure that Lydia understands her message and has time to think and respond. Special care is taken to provide Lydia with written instructions for prescriptions and for following through on home care.

CASE STUDY REVIEW QUESTION

1. What are the special communication needs of the patient with hearing impairment in the ambulatory care setting?

_____

_____

_____

_____

_____

_____

_____

2. How can the medical assistant's actions make a direct impact on the quality of care given to patients with hearing impairment?

_____

_____

_____

_____

3. Suppose that Lydia is an elderly woman who is embarrassed and sensitive about her hearing loss and will not admit that she has trouble hearing others. How might the medical assistant accommodate the special needs of this patient?

_____

_____

_____

_____

_____

_____

Role-Play Exercises

The administrative medical assistant is the person who sets the social climate for the interchange between the patient and the health care team. A friendly, reassuring demeanor and an ability to screen situations are essential skills. With another student, role-play as a patient and an administrative medical assistant. Have the "patient" say each of the phrases below. When you are finished role-playing, write what you have said and done in response to each statement below.

1. A patient with intense stomach pain doubles over and then bolts up to the reception desk, saying, "I'm going to throw up."

   _____

   _____

   _____

   _____

   _____

2. When presented with a bill, the patient exclaims, "I can't pay for all of this now! Every time I come here it seems like the doctor bill goes up a hundred dollars."

   _____

   _____

   _____

   _____

   _____

3. A patient is looking for the correct exit from the examination area to the waiting area and makes a wrong turn into the administrative medical assistant's area. He asks, "Where do I go?"

   _____

   _____

   _____

Web Activities

1. Using your favorite search engine, key in "ADAAG" or "ADA Accessibility Guidelines for Buildings & Facilities." You will find a number of sites to research.

   a. Determine the correct placement for drinking fountains, wall mirrors, and sinks.

   b. What would you need to do to accommodate someone in a wheelchair in your own home? In your classroom?

CHAPTER POST-TEST

Perform this test without looking at your book.

1. A reception area should:
   a. be comfortable, clean, and uncluttered
   b. contain current reading materials for all ages
   c. have adequate lighting for reading
   d. contain accommodations for patients with disabilities
   e. All of the above

2. At least _____ accessible entrance(s) must comply with ADA guidelines at a medical facility.

   a. four

   b. three

   c. two

   d. one

3. Keeping the reception area clean is a responsibility of:

   a. the administrative medical assistant

   b. the bookkeeper

   c. the laboratory technician

   d. the office manager

   e. all employees

4. The acronym ADA stands for:

   a. American Disabled Act

   b. Americans with Disabilities Act

   c. American Disability Act

   d. American Disability Association

5. Space planners indicate that the reception area should accommodate at least _____ worth of patients per provider and a friend or relative who may accompany the patient.

   a. 30 minutes

   b. 1 hour

   c. 45 minutes

   d. 90 minutes

SELF-ASSESSMENT

1. Visualize your last visit to a medical facility. Was the reception area clean, tidy, welcoming, and comfortable? What would you do to improve it?

   _____

   _____

   _____

   _____

2. List at least three things you would add to any reception area to make it even more accommodating. Think of items not mentioned in the textbook.

   _____

   _____

   _____

   _____

CHAPTER **11**

Computers in the Ambulatory Care Setting

CHAPTER PRE-TEST

Perform this test without looking at your book.

1. The keyboard and the mouse are considered to be:
   a. The most common types of input devices
   b. The most common types of output devices
   c. Portable memory storage devices
   d. Read-write devices

2. To ensure that your work in the computer is safe from hackers, you should:
   a. Store all work on data storage devices
   b. Defragment frequently
   c. Use firewalls
   d. Back up frequently

3. Circle each of the following tasks that are performed by a computer as part of a total practice management system:
   a. Keeping track of appointments
   b. Writing and forwarding prescriptions to the patient's pharmacy
   c. Creating patient statements
   d. Processing insurance claims
   e. Reading directions on how to download a software program

4. The "brain" of the computer is called the:
   a. Motherboard
   b. Modem
   c. Video card
   d. Central processing unit (CPU)

5. To prevent unauthorized use of your clinic computers, you should:
    a. Keep the computer in a locked cabinet at all times
    b. Keep the computer in a locked cabinet at night
    c. Assign every employee a password
    d. Have only one person on the computer at a time

VOCABULARY BUILDER

Misspelled Words

Find the words below that are misspelled; circle them, and correctly spell them in the spaces provided. Then insert the correct vocabulary terms from the list that best fit the descriptions below.

electronic medical records   hardware   RAM

erganomics   Internet   total practice management system

fishing   modom

_____   _____   _____

1. _____   A device used by a computer to communicate with a remote computer through phone lines

2. _____   Maximizing the user's safety when setting up a workstation that involves preventing back, neck, and eye strain

3. _____   Acronym for *random access memory*, a type of computer memory that can be written to and read from

4. _____   The physical equipment used by the computer system to process data

5. _____   The practice of attempting to acquire sensitive information (such as passwords or bank account numbers) by masquerading as a trusted source through email communication

6. _____   Electronic patient records from a single medical practice, hospital, or pharmacy

7. _____   A worldwide computer network available via modem

8. _____   A category of software that deals with the day-to-day operations of a medical practice

LEARNING REVIEW

Short Answer

1. List the tasks that should be performed by members of the health care team when maintaining the computer.

_____

_____

2. What precautions must be taken to ensure that data are not lost during a power outage?

   _____

   _____

   _____

3. What are the three most common networks encountered in the medical clinic?

   _____

4. Name several hardware connections to a network.

   _____

5. Name several wireless connections to a network.

   _____

6. Name the two different techniques used by antivirus software to scan files to identify and eliminate computer viruses and malware.

   _____

   _____

7. List at least six of the defenses that should be used in protecting the health care facility's computer system.

   _____

   _____

   _____

8. The four fundamental elements of all computer systems are:

   _____

9. List the HIPAA compliance measures to be taken that will ensure that all PHI data are accurate and not altered, lost, or destroyed.

   _____

   _____

   _____

   _____

10. The identifying characteristics of a secure site are *(circle all that apply):*
    a. small padlock icon in the Web browser window
    b. site address: https://
    c. an "S" in the upper left corner of the screen
    d. site address: http://

11. What is meant by "electronic medical record" and "electronic health record"? Distinguish between the terms.

    _____

    _____

    _____

CERTIFICATION REVIEW

These questions are designed to mimic the certification examination. Select the best response.

1. A flash drive is a:
   a. memory device
   b. type of software device
   c. DVD drive
   d. safety warning

2. What step(s) should be followed when selecting software?
   a. Choose a knowledgeable vendor.
   b. Determine what tasks will be computerized.
   c. Software available for each task should be identified and evaluated on a trial basis.
   d. All of the above

3. A personal digital assistant is classified as a:
   a. supercomputer
   b. mainframe computer
   c. minicomputer
   d. microcomputer

4. Computers in the medical office or clinic are used to perform:
   a. routine office tasks
   b. maintenance of electronic medical records and management of the clinic or practice
   c. clinical laboratory applications
   d. a and b only
   e. a, b, and c only

5. Defragmenting gets rid of:
   a. fragments of information that you do not need anymore
   b. old information no longer needed
   c. empty spaces on the hard drive
   d. removal of software that you do not use

6. The fastest, most complex, and most expensive computer that is also used in medical research is the:
   a. mainframe
   b. supercomputer
   c. minicomputer
   d. personal digital assistant

7. The smallest but most widely used type of computer in today's heath care facility is the:
   a. microcomputer
   b. supercomputer
   c. mainframe computer
   d. minicomputer

8. Examples of output devices would be:
   a. printers, fax machines, monitors
   b. keyboard, mouse
   c. scanners, electronic tablets
   d. touch screens, digital cameras

9. What step(s) should be taken in the changeover to a computer system?
   a. Schedule during a down period, such as a long holiday or vacation period.
   b. Introduce the new system while continuing to use the old system.
   c. Transfer files and data and when the staff is comfortable with the system and their computer skills, then make the changeover.
   d. All of the above

10. Manuals and documents that define how programs operate are called:
    a. the operating system
    b. system software
    c. computer system documentation
    d. application software

11. Compact disks and digital video versatile disks are two types of:
    a. hard drives
    b. optical drives
    c. flash drives
    d. tape drives

12. Data storage device capacity is often referred to as:
    a. hardware
    b. the operating system
    c. memory
    d. algorithms

13. Portable memory storage devices from which the storage media can be readily removed and transported are called:
    a. flash drives
    b. ROM
    c. RAM
    d. optical drives

LEARNING APPLICATION

Critical Thinking

1. Assume you work in an ambulatory care setting that operates on a manual system. Identify the functions you would have a computer perform in the clinic.

_____

_____

_____

_____

_____

_____

_____

2. The same clinic is now going to make the transition to a computerized system. What steps would you take to make the transition as smooth as possible?

_____

_____

_____

_____

_____

_____

_____

_____

3. Discuss the study of ergonomics and identify the steps to take in order to decrease or prevent computer-related injury.

_____

_____

_____

_____

_____

_____

_____

_____

_____

_____

_____

_____

_____

_____

_____

_____

_____

_____

_____

_____

_____

_____

_____

_____

_____

_____

4. Protection of a computer system from unauthorized access requires defense in depth. Using the Internet, identify as many defenses as you can find to protect the clinic and prioritize the order of importance.

_____

5. Your provider-employer has asked you to research a particular medical topic using the computer. How do you proceed?

_____

_____

_____

_____

_____

_____

_____

6. Discuss the importance of patient confidentiality in medical computing. What measures are you required to take to be HIPAA compliant? How are these documented?

_____

_____

_____

_____

_____

_____

_____

_____

_____

_____

_____

_____

_____

Case Studies

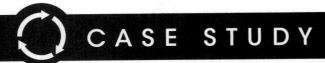

CASE STUDY

Due to an influx of patient volume, the practice of Drs. Lewis and King will have to hire more administrative staff and expand their office space. Three more computers have been installed, with updated software programs. Shirley Brooks, CMA (AAMA), practice manager, is trying to avoid any future safety issues in the workplace.

CASE STUDY REVIEW QUESTION

1. What factors should she take into consideration when setting up each workstation to be "ergonomically correct"?

_____

_____

_____

_____

_____

_____

_____

_____

_____

_____

_____

Web Activities

Go to the Web site of the supplier of the hardware and software used by your computer system. For example, hardware could be your printer; software could include Microsoft Office. Determine whether new drivers for the hardware or service updates for the software are available. Download and save the files to a temporary file folder. (Do not install the downloads unless instructed to do so by your computer system administrator or classroom instructor.)

CHAPTER POST-TEST

Perform this test without looking at your book.

1. The most common type of input device is the:
   a. USB port
   b. flash drive
   c. monitor
   d. keyboard

2. To ensure that your computer information is safe from unauthorized viewing within the clinic:
   a. use firewalls
   b. defragment frequently
   c. use passwords
   d. back up frequently

3. Which of the following is *not* a function of a total practice management system?
   a. Keeping track of appointments
   b. Keeping track of accounts receivable
   c. Keeping track of accounts payable
   d. Processing insurance claims
   e. Reading directions on how to download software

4. The part of the system that carries out instructions defined by the program software or the data input and then sends the results to the selected output devices is called the:
   a. motherboard
   b. modem
   c. video card
   d. CPU

5. To prevent unauthorized use of your clinic's computers, you should:
   a. establish only one person who has access to the computer
   b. keep the computer in a locked cabinet at night
   c. assign every employee a password
   d. have only one person on the computer at a time

SELF-ASSESSMENT

How comfortable are you with moving a computer from one area to another and hooking up all the cords, connections, and wires? What do you think you could do to become more comfortable with computer hardware connections? Look at the connections of your computer and its accessory hardware. Is it color coded or marked in some way?

_____

_____

_____

_____

_____

_____

_____

_____

CHAPTER **12**

Telecommunications

CHAPTER PRE-TEST

Perform this test without looking at your book.

1. _____ involves saying words correctly.
   a. Enunciation
   b. Pronunciation
   c. Articulation
   d. Personification

2. Guidelines that ensure successful transfer of calls include:
   a. Getting the caller's full name, telephone number, and date of birth
   b. Following up to be sure the call transferred directly to the clinic manager
   c. Determining who would be the best person to assist with the situation
   d. Following your telephone system's procedure for transferring the call
   e. All of the above
   f. c and d only

3. A telephone call concerning a complaint about medical service should be routed to the:
   a. Provider
   b. Clinical medical assistant
   c. Administrative medical assistant
   d. File clerk

4. The act of evaluating the urgency of a medical situation and prioritizing the call is known as:
   a. Screening
   b. Triage
   c. Delegation
   d. Enunciation

5. Advantages of using a fax machine include:

   a. Documents are transmitted immediately

   b. The receiver has the hard copy document versus relying on verbal information

   c. The cost of a fax is the approximate cost of a telephone call

   d. All of the above

VOCABULARY BUILDER

Misspelled Words

Find the words below that are misspelled; circle them, and correctly spell them in the spaces provided. Then fill in the blanks in the following paragraph with the appropriate terms. (Hint: not all terms will be used.)

answering services	etiquette	modulated
articulate	faximile	pronounciation
automated routing unit	fluent	screening
buffer words	Good Samaritan laws	
clincial email	handheld devices	
enuncate	jargine	

_____ _____ _____

_____ _____

When speaking on the telephone, medical assistants must use proper telephone _____, which means being courteous and professional to others. To ensure that listeners understand what is said, it is important to _____, or say the words clearly. Simple terms rather than medical _____ promote mutual understanding rather than confusion. The use of slang words and expressions is considered unprofessional and disrespectful. When speaking with a caller who is not _____ in English, it is helpful to speak slowly and use short sentences. Proper _____ of all words in a carefully _____ voice will also help people understand what you are saying, especially non–English-speaking people. Good communication skills are of real benefit to a medical assistant when using the telephone and when speaking directly to patients.

Matching

Match the following devices or services listed in Column A with corresponding descriptions in Column B.

_____ 1. answering service   A. Takes calls when the clinic is closed

_____ 2. cellular phone   B. Sends a message via computer networks to an electronic mailbox located in another person's computer

_____ 3. automated routing unit   C. A portable telephone

_____ 4. fax   D. A document sent over telephone lines from one facsimile machine or modem to another

_____ 5. email   E. A system that allows callers to reach specific people or departments by pressing a specified number on a touch-tone telephone

LEARNING REVIEW

Short Answer

1. Name four reasons why a potential patient will contact an ambulatory care facility by telephone.

     _____

     _____

     _____

2. Many hospitals and ambulatory care settings have telephone systems to manage heavy telephone traffic; these are called automatic routing units.

3. No call should be left unattended for more than 20–30 seconds.

4. What is the difference between enunciation and pronunciation?

     _____

     _____

5. Name the three different types of Voice-over-Internet Protocol (VoIP) services in use.

     _____

     _____

6. List three advantages of email and three disadvantages of email.
     Advantages:

     _____

     _____

     _____

     Disadvantages:

     _____

     _____

     _____

7. Explain the difference between email and clinical email.

     _____

     _____

     _____

8. Why is it important for email to be encrypted?

     _____

     _____

9. List six questions that should be asked during telephone screening.

     _____

     _____

     _____

     _____

10. Telephone documentation should include what seven pieces of information?

_____

_____

_____

Scope of Practice Review

Indicate the calls described below that fall within the scope of practice for a medical assistant (MA) to respond to and the calls that should be directed to the provider (P).

Type of Call	Who Should Handle
Insurance questions	
Scheduling patient testing and clinic appointments	
Medical advice	
Requests for prescription refills	
Provider's family members	
General information about the practice	
Poor progress reports from a patient	
Requests for medications other than prescription refills	
Other providers	
Salespeople	
STAT reports	

Patient Confidentiality Activity

Because medical assistants must observe laws regarding both patient confidentiality and the patient's right to privacy, it is crucial for the medical assistant to understand and comply with legal and ethical principles and the restrictions governing the issues of patient confidentiality. Indicate by checking off the appropriate box whether the medical assistant may discuss a patient's medical condition or reveal details from the medical record.

	Yes	No	Yes, with signed release
Patient's spouse or family member			
Patient's employer			
Patient's attorney			
Another health care provider			
Patient's insurance carrier			
Referring provider's clinic			
Credit bureau or collection agency			
Member of the clinic staff, as necessary for patient care			
Other patient			
People outside the clinic (friends, acquaintances)			
Patient's parent or legal guardian, except concerning issues of birth control, abortion, or STDs			

CERTIFICATION REVIEW

These questions are designed to mimic the certification examination. Select the best response.

1. Telephone calls that may be handled by the medical assistant include all but which one of the following?
   a. Billing questions
   b. Appointment changes
   c. Requests for prescription refills
   d. Calls from other providers

2. When a medical assistant is talking to a patient on the telephone and another line rings, what should the medical assistant do?
   a. Ask permission from the first caller to put her on hold, answer the second call and then ask permission from that caller to put him on hold, and go back to the first caller to finish up.
   b. Put the first call on hold, answer the second call and handle that issue, then go back to the first caller.
   c. Let the second line ring; it will be picked up by an answering system.
   d. Finish with the first caller, then answer the second line.

3. Which of the following is *not* a good idea in a medical clinic?
   a. Using a speaker phone to listen to voice messages
   b. Speaking quietly on the telephone so other patients cannot hear
   c. Using a privacy screen to reduce the chance of being overheard on the telephone
   d. Using only email so you will not be overheard

4. After-hours telephone messages are usually directed to:
   a. the provider's home
   b. the medical manager's home
   c. a voice mail system or answering service/machine
   d. an email system

5. When talking to older adult patients on the phone:
   a. if the patient is hearing impaired, speak slower, clearer, and a little louder
   b. assume that they are senile or at least forgetful and repeat all the information several times
   c. if the person has difficulty understanding, simplify the information, ask if there are any questions, and try to explain patiently in simple terms
   d. all of the above
   e. a and c only

6. Guidelines of the Health Insurance Portability and Accountability Act (HIPAA) for telephone communication include:
   a. determine if patients have specific instructions on who has been granted privilege to their private medical information
   b. determine if patients have a particular number they want called for confidential communications
   c. ask if it is acceptable to leave a message if patients are not at the number provided
   d. all of the above

7. The best solution for handling a caller who refuses to give information after gentle prodding is:
   a. tell the patient to call back when he is ready to cooperate
   b. hang up on the caller
   c. take a message and then give it to the provider
   d. argue with the patient, telling him that he is being unreasonable and that you need the information

8. The administrative medical assistant should always try to answer a call:

    a. by the end of the first ring if possible but definitely within three rings

    b. after five rings

    c. after two rings and before five rings

    d. within a minute

9. Before transferring a call to the appropriate party, a guideline to follow is:

    a. put the caller on hold, then transfer the call

    b. put the caller on hold and contact the person to whom the call is going, to see if the person can speak to the caller

    c. transfer the call immediately

    d. get the caller's name, number, and any pertinent information

10. If a call is a medical emergency, what protocol should be followed in handling that type of situation?

    a. Tell the patient to go to the emergency room.

    b. Keep the caller on the line and call 911 on another line.

    c. Put the caller on hold and try to get the provider on the phone.

    d. Tell the patient that you will call 911 for her and then call her back.

11. To ensure sensible risk management when making calls, you should protect the patient's privacy at all times; this is referred to as:

    a. confidentiality

    b. jargon

    c. elaboration

    d. screening

LEARNING APPLICATION

Critical Thinking

1. Answering the telephone professionally is critical in the health care profession. Meet with several classmates who each have written a scenario appropriate for an ambulatory care setting phone call. Now take turns being the caller and the medical assistant answering the clinic phone. Follow the steps outlined in Procedure 12-1 to cultivate your skills.

    _____

    _____

    _____

2. You are the medical assistant assigned to answering the telephone today. You receive a call from an angry patient. He wants to know why his bill was so high when he was only in the clinic with the provider for five minutes. What will happen if you become angry in retaliation? How should you handle this call in a professional manner?

    _____

    _____

    _____

3. How would you go about writing a policy concerning the use of clinical email in your clinic? What legal and ethical considerations must you consider? What information might be addressed in a disclaimer related to clinical email use?

_____
_____
_____
_____
_____
_____
_____
_____
_____
_____
_____
_____
_____

Case Studies

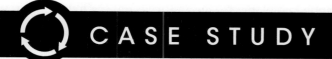

CASE STUDY

As Inner City Health Care, an urgent care center, continues to grow, increasing both patient load and staff, the existing telephone system, consisting of a simple intercom and four telephone lines, is no longer sufficient to handle the call volume and allow for full, immediate accessibility for all staff members. Callers are frustrated by the length of time it takes to get through and by long amounts of time spent on hold. Messages are often late in getting properly routed. Administrative medical assistant Karen Ritter suggests to clinic manager Jane O'Hara that an automated routing unit (ARU) might be more efficient for the growing clinic's needs. At the next regularly scheduled staff meeting, the provider-employers give the go-ahead to research an ARU.

CASE STUDY REVIEW QUESTIONS

1. ARU systems provide several options for callers that identify specific departments or services that callers can be connected with directly. What kinds of caller options might be appropriate for Inner City Health Care?

_____
_____
_____
_____
_____

2. What can be done so the patient with an emergency or the hearing-impaired patient can speak automatically to a "live" operator?

_____
_____
_____

3. How can an ARU help staff members receive their calls more efficiently?

_____
_____
_____

Role-Play Exercises

Effective telephone communication requires prompt and professional responses from medical assistants. With another student, role-play the following scenarios as patient and as medical assistant. When you are finished role-playing, write below what you said as the "medical assistant."

1. Patient Nora Fowler calls with a question about medication prescribed for her rheumatoid arthritis and insists on a call back from Dr. Elizabeth King. Dr. King is presently on rounds at the hospital and will not be available until 4:30 PM. Nora's tone of voice indicates that she is upset, and she states that her medication is not helping her discomfort. It is clear from the conversation that Nora has discontinued taking her medication.

   _____

   _____

   _____

   _____

   _____

2. While speaking on telephone line 1 with patient Bill Schwartz, who is calling to schedule a physical examination, medical assistant Wanda Slawson receives another call on line 2 from a laboratory with a summary of emergency test results for another patient. Wanda knows that Dr. Susan Rice is waiting for the test results.

   _____

   _____

   _____

   _____

3. Medical assistant Bruce Goldman takes a call from patient Juanita Hansen. Juanita is inquiring about a bill and indicating that her insurance carrier, Blue Cross, did not pay the entire fee for her son's last examination, which left her with a balance owed to Inner City Health Care. Clinic manager Walter Seals is responsible for managing insurance claims and inquiries.

   _____

   _____

   _____

Hands-on Activities

1. Each morning, medical assistant Ellen Armstrong is responsible for transcribing messages left on the medical practice's answering machine the evening before. Using the message pad slips below, transcribe each message completely and appropriately. In the space for "Attachments," list any records, files, or documents that should be attached to the message slip for the recipient's review.

   A. "Ellen, this is Anna Preciado. Can you tell Marilyn Johnson, the clinic manager, that I won't be in tomorrow for the afternoon shift? I have a 101-degree temperature and bad flu symptoms. Check with Joe Guerrero to see if he can come in to sub for me as the clinical medical assistant. Yesterday he told me he would be available if I wasn't feeling well enough to come in. I know Dr. Lewis has several patients scheduled for clinical testing in the afternoon. I can be reached at 555-6622."

   B. "This is Charles Williams. Dr. Lewis put me on a Holter monitor today. It's about 11:00 PM and one of the leads came off. I put it back on, but I am worried about whether I will have to do this test again. Can you call me tomorrow at home before 8:00 AM at 555-6124 or at the office after 9:00 AM at 555-8125? Thanks."

To: _____   Date: _____

From: _____   Time: _____

Telephone #: _____

Message: _____
_____
_____
_____
_____

Initials: _____

Attachments: _____
_____
_____

© Cengage Learning 2014

To: _____   Date: _____

From: _____   Time: _____

Telephone #: _____

Message: _____
_____
_____
_____
_____
_____
_____

Initials: _____

Attachments: _____
_____

© Cengage Learning 2014

Web Activities

Using the Internet, search for current information relative to legal and ethical considerations when using telecommunications in the ambulatory care setting. Compile your information into a one-page report, and list your URL addresses for your instructor.

CHAPTER POST-TEST

Perform this test without looking at your book.

1. A digital ID is composed of a:
   a. digital signature
   b. private key
   c. password
   d. a. and b. only

2. The advantages of using email as a means of communication include:
   a. avoiding talking to the recipient face-to-face
   b. creating a documentation trail of interactions between provider and patient
   c. lack of real-time interaction and feedback
   d. lack of body language or vocal inflection

3. A disadvantage of VoIP telecommunication is that:
   a. emergency services through 911 may not be available
   b. emergency services through 911 are always available
   c. most VoIP services will still work during a power outage
   d. directory assistance/white page listings are available on a consistent basis

4. Examples of operator-assisted calls include:
   a. international calls
   b. conference calls
   c. collect calls
   d. all of the above

5. Using professional _____ is not advised if simpler terms will convey a message appropriately to a patient.
   a. etiquette
   b. jargon
   c. buffer words
   d. pronunciation

SELF-ASSESSMENT

1. Discuss the following questions with another classmate or in a small group. During the discussion, consider how different people react in different ways, depending on their personalities, their patience, and their confidence levels. After the discussion, spend a moment in self-reflection to think of ways you can improve your telephone communication skills.

   (1) Have you ever conversed with someone on the telephone whom you could not understand?

   _____

   _____

   (2) Was the problem the language of the individual, or his or her accent, enunciation, or volume?

   _____

   _____

   (3) Would it have been easier to understand the individual if you were face-to-face with that person?

   _____

   _____

   (4) How did you handle the situation? Did you ask the person to speak louder, slower, or more clearly?

   _____

   _____

(5) How do you think most people would handle a situation in which they could not hear the speaker clearly? What if the speaker were an older adult? A non–English speaker? A person in pain or very ill?

_____

_____

2. Of the following telecommunication devices and methods, with which are you most familiar and which will you need to learn more about? What do you think is the best way to become more familiar with the following devices and methods?

- Email
- Multiline phones
- Cell phones
- Fax machines
- Answering services

_____

_____

_____

_____

CHAPTER **13**

Patient Scheduling

CHAPTER PRE-TEST

Perform this test without looking at your book.

1. Circle the letter that lists correct types of scheduling systems:
   a. Wave, modified wave, double booking, mile-a-minute
   b. Open hours, wave, clustering, stream, double booking
   c. First-come, first-served; open hours; clustering

2. Below are guidelines to scheduling. Which one is correct?
   a. Urgent calls should be sent to the hospital, which is better equipped to handle them.
   b. Urgent calls should be assessed before determining the best course of action.
   c. Referrals by other providers need to be seen immediately.
   d. Appointments for pharmaceutical and medical supply representatives should be referred to the provider.

3. Information that should be obtained from all new patients includes all but which one of the following?
   a. The patient's full legal name
   b. The patient's birth date
   c. The patient's address and telephone numbers
   d. The reason for the visit
   e. The patient's insurance information
   f. The patient's family health history

4. The appointment _____ provides a current and accurate record of appointment times available.
   a. schedule
   b. screening
   c. matrix
   d. referral

5. What type(s) of information are necessary for the patient to provide when scheduling their own procedure?
   a. Name of the provider
   b. Insurance information
   c. Social Security number
   d. All of the above

VOCABULARY BUILDER

Misspelled Words

Find the words below that are misspelled; circle them, and correctly spell them in the spaces provided. Then insert the correct vocabulary terms from the list that best fit the scenarios below.

clustering

double booking

encription technology

matrics

modified wave scheduling

no-show

open hours

practice based

screaning

stream scheduling

wave scheduling

_____

_____

_____

1. _____ Inner City Health Care reserves 9 am to 12 pm on Thursday mornings for walk-in patients who are seen on a first-come, first-served basis within that time frame.

2. _____ At the clinic of Drs. Lewis and King, Ellen Armstrong, CMA (AAMA), schedules Mary O'Keefe for a 1:00 pm appointment for some blood work and Martin Gordon for a 1:00 pm appointment for a blood pressure check so Dr. King can assess whether his medication is at the proper level.

3. _____ Lenny Taylor, an older adult patient with mild dementia, forgets his third appointment with Dr. James Whitney.

4. _____ At Inner City Health Care, vaccinations are scheduled every 10 minutes from 10 am to 12:20 pm on Mondays; Tuesday office hours are reserved for new patients only.

5. _____ Three patients are scheduled to receive treatments in the first half hour of every hour.

6. _____ Dr. Elizabeth King prefers to see patients for regular gynecologic examinations in consecutive appointments scheduled from 8:30 am to 11:30 am and obstetric patients from 1:00 pm to 3:30 pm.

7. _____ When patient Herb Fowler calls to set up an appointment with Dr. Winston Lewis for his chronic cough, Ellen Armstrong, CMA (AAMA), asks Herb a series of questions to ascertain the nature, extent, and urgency of his condition.

8. _____ Dr. Winston Lewis prefers that each patient be assigned a specific time, scheduling at 30- or 60-minute intervals on a continuous basis throughout the day.

9. _____ An ophthalmologist schedules three patients at the beginning of each hour for comprehensive examinations, followed by single appointments every 10 to 20 minutes during the rest of the hour for quick, follow-up procedures such as removing eye patches or instilling eye drops.

10. _____ On the 15th day of each month, clinic manager Walter Seals, CMA (AAMA), who is responsible for efficient patient flow at Inner City Health Care, asks each of the urgent care center's five providers to confirm their scheduling commitments for the upcoming month to block off unavailable times in the appointment book.

11. _____ The medical assistant uses software to protect patients' confidentiality in electronic format.

LEARNING REVIEW

Short Answer

1. Appointment books are legal documents recording patient flow. For a manual appointment system, where pencil is used for ease in rescheduling, what can the medical assistant do to ensure that a permanent record is secured?

_____

_____

2. For a computerized appointment system, what can a medical assistant do to ensure that a permanent record of patient flow is secured?

_____

_____

3. Name two primary goals in determining the best method for scheduling patient appointments.

_____

_____

4. What is the typical scheduling time for each of the following types of clinic visits for an internal medicine practice?

    (1) Patient consultation:

    (2) Established patient routine follow-up:

    (3) New patient:

    (4) Complete physical examination:

    (5) Cold/flu symptoms:

    (6) Vaccination:

5. What are six variables involved in the process of scheduling appointments for patients and other visitors to the ambulatory care setting?

_____

_____

_____

_____

6. Patient flow analysis sheets help medical practices determine the effectiveness of patient scheduling and devise plans for improving a smooth patient flow through the ambulatory care setting. What kinds of issues can a study of these data reveal?

_____

_____

_____

7. What are the five steps of scheduling a specific appointment time for a patient?

_____

_____

_____

_____

_____

8. Two ways of reminding patients of upcoming appointments are to give the appointment card personally to the patient and to mail the card to the patient. Identify a third reminder system. What procedures must be observed to protect patient confidentiality when using this third method?

_____

_____

_____

9. Identify seven scheduling styles.

_____

10. Identify the best scheduling system for the examples below, and explain the reasoning behind your choice.

(1) Hospital emergency room: _____

_____

(2) Laboratory for blood testing: _____

_____

_____

(3) Two or more patients are given a particular appointment time: _____

_____

(4) Best-known and widely used scheduling system: _____

_____

CERTIFICATION REVIEW

These questions are designed to mimic the certification examination. Select the best response.

1. Scheduling outpatient procedures:
   a. is done at the end of each day
   b. is best done with the patient present
   c. will be easier with a calendar for visualization of days discussed
   d. b and c

2. One principle above all else in scheduling for the clinic is:
   a. flexibility
   b. neatness
   c. accountability
   d. estimation

3. The type of scheduling that requires visits to be set up around patients with specific chronic ailments such as diabetes and hypertension is called:

   a. screening

   b. referral appointments

   c. group scheduling

   d. stream appointments

4. The general rule for no-shows and cancellations is that after ___ consecutive missed appointments, the provider will review the patient's record and could terminate care.

   a. five

   b. three

   c. two

   d. ten

5. What, more than anything else, determines the success of a day in the ambulatory care setting?

   a. Patient care

   b. Efficient patient flow

   c. Operational functions

   d. Interpersonal skills

LEARNING APPLICATION

Critical Thinking

1. Why is there no one best system of scheduling?

   _____

   _____

   _____

   _____

2. For the following situations, briefly explain which type of scheduling system you would choose and why.

   a. A four-provider practice has only two providers seeing patients at any one time. Three medical assistants share front- and back-office duties for all of the providers.

   b. An obstetrics practice specializes in problem pregnancies. There is one administrative and one clinical medical assistant.

   _____

   _____

   _____

   _____

3. With another person in your class, identify two or three public encounters where you feel ignored or rushed as a customer. How does it make you feel? What suggestions would you make to the business to change that feeling?

   _____

   _____

   _____

   _____

   _____

   _____

Case Studies

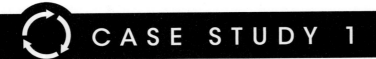

CASE STUDY 1

When patient Lenore McDonell falls from the examination table and lacerates her arm while attempting an independent transfer from the table to her wheelchair, clinical medical assistant Joe Guerrero alerts Dr. Winston Lewis, and the two begin to implement emergency procedures to control Lenore's bleeding and assess damage to the arm. Lenore's fall occurred at the end of her appointment, a routine checkup with Dr. Lewis.

Administrative medical assistant Ellen Armstrong must adjust Dr. Lewis's schedule to accommodate the emergency situation. Martin Gordon, a man in his mid-60s, diagnosed with prostate cancer, waits in the reception area for Dr. Lewis's next appointment. Mr. Gordon's appointment, a 6-month follow-up, is expected to take 30 minutes. Mr. Gordon is also being rated for depression related to his cancer diagnosis. Hope Smith, a new patient in good general health, is scheduled for a complete examination; she is due to arrive at the clinic of Drs. Lewis and King at the Northborough Family Medical Group within 20 minutes. Jim Marshall, an impatient and aggressive businessman, is scheduled for the first afternoon appointment after Dr. Lewis's lunch commitment. Mr. Marshall's appointment for a physical examination and ECG to investigate chest pains he has experienced recently is expected to take 45 minutes. Dr. Lewis's schedule is completely booked for the rest of the day.

CASE STUDY REVIEW QUESTIONS

1. What scheduling alternatives will Ellen offer Mr. Gordon, who is already waiting in the reception area? What special considerations regarding Mr. Gordon should Ellen take into account and why?

_____

_____

_____

_____

_____

_____

2. What is Ellen's first action regarding Ms. Smith, Dr. Lewis's next patient due to arrive? What scheduling alternatives should Ellen offer her?

_____

_____

_____

_____

3. What scheduling alternatives, if any, should Ellen present to Mr. Marshall? Explain your logic.

_____

_____

_____

Hands-on Activity

Patient Martin Gordon has a 30-minute appointment scheduled with Dr. Lewis on Wednesday, February 7, 2012 for routine follow-up for prostate cancer. He calls the clinic on January 30 and would like to reschedule his appointment for two weeks later at 3:00 pm, the same time. You mark through his name on the appointment schedule with a single line in red pen, and document the change in the patient's chart. Now, complete the appointment card below to be mailed to Mr. Gordon as a reminder of his new appointment time.

LEWIS & KING, MD
2501 CENTER STREET
NORTHBOROUGH, OH 56789

Patient: _____

has an appointment on

Mon. _____ at _____
Tues. _____ at _____
Wed. _____ at _____
Thurs. _____ at _____
Fri. _____ at _____

If unable to keep appointment, kindly give 24 hours' notice.

© Cengage Learning 2014

Web Activities

1. Go to http://www.physicianpractice.com, and look for any information you can find regarding online patient scheduling. Identify advantages and disadvantages of online scheduling.

2. Go to your favorite search engine and key in "patient scheduling." Numerous sites will appear. Many offer a free download to examine their components. What particular components seem most helpful? How many are separate software pieces as compared with the software in connection with a total practice management program? How many require specialized training? Recommend two or three packages to examine more closely.

CHAPTER POST-TEST

Perform this test without looking at your book.

1. Circle the letter that lists correct types of scheduling systems.
   a. Modified wave, wave, clustering, mile-a-minute
   b. Stream, open hours, wave, grouping, separating
   c. First-come, first-served; open hours; clustering
   d. Open hours, wave, clustering, stream, double booking

2. Below are guidelines to scheduling. Which one is correct?
   a. Urgent calls should be scheduled for the next available appointment time.
   b. Urgent calls should be sent to the hospital, which is better equipped to handle them.
   c. If a referral patient calls, it is best to obtain information from the referring provider's clinic to determine the urgency of the appointment.
   d. Appointments for pharmaceutical and medical supply representatives should be referred to the provider.

3. Information that should be obtained from all new patients includes all but which one of the following?

   a. The patient's full legal name

   b. The patient's birth date

   c. The patient's address and telephone numbers

   d. Family health history

   e. Reason for the visit

   f. The patient's insurance information

4. The appointment _____ provides a current and accurate record of appointment times available.

   a. referral

   b. schedule

   c. screening

   d. matrix

5. What type(s) of information are necessary for the patient to provide when scheduling their own procedure?

   a. Patient's address and phone number

   b. Insurance information

   c. Social Security number

   d. All of the above

   e. a and b only

SELF-ASSESSMENT

1. When you call a provider's clinic, do any of the following aggravate you? Do you think other people are aggravated by these?

   a. Being put on hold right away or too often

   b. The administrative medical assistant asking too many questions

   c. Not enough appointment time choices; that is, you have to wait too long for an appointment

   d. Not getting a real person; that is, having to listen to menu choices and make selections

   e. Other (add your own idea) _____

2. Now go to each of the situations in question 1 and determine an action that could alleviate all or some of the aggravation. Keep in mind that the situation might still exist (e.g., the receptionist might still have to ask a lot of questions), but how might he or she make the experience more pleasant?

3. When you visit a provider's clinic, do any of the following aggravate you?

   a. The administrative medical assistant does not acknowledge you right away

   b. The wait is too long

   c. The waiting room is noisy, messy, or uncomfortable

   d. There are no magazines of interest to you

   e. Other (add your own idea) _____

4. Similar to the instructions in question 2, go to each of the situations in question 3 and determine solutions that could alleviate all or some of the causes of aggravation. Keep in mind that the solutions in this case are obvious and doable.

CHAPTER **14**

Medical Records Management

CHAPTER PRE-TEST

Perform this test without looking at your book.

1. In the SOAPER approach, the letter "E" stands for:
   a. Equipment needed
   b. Education for patient
   c. Eliminated medications
   d. Education for staff

2. Which of the following is *not* an important skill to have when filing?
   a. You should know the alphabet.
   b. You should know the basic rules of filing.
   c. You should pay attention to details.
   d. You should be good at math.

3. Which of the following is not an advantage of a manual medical record?
   a. Can be used by only one person at a time
   b. Easier to protect confidentiality
   c. No worry of computer malfunction
   d. Currently established and understood

4. Which of the following patients would be filed first if the method of alphabetic filing by last name were used?
   a. Betty Donaldson
   b. Bradley Donalds
   c. Annette Dunn
   d. Amber Davidson

5. The standard in court is that if there is no record of any piece of information related to a patient and that patient's care and treatment:

   a. The record must have been misfiled and must be produced immediately

   b. The treatment did not happen

   c. The record is assumed as being destroyed

   d. The patient declined the treatment and therefore no record exists

VOCABULARY BUILDER

Misspelled Words

Find the words below that are misspelled; underline them, and correctly spell them in the space provided. Then, fill in the blanks in the following sentences with the appropriate terms. (Hint: not all words will be used).

accession record	out-gide	source-orientated medical record
captions	perging	tickler file
coding	problem-orientated medical record	unit
cross-reference		
key unit	SOAP	

_____   _____

_____   _____

1. To remember to check with the reference laboratory on Friday to obtain patient Martin Gordon's test results, Ellen Armstrong, CMA (AAMA), places a note in her _____.

2. Every six months, Marilyn Johnson follows clinic policy and procedures for _____ in-active files to remove and archive those not in active use.

3. The organized method of identifying and separating items to be filed into small subunits is accomplished with the use of _____ units.

4. When Liz Corbin, CMA (AAMA), retrieves Annette Samuels's chart for Dr. Woo, she places an _____ in the filing cabinet to show that the file has been removed from storage.

5. The _____ is a journal (or computer listing) where numbers in a numeric filing system are pre-assigned. The log sequentially lists numbers to be used to assign to numeric records.

6. The file for Kent Memorial Hospital contains three indexing _____ to be considered when preparing the filing label.

7. If a _____ card is required in the alphabetic card file of a numeric filing system, such as when making note of an established patient's married name, a card is prepared that includes an *X* next to the file number to indicate that this card does not designate the primary location card for the file.

8. In the _____ system of recordkeeping, patient problems are identified by a number that corresponds to the charting relevant to that problem number; that is, asthma #1; dermatitis #2; and so on.

9. When a filing system other than alphabetic is being used, the proper _____ must be determined for the chart or file so it can be retrieved.

10. _____ are used to identify major sections of file folders by more manageable subunits, such as GA–GE, or Miscellaneous. They are marked on the tabs of the guides.

11. Inner City Health Care uses the _____ method of recordkeeping, which groups information according to its origin—for example, laboratories, examinations, provider notes, consulting providers, and other types of information.

12. Some medical facilities have added two additional letters, *E* and *R*, to the _____ approach, which stand for "Education for patient" and "Response of patient to education and care given."

LEARNING REVIEW

Short Answer

1. Why is accurate, up-to-date, complete documentation in patient medical records essential in the ambulatory care setting?

   _____

   _____

   _____

   _____

2. Why is the POMR system commonly used by family practice clinics?

   _____

   _____

3. Why is a color-coding system effective in the ambulatory care setting?

   _____

4. How important is an effective, easy-to-use, and easy-to-access filing system to the efficiency of the ambulatory care setting?

   _____

   _____

   _____

   _____

5. List at least four advantages of EMRs.

   _____

   _____

   _____

6. What does the acronym SOAPER stand for?

   _____

   _____

7. List three numeric filing systems that are used in medical facilities.

   _____

Indexing Units Exercise

Assign the correct units to the following items to be filed using the rule for filing patient records that is listed for each.

1. Names that are hyphenated are considered one unit.
   A. Jackson Hugh Levine-Dwyer

   unit 1 _____   unit 2 _____   unit 3 _____

   B. Leslie Jane Poole-Petit

   unit 1 _____   unit 2 _____   unit 3 _____

2. Seniority units are indexed as the last indexing unit.
   A. Keith Wildasin Sr.

   unit 1 _____   unit 2 _____   unit 3 _____

   B. Gerald Maggart III

   unit 1 _____   unit 2 _____   unit 3 _____

3. Titles are considered as separate indexing units. If the title appears with first and last names, the title is considered the last indexing unit.
   A. Dr. Louise Udolf

   unit 1 _____   unit 2 _____   unit 3 _____

   B. Prof. Valerie Rajah

   unit 1 _____   unit 2 _____   unit 3 _____

4. The names of individuals are assigned indexing units respectively: last name, first name, middle, and succeeding names.
   A. Lindsay Adair Martin

   unit 1 _____   unit 2 _____   unit 3 _____

   B. Abigail Sue Johnson

   unit 1 _____   unit 2 _____   unit 3 _____

5. Foreign language units are indexed as one unit with the unit that follows. Spacing, punctuation, and capitalization are ignored.
   A. Joseph Jack dela Hoya

   unit 1 _____   unit 2 _____   unit 3 _____

   B. Maurice John van de Veer

   unit 1 _____   unit 2 _____   unit 3 _____

Multiple Choice

Circle the right answer(s) from the choices below.

1. The most important reason for using numeric filing is that:
   a. it preserves patient confidentiality
   b. a larger number of records can be easily filed
   c. a computer can more readily read numeric filing labels

2. Walter Seals, CMA (AAMA), is filing using a terminal digit filing system. For the patient file labeled 67 84 30, what is unit 1?
   a. 67
   b. 30
   c. 80

3. Outgoing correspondence is:

    a. friendly correspondence

    b. correspondence sent out of the medical clinic

    c. correspondence to be thrown away

4. Karen Ritter, RMA (AMT), is filing patient files using a numeric filing system. She comes across a file for a patient who has not yet been assigned a number. Karen should put the file:

    a. in the miscellaneous numeric file section

    b. in a pending filing bin until the provider can assign a number

    c. directly behind the rest of the files

5. An out guide in paper or manual records should contain:

    a. a record of when the chart was removed

    b. the signature of the patient's provider

    c. a record of when the file is expected to be returned

6. State statutes have ruled that medical records are the property of the:

    a. state medical society

    b. ones who create them

    c. patient only

7. Any information to be released from the medical record:

    a. goes to medical insurance

    b. requires a provider's signature

    c. requires patient notification and approval

    d. requires a subpoena

8. Filing equipment:

    a. should have a locking capability

    b. is available in vertical or lateral styles

    c. is to be stored in an area accessible only to authorized personnel

    d. all of the above

9. EMR stands for:

    a. emergency room

    b. a popular color-coding system's trade name

    c. electronic medical records

    d. emergency medical rules

10. Release marks include:

    a. date stamp and initials

    b. out guides

    c. tabs

    d. SOAP/SOAPER

CERTIFICATION REVIEW

These questions are designed to mimic the certification examination. Select the best response.

1. The POMR is also known as:
   a. a source-oriented medical record
   b. a SOAP/SOAPER system
   c. a traditional method
   d. a problem-oriented medical record
   e. none of the above

2. The SOAP/SOAPER format is:
   a. a way to sanitize instruments
   b. a form of patient electronic records
   c. a type of filing system
   d. a specific charting system
   e. none of the above

3. If a patient needs to return for another examination in six months, you might use a reminder system. What is the name of that system?
   a. Reminder system
   b. Recall system
   c. Phone log
   d. Tickler system
   e. Out guide

4. The most common method of filing in today's medical clinic is:
   a. alphabetically
   b. numerically
   c. by insurance
   d. by subject
   e. color coding

5. If a medical document is filed in multiple places, you might use a(n):
   a. index
   b. out guide
   c. cross-reference
   d. multiple reference
   e. cross-filed card

6. The best method to use for making a correction in a paper medical record is:
   a. use a "white out" product
   b. scribble over the error with a magic marker
   c. put *X*'s through the error
   d. draw a single line through the error, make the correction, write "**CORR**" or "**CORRECTION**" above the area corrected, and add your initials and date

7. Identifiable patient information that should *not* appear on the outside of the chart would include:
   a. patient's address
   b. patient's social security number
   c. patient's birth date
   d. patient's phone number
   e. all of the above

8. Closed files are usually kept:
   a. 3 to 6 years beyond the statute of limitations
   b. 2 to 5 years
   c. indefinitely
   d. 10 years

9. The three types of cabinets used in medical clinics are:
   a. vertical, lateral, and movable
   b. metal, hanging, and color coded
   c. horizontal, lateral, and movable
   d. open, locked, and movable

10. Captions are used:
    a. to separate file folders
    b. to identify major sections of file folders
    c. in vertical and lateral systems
    d. a and c only

LEARNING APPLICATION

Filing Order Review

Using the numbers 1, 2, and 3, label the patient names in each group according to the correct filing order of names in an alphabetic filing system.

L. Sanders

Larry Paul Samuels

Lawrence P. Sanders

James Edward Reed Sr.

James Edward Reed

James Edward Reed Jr.

Lynn Elaine Brenner

Lynn Ellen Brenner

Lynn Eloise Brenner

Patrick Sam Saint

Patrick Sam St. Bartz

Paul Sam Saint

Critical Thinking

1. A patient's chart has been subpoenaed for pending malpractice litigation. In preparing the chart, you discover an error that was made when the results of the laboratory report were incorrectly documented in the chart. You have the original laboratory report. What should you do?

_____

_____

_____

_____

_____

_____

_____

2. Research the statute of limitations in your state for medical records to determine how long a medical record should be kept. The statute will also tell you what triggers activity on a medical file that might dictate it be kept longer than normally indicated.

_____

_____

3. Identify the steps you might take in "inspecting" the charts before filing. What would you do if you found something missing or an unsigned report?

_____

4. It has been said that filing records is the easiest task the medical assistant will perform, yet it is often the most difficult. What reasons can you give for this statement?

_____

_____

_____

Web Activities

1. Using your favorite search engine, key in "medical record authorization for release of information." Are you able to find a site that has a sample blank form to be completed? Are there any surprises? For how long is the authorization valid?

2. Search for information on electronic medical records. Identify the number of sites that come up. Select two or three sites that allow you to view or download a sample of the product software. Identify your likes and dislikes and give your rationale. What would influence you if you were helping to select electronic medical record software for a medical facility where you are employed?

CHAPTER POST-TEST

Perform this test without looking at your book.

1. Certain indexing rules have been developed by the Association of Medical Records Administrators (AMRA) to:
   a. facilitate the alphabetic process in maintaining files
   b. facilitate the indexing process in maintaining files
   c. facilitate the storage process in retrieving files
   d. facilitate the numeric process in tracking files

2. When filing, you need to be skilled in all but which one of the following?
   a. Knowing the alphabet
   b. Knowing the basic rules of filing
   c. Being able to pay attention to details
   d. Being good at math

3. The three major filing systems that are commonly used in the ambulatory care setting are alphabetic, numeric and _____.
   a. color coding
   b. subject
   c. alphanumeric
   d. indexing

4. A method that serves as a reminder that some action needs to be taken at a date in the future is:
   a. tickler file
   b. alpha file
   c. reminder file
   d. indexing file

5. In terminal digit filing:
   a. the middle digits are the primary units
   b. the first two digits are the primary units
   c. the last two digits are the primary units
   d. none of the above
   e. a and c only

SELF-ASSESSMENT

To perform this self-assessment, you must first perform an exercise: Go to your spice drawer; a stack of magazines; a bunch of bills/statements; or even your clothes closet, drawers, or the shelves you keep your towels on. (Maybe organize something in your medical assisting classroom or laboratory area!)

1. Think of the best way to organize them. Is it by size, color, or both? Alphabetically? By date? Frequency of use?

   _____

   _____

2. Perform the organization. What was the most difficult part: planning how to best accomplish it, or actually doing it? Did you have to take everything out and place it back in order, or were you able to just move things around? Was this a time-consuming exercise? Is the order now a useful tool? Did you have any decisions to make, such as do you file red pepper under red or pepper? Should your pants be organized with their matching tops, or should all the pants be together and all the tops together? Should the medications be organized in alphabetic order, or by classification (type of action)?

_____

_____

3. Now choose another item to organize in a different way. How did this second exercise differ? (For example, towels might have been organized by size or by color, whereas your spices would be organized alphabetically.) Do you think another person would have chosen a different method?

_____

_____

4. Who do you think decides in an office how a particular area is to be organized? Do you think there might be different ways?

_____

_____

5. Pretend that your provider's clinic has its patients' charts filed alphabetically, but now they are moving to more computerized records and want to change their files to a numeric system. Make a list of the supplies the staff will need, calculate the time it might take, and make up a plan on how to accomplish this (remember the files are still being used every day). Does this seem like a major undertaking? Could any files be purged (pulled out of circulation) during this reorganization?

_____

_____

CHAPTER **15**

Written Communications

CHAPTER PRE-TEST

Perform this test without looking at your book.

1. The four major letter styles are (*circle four of the following*):
   a. Full block
   b. Modified block, standard
   c. Facilitated block
   d. Simplified block
   e. Simplified
   f. Modified block, indented

2. The part of a letter that includes a specially designed logo with the address and phone numbers is called the:
   a. Salutation
   b. Inside address
   c. Letterhead
   d. Reference heading
   e. Enclosure

3. The process of reading a document and checking for accuracy is known as:
   a. Referencing
   b. Proofreading
   c. Verification
   d. Rationalizing

4. This part of a letter should begin on the second line below the salutation unless a subject line is used that precedes two lines above the body:
   a. Postscript
   b. Copy notation
   c. Complimentary closing
   d. Body of the letter

5. A computerized feature that allows you to send the same letter, although personalized, to many different people using a database is called:

   a. Word processing letters

   b. Mail merge

   c. Database letters

   d. Merge correspondence

VOCABULARY BUILDER

Misspelled Words

Find the words below that are misspelled; underline them, and correctly spell them in the space provided. Then, fill in the blanks in the passage below with the correct vocabulary terms. (Hint: not all terms will be used.)

bond paper	mail merge	proofread
form letters	modified block letter	simplified letter
full block letter	optical character reader	watermarque
keed	portfoleo	ZIP+4

_____ _____ _____

There are four major types of letter styles in which medical assistants commonly write. Of these, the _____ _____ style is the most time-efficient, because it does not use excessive tab indentations for the address, complimentary closure, or keyed signature. In the _____ style, all lines begin at the left margin with the exception of the date line, complimentary closure, and keyed signature. Medical assistants may choose to use the _____ style, which is the style of letter recommended by the Administrative Management Society. In this style, all lines are _____, or input by keystroke, flush with the left margin. When selecting paper supplies, the medical assistant should choose _____ with a _____, or image imprinted during the papermaking process that is visible when a sheet is held up to the light. When preparing letters for outgoing shipments, it is important for the medical assistant to pay attention to several factors, including addresses. Medical assistants should machine-print addresses (including the _____ code) with a uniform left-hand margin so that the addresses can be read by the U.S. Postal Service's _____ (OCR). One creative approach to letter composition is to create a _____ or database of frequently used form _____.

LEARNING REVIEW

Abbreviations Exercise

Write what each abbreviation stands for.

1. Enc. _____

2. c _____

3. P.S. _____

4. OCR _____

5. CAP _____

6. ROM   _____

7. LC   _____

8. WF   _____

MATCHING

Match the common proofreader's mark in column 1 to its meaning in column 2.

_____ 1. #   A. "Let it stand"

_____ 2. ^   B. Paragraph indent

_____ 3. BF   C. Insert space

_____ 4. STET   D. Move left

_____ 5.]   E. Italic type

_____ 6. [F. Align type horizontally

_____ 7. :| G. Insert

_____ 8. =   H. Boldface type

_____ 9. ITAL   I. Move right

_____ 10. ¶   J. Insert colon

Processing Mail Exercise

For each type of mail below, list the action the medical assistant should take or to what department or person the medical assistant should forward the mail.

Type of Mail	Action Taken
Invoices for supplies and equipment	
Magazines for reception area	
Insurance forms	
Patient payments	
Medical journals	
Personal or confidential letters	

CERTIFICATION REVIEW

These questions are designed to mimic the certification examination. Select the best response.

1. The "salutation" of a letter is the:
   a. signature
   b. greeting
   c. return address
   d. closing remark (such as "Sincerely")
   e. the recipient's name, title, and address

2. When addressing an envelope, the proper way to list the state is:
   a. to write it out completely
   b. to abbreviate it using at least the first four letters
   c. to capitalize it using the official two-letter abbreviation
   d. to use any of the above so long as it is in uppercase letters and is written clearly

3. Which of the following would be incoming mail to a provider's office?
   a. Email
   b. Insurance forms
   c. Medical journals
   d. Letters from patients
   e. All of the above

4. The medical assistant may, with the provider's permission, sign certain letters such as:
   a. the ordering of supplies or subscriptions
   b. notification of collection procedures and reminder of payments
   c. dismissal letters
   d. a and b

5. When addressing an envelope:
   a. the address should be machine-printed with a uniform left margin
   b. all punctuation should be eliminated
   c. use dark ink on a light background using uppercase letters
   d. all of the above

6. The types of envelopes most often used are:
   a. number 7
   b. number 6¾
   c. number 10
   d. b and c

7. Periodical is the new classification for:
   a. second class mail
   b. third class mail
   c. priority mail
   d. parcel post mail

8. Before presenting any correspondence to the provider for signature, the document should be:

   a. date stamped

   b. checked for accuracy

   c. folded and put in an envelope

   d. typed on plain white paper

9. The most secure service the USPS offers is:

   a. priority mail

   b. express mail

   c. registered mail

   d. certified mail

LEARNING APPLICATION

Critical Thinking

1. With a group of classmates, organize a spelling bee of commonly misspelled medical words. Include some nonmedical English words that are often misspelled also. Conduct the spelling bee.

2. Practice how to compose business correspondence using all components. Procedure 15-1 is a helpful guide. Print a draft copy of your letter and use common proofreader's marks to indicate any corrections.

3. Rekey the above letter and practice how to fold it correctly. Procedure 15-3 provides step-by-step instructions.

4. Practice how to address an envelope with all address elements in proper format for expeditious handling by the U.S. Postal Service. Procedure 15-2 provides step-by-step instructions for addressing envelopes. Now place your letter into the envelope correctly. Refer to Procedure 15-3 if you have forgotten how to insert the letter properly.

Case Studies

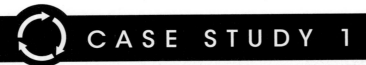

CASE STUDY 1

Ellen Armstrong, CMA (AAMA), enjoys working on correspondence for Drs. Lewis and King and takes pride in her written communication skills. As an ongoing project, clinic manager Marilyn Johnson asks Ellen to make suggestions for updating and revising the style manual used in the medical office for written communication guidelines. Ellen suggests the addition of a section in the style manual to discuss bias in language. Bias-free language is sensitive in applying labels to individuals or groups and uses sex-specific words and pronouns appropriately. For example, "dementia" is used instead of "crazy" or "senile." Instead of using "layman," consider using "layperson." Apply "he or she" only in sex-specific usage. Marilyn and the provider-employer ask Ellen to implement the addition to the style manual.

CASE STUDY REVIEW QUESTIONS

1. Why is bias-free language an important consideration in written communication for the ambulatory care setting?

_____

_____

_____

_____

2. List other examples of biased language and give suggestions for bias-free alternatives.

_____

_____

_____

_____

Proofreading Exercise

Proofread the letter below, correcting all errors by inserting the proper proofreader's marks directly onto the text. (Consult your textbook for a list of common proofreader's marks and refer to a medical dictionary, if necessary.)

JAMES CARTER, MD, NEUROLOGY

Metropolitan University Medical Center, 8280 Wright Avenue, Northborough, OH 12382

```
February 2, 20XX

Elizabeth Kind, M.D
Northborough Medical Family Group
The offices of Lewis & King, MD
2501 Center Street
Nrothborough, OH 12345

RE: MARGARET THOMAS

Dear Dr. King:

Thank you for refering Margaret Thomas to my neurological practice. Margaret come to you recently
as a new patient for a comprehensive physical examination to evaluate troubling symptoms she had
been experiencing for several months. Margaret notices symtoms of tremor, difficulty walking, de-
fective judgement, and hot flushes; she is not able to poinpoint the exacttime symptoms began. Your
```

physical examination suggested the possible diagnoisis of parkingson's Disease. Margaret presented today for a complete nuerological evaluation.

MEDICAL/SURGICAL HISTORY. The patient is posiitive for the usual childhood diseases and the births of three children, following normal pregnancies. Her surgical history includes an Appendectomy performed 10 years ago. She has a food allergy to shellfish, but no known allergies to medications. She takes Pepto-Bismol and Metamusil for frequent stomach upset and constipation. She is a widow with two children, ages twenty three, twenty-five, and 29, and is a retired homemaker. She does not smoke and has an occassional glass of wine. Her family history is positive for colon cancer in her mother and parenteral grandfather and for lung cancer in her father.

PYHSICAL EXAMINATION. VITAL SIGNS: The patient has normal vital signs for a 52-year old Caucasian female. HEENT: The patient had a normacephalic and atraumatic exam. There is mild bobing of the head and facial expressions appear fixed. Pupils equal, round, react to light and acommodation. The fundi were benign. There was normal cup to disc ratio of 0.3. Tympanic Membranes were both clear and mobile. Her nose was clear. the oropharynz ws clear without any evidence of lezions. There was not cervical adenopathy, no thyromegely, or other masses. NECK: Musles of the neck are quite rigid and stiff. CHEST: Cear to percussion and auscultation. HEART: Regular rate and rhythm without murmurs or gallops. there was no jugular venous distention, no peripheral edema, no carotid buits. Pulses were 2+ and symetrical. ABDOMEN: Some what obese, but benigh. There was not organomegaly or masses. Bowel tones were normal. There was no rebound tenderness. BACK: Examination reveals loss of postural reflex and patient stands with head bent forward and wals as if in danger of falling forward. There is difficulty in pivoting and loss of balance. GENITOURINARY: Normal. EXTREMITIES: Thre is moderate bradykinesia. Chracteristic slow, turning motion (pronation-supination) of the forearm and the hand. a motion of the thumb against the fingers as if rolling a pill between the fingers is noted. This condition seems to worsen when the patient is concentrating or feeling anxious.

NEUROLOGICAL. The patient was cooperative and answered all questions. There is no history past of mental disorders or cardiovascular disease. There is muscle weakness and rigidity in all four extremities. Intellect remains intact.

LABORATORY DATA: Urinanalysis reveals low levels of dopamin. Cat scan reveals degeneration of nerve cells occuring in the basel ganglia.

ASSESSMENT. Based on the patient history and neurologic examination, it appears most likely that the patient has mild to moderate Parkinsons Disease.

PLAN. 1. Recommend physical therapy focussed on learning how to manage difficult movements such as descneding stairs safely.
2. Exercises to maintain flexibility, motility, and mental well-being.
3. Levadopa to increase dopamine levels in the brain to control symptoms. Please advise the patient that alchohol consumption shoudl be limited because it acts antegonistically to levodopa.
4. Relaxation and stress management counseling.

PROGNOSIS. Parkinson's disease progresses slowly. Patient should be follow on a regular basis and observed for any signs of damentia which may result in about one-third of cases.

Sincerely,

James Carter, MD

DD: February 2, 2012
DT: February 3, 2012
JC/bl

Web Activities

Use the Internet to research the most economical and expedient method of mailing paperwork in a 15 × 12 × 0.75 inch envelope from your school's address to Lancaster, Pennsylvania. Also find the most economical and expedient method of mailing a parcel, boxed and weighing 62 pounds, from your school's address to Anchorage, Alaska. Follow your instructor's instructions on completing and turning in your results.

CHAPTER POST-TEST

Perform this test without looking at your book.

1. The most commonly used of the four major letter styles in the ambulatory care setting is:
    a. full block
    b. modified block, standard
    c. facilitated block, indented
    d. simplified

2. The part of a letter that includes the return address and perhaps a logo is the:
    a. salutation
    b. inside address
    c. letterhead
    d. reference heading
    e. enclosure

3. Whenever documents are to be included in a mailed letter, the word *enclosure* should be indicated by:
    a. Enclosures
    b. Enc.
    c. 1 Enc.
    d. 2 Enclosures
    e. Enclosures (2)
    f. any of the above

4. In which type of letter format are paragraphs indented five spaces?
    a. Simplified letter
    b. Modified block
    c. Indented modified block
    d. Standard modified block

5. When it is desirable to send the same letter, although personalized, to many different people, a computerized feature that can be used is called:
    a. word processing letters
    b. mail merge
    c. database letters
    d. merge correspondence

SELF-ASSESSMENT

In your written communications, are you able to express yourself accurately and concisely? Able to communicate ideas effectively? Capable of proofreading and editing for content? Use this simple self-assessment to gauge your comfort and proficiency in written communications by identifying strengths and pinpointing any weak areas that could use improvement. For each statement below, circle the corresponding letter to the response that best describes you.

1. When writing a letter, I generally feel
    a. confident. I communicate effectively on the page and enjoy writing letters.
    b. at ease. My written communication skills are acceptable.
    c. uncomfortable. I would rather communicate orally than through writing.

2. As far as content goes, when I am given the required information and asked to compose a letter, I

   a. almost always understand exactly what I am being asked to communicate and am able to convey it precisely in letter form.

   b. generally understand what I am being asked to communicate, but sometimes have to fine-tune my letters.

   c. often have trouble understanding what I am being asked to communicate and usually have to go back and ask questions about the letter's content.

3. In general, when choosing words for written correspondence, I feel

   a. secure about my ability to select appropriate language and use medical terminology accurately.

   b. pretty confident, although my general vocabulary and knowledge of medical terminology could use some improvement.

   c. frustrated; I always seem to confuse words and medical terms no matter how hard I try not to.

4. As far as spelling goes, I am

   a. a top-notch speller; I always keep both a standard and medical dictionary on hand for the words I am not sure of.

   b. an adequate speller; sometimes I confuse a word here or there; I always have to proofread carefully for spelling errors.

   c. a below-par speller; my letters are always littered with misspellings and someone else has to proofread my work.

5. Grammatically speaking, I am

   a. above average; I routinely find mistakes in my colleagues' work.

   b. passable; I make minor mistakes but usually catch them while proofreading.

   c. hopeless; people find mistakes in my work even after I have checked it twice.

6. Regarding proofreader's marks, I am

   a. highly capable of proofreading my work; if colleagues need someone to proof their work, I am first on their list.

   b. an okay proofreader; I occasionally overlook a mistake, but nobody's perfect.

   c. frightened; proofreading marks are just a bunch of meaningless squiggles to me.

7. How would you describe your formatting skills?

   a. Exemplary. I understand all basic letter forms, and all of my letters are rigorously formatted according to correct specifications.

   b. Satisfactory. Every so often, I confuse styles or forget an annotation; but in general, all my letters are formatted correctly.

   c. Fair to nonexistent. I have trouble understanding why every letter has to be so formally constructed.

8. When adhering to clinic style guidelines, I

   a. always follow the guidelines.

   b. usually have no problem sticking to style guidelines; when I make a mistake, it is a rare event.

   c. need improvement; my letters are frequently littered with style inconsistencies, and I do not understand the need for a clinic style as long as each letter is written with accurate information.

9. Overall, I think of writing letters in the health care environment as

   a. one of my strong suits.

   b. a task that I am able to accomplish, just not one I particularly enjoy.

   c. a necessary evil.

Scoring

If your answers were mostly "a" responses, you have strong written communications skills and enjoy writing letters. If your responses were mostly "b", your written communications skills are good but could stand some improvement. Try reviewing pertinent information in this chapter to strengthen areas that need it. If your answers were mostly "c," you need to work on your written communication skills. Volunteer to take on as many written correspondence assignments as you can—practice may help you overcome your apprehension about writing letters and will almost certainly raise the quality of your work.

_____

_____

_____

_____

_____

_____

_____

_____

CHAPTER **16**

Medical Documents

CHAPTER PRE-TEST

Perform this test without looking at your book.

1. The practice of contracting with a service outside the clinic or hospital to a company where the task can be accomplished at a lower cost and with a faster turnaround time is known as:
   a. Delegating
   b. Outsourcing
   c. Biometrics
   d. Risk management

2. The abbreviation EMR stands for:
   a. Electronic medical report
   b. Electronic medicine record
   c. Electronic medical record
   d. Electronic medication record

3. Voice recognition software is also known as:
   a. Automatic speech recognition
   b. Natural language recognition
   c. Speech recognition
   d. All of the above
   e. a and b only

4. Treating the patient's medical information as private and not for publication is known as:
   a. Confidentiality
   b. Privacy
   c. Privileged
   d. Concealment

5. A concise description of the patient's encounter with the medical clinic is known as:

   a. Chief complaint

   b. History of present illness

   c. Review of systems

   d. Progress notes

6. The _____ chronicles the details of a surgical procedure performed in a hospital, outpatient surgical center, or clinic.

   a. radiology report

   b. pathology report

   c. operative report

   d. consultation report

VOCABULARY BUILDER

Misspelled Words

Find the words below that are misspelled; circle them, and correctly spell them in the spaces provided. Then insert the correct vocabulary terms from the list that best fit the descriptions below.

athentication	discharge summery	priveliged
autapsy report	editor	progress notes
chart notes	electronic medical records	proofreading
chief complaint	gross examination	quality assurence
confidentiality agreement	history and physical	review of systms
consultation reports	medical transcriptionist	turnaround time
correspondence	outsourcing	voice recognition software
currant reports	patholigy	

_____   _____   _____

_____   _____   _____

_____   _____   _____

1. Today, the _____ may be more involved with quality assurance than actually transcribing medical records, notes, letters, and documents.

2. The part of the pathology report that describes the size and shape of a biopsy specimen is called a _____.

3. The part of patients' hospital records that describe their entire hospital stay, progress, and condition on release is called a _____.

4. The part of the patient's medical record that contains information related to the main reason for the encounter, as well as a synopsis of the patient's previous medical information, is called the _____.

5. Reports such as history and physical examinations that should be completed within 24 hours are called _____ reports.

6. A type of signature that may use various computer key entries as identification is referred to as _____.

7. Software that translates spoken sounds into written words is called _____.

8. A medical report generated to describe the examinations of tissues or cells obtained through a surgical or medical procedure is the _____ report.

9. The practice of contracting transcription with a service outside the clinic or hospital to a company where it can be done at a lower cost and with a faster turnaround time is called _____.

Definitions

Define the following terms.

1. Joint Commission:

_____

_____

2. Consultation report:

_____

_____

_____

3. Editing:

_____

4. Flag:

_____

_____

5. Turnaround time:

_____

_____

_____

LEARNING REVIEW

Short Answer

1. List five personal attributes of the medical transcriptionist.

_____

_____

_____

2. List at least four advantages of outsourcing.

_____

_____

_____

_____

3. Identify four ways the medical transcriptionist can be compliant with HIPAA.

_____

_____

_____

_____

_____

4. Define the following types of medical documents.

   a. Chart notes (progress notes):

   _____

   b. History and physical examination (H&P) report:

   _____

   c. Radiology report:

   _____

   _____

   d. Operative report:

   _____

   e. Pathology report:

   _____

   _____

   f. Consultation report:

   _____

   g. Discharge summary:

   _____

   h. Autopsy report:

   _____

5. Clinics using electronic medical records may delegate much of the medical transcriptionist's responsibility to other medical personnel. Identify the items below that may be entered into an electronic medical record by the medical assistant by writing "MA" next to the entry, and those items that may be entered by the provider as "P."

Reason for the patient's visit   ____

Entering chart notes   ____

Entering vital signs   ____

Entering and transmitting prescription to a pharmacy   ____

Transmitting the medical record to another provider   ____

Entering current medications   ____

Entering the chief complaint   ____

Abbreviations Exercise

Write what each abbreviation stands for.

1. EHR   _____

2. MT   _____

3. TAT   _____

4. QA   _____

5. VRS   _____

6. CMT   _____

7. CC   _____

8. ROS   _____

9. H&P   _____

10. DS   _____

11. OR   _____

12. HIPAA   _____

CERTIFICATION REVIEW

These questions are designed to mimic the certification examination. Select the best response.

1. Association for Healthcare Documentation Integrity (AHDI) credentials _____.
   a. MTs
   b. CMTs
   c. CMTs and RMTs
   d. CMAs and RMAs

2. A digital dictation system allows you to measure to:
   a. the 30th or 90th of a minute
   b. 60 seconds
   c. the 10th or 100th of a minute
   d. 30–40 seconds

3. The medical report must be:
   a. dated correctly
   b. signed or initialed by the dictator
   c. legible
   d. all of the above

4. The specific time period in which a document is expected to be completed from the time it is received by the transcriptionist until it is returned to the provider and made part of the permanent medical record is called:
   a. filing time
   b. turnaround time
   c. completion time
   d. return time

5. Radiology, pathology, and laboratory reports are usually termed as _____ to indicate the need for immediate turnaround.

    a. ASAP

    b. current

    c. old

    d. stat

LEARNING APPLICATION

Critical Thinking

1. You have excellent keyboarding skills and understand word processing programs well. Your spelling and medical terminology skills, however, are poor. How will this impact your medical transcription productivity?

_____

_____

_____

_____

_____

2. List a minimum of three HIPAA confidentiality regulations that apply to medical transcription. What are the consequences of not being compliant?

_____

_____

_____

_____

3. Turnaround time is an important issue in medical transcription. What happens when the transcriptionist does not complete medical documents within the turnaround time limits? What steps could be taken to ensure compliance with turnaround time?

_____

_____

_____

_____

4. What if a serious error is made when transcribing a discharge summary and the court subpoenas the document because of litigation? What legal responsibility does the transcriptionist have for the accuracy of the document?

_____

_____

_____

_____

Case Studies

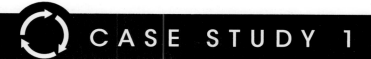

CASE STUDY 1

You are transcribing a report when you notice it is a report about your neighbor. The report states that the test run for multiple sclerosis is positive. You had just spoken to your neighbor yesterday and she was concerned that she hadn't heard from her provider and was wondering about the results of her tests.

CASE STUDY REVIEW QUESTIONS

1. What should you do?

_____

_____

_____

_____

Proofreading Exercise

Correct the following paragraph.

her past medical history is postivie for the usual childhood diseases and the births of to children following normal pregnancies. she has a negative pasts urgical history. she has no allergies To medications and takes tylenol for occasional headashes. She is married and has to children, ages 3 and 12 months. She does not smoke or drink.

Web Activities

Using the Internet, locate the AHDI website (http://www.ahdionline.org) and search through the web pages to locate the *Medical Transcriptionist Job Description* and *AHDI Statement on Quality Assurance for Medical Transcription.* Download these items.

a. Study the difference between Professional Levels 1, 2, and 3 provided on the job description. Where do you fit? Where would you like to be in 5 years? What will you have to do to achieve your goals?

b. Now locate the MT QA manager job description and read through the *AHDI Statement on Quality Assurance for Medical Transcription* (http://www.ahdionline.org).

c. Write a summary report responding to the three questions related to the job description and the QA statement. Follow your instructor's directions related to this activity.

CHAPTER POST-TEST

Perform this test without looking at your book.

1. The discharge summary includes:

   a. the reason for hospital admission

   b. the final diagnosis

   c. follow-up instructions

   d. all of the above

2. The abbreviation CMT stands for:

    a. certified medical technician

    b. certified medical transcriptionist

    c. certified medical transcriber

    d. certified medical technologist

3. A description of symptoms, problems, or conditions that brought the patient to the clinic:

    a. current medical issue

    b. chief complaint

    c. present problem

    d. b and c only

4. Information that may only be communicated with the patient's permission or by court order is known as:

    a. privileged

    b. private

    c. confidential

    d. disclosed

5. Gross and microscopic examinations may be performed on:

    a. tissue

    b. organs

    c. body fluid

    d. a and b only

    e. all of the above

SELF-ASSESSMENT

1. Do you think you would enjoy working as a transcriptionist? What is it about the profession that appeals to you? What is it about the profession that does not appeal to you?

_____

_____

_____

_____

_____

_____

_____

_____

_____

_____

_____

_____

_____

_____

C H A P T E R **17**

Medical Insurance

CHAPTER PRE-TEST

Perform this test without looking at your book.

1. Managed care organizations were established in an attempt to _____ and provide for more efficient use of medical resources.
   a. control treatment plans
   b. curb medical costs
   c. avoid conflicts of interest
   d. recognize a profit

2. The MCO can be a health care plan, hospital, _____, or health system.
   a. delivery system
   b. participating provider
   c. provider group
   d. exclusive contract

3. Outpatient expenses such as physical therapy, laboratory tests, ambulance services, and charges for durable medical equipment (DME) are covered by:
   a. Medicare Part A
   b. Medicare Part B
   c. Medicare Part C
   d. Medicare Part D

4. Which of the following is true about a coordination of benefits?
   a. A referral is always required.
   b. A deductible does not apply.
   c. The final total benefit is greater than the original charge.
   d. The final total benefit is not greater than the original charge.

5. Most traditional insurance plans have a coinsurance amount that is:

   a. 80%

   b. 100%

   c. 50%

   d. 60%

VOCABULARY BUILDER

Misspelled Words

Find the words below that are misspelled; circle them, and correctly spell them in the spaces provided. Then, insert the correct vocabulary terms from the list that best fit the descriptions below.

adjustmint

benefit period

Medicare Part D

point-of-service plan

preautherization

prefered provider organization

primary care provider

referral

resourse-based relative value scale

self-insurance

usual, customarry, and reasonable

_____   _____   _____

_____   _____

1. The _____ is a doctor chosen by the patient who is the first doctor the patient sees and is responsible for making referrals for further treatment by a specialist or for hospitalization.

2. A _____ allows the enrollee to have the freedom to obtain medical care from an HMO provider or to self-refer to a non-HMO provider at a greater cost.

3. The _____ was developed using values for each medical and surgical procedure based on work, practice, and malpractice costs and factoring in the regional differences.

4. _____ means that prior notice and approval need to be obtained before services will be covered.

5. A _____ is an organization of providers who network together to offer discounts to purchasers of health care insurance.

6. The _____ is the specified time during which benefits will be paid under certain types of health insurance coverages.

7. The amount a provider writes off the patient's account is known as an _____.

8. _____ is prescription drug coverage by Medicare.

LEARNING REVIEW

Short Answer

1. What questions should the medical assistant ask when screening for medical insurance coverage?

_____

_____

2. What measures do managed care organizations employ to ensure cost-effective services?

_____

_____

3. List and describe the six models of managed care organizations.

_____

_____

_____

_____

_____

_____

_____

_____

_____

_____

_____

_____

4. List seven pieces of information that should be maintained in a log regarding preauthorization, precertification, or referral procedures for various insurance carriers.

_____

_____

_____

_____

5. List and describe the three elements that should be considered when a provider's fee schedule is being created.

_____

_____

_____

_____

_____

_____

_____

_____

6. The insurance carrier generates an EOB and an RA. Explain what these are and who they are sent to.

_____

_____

_____

_____

7. List three examples of insurance fraud and three examples of insurance abuse.

   A. Fraud:

   _____

   _____

   _____

B: Abuse:

_____

_____

8. Discuss the importance of workers' compensation insurance.

_____

_____

_____

9. Define the following types of managed care insurance.

   A. Exclusive provider organization:

_____

_____

   B. Integrated delivery system:

_____

   C. Point-of-service (POS) plan:

_____

_____

_____

   D. Preferred provider organization (PPO):

_____

_____

   E. Triple option plan:

_____

Matching

Match the statements below to the appropriate Medicare Part.

_____ 1. Covers outpatient expenses including providers' fees, lab tests, and radiologic studies

_____ 2. Covers hospital admission and stays

_____ 3. Offers prescription drug coverage for everyone covered by Medicare

_____ 4. Referred to as Medicare advantage plans

_____ 5. Does not require a monthly premium

_____ 6. Has a "donut hole" or coverage gap

_____ 7. Will start paying for services after a $131 deductible has been met

_____ 8. Requires a monthly premium

_____ 9. Covers hospice care

_____ 10. Covers charges for durable medical equipment

A. Medicare Part A

B. Medicare Part B

C. Medicare Part C

D. Medicare Part D

CERTIFICATION REVIEW

These questions are designed to mimic the certification examination. Select the best response.

1. The portion of the medical fees that the patient needs to pay at the time of services is called:
   a. co-payment
   b. fee for service
   c. out-of-pocket expenses
   d. premium

2. The largest medical insurance program in the United States is:
   a. Blue Cross/Blue Shield
   b. Medicaid
   c. Medicare
   d. TRICARE

3. The cost that patients must pay each month (sometimes provided by their employers) is called the:
   a. out-of-pocket expense
   b. co-payment
   c. premium
   d. relative value scale

4. Which of the following describes HIPAA?
   a. It is about confidentiality, patient privacy, and security of personal health information.
   b. It protects health insurance coverage for workers and their families when they change or lose their jobs.
   c. It includes national standards for electronic health care transactions.
   d. It establishes rules for national identifiers for providers, health plans, and employers.
   e. a and c only

5. Noncovered services are also known as:
   a. nonallowed services
   b. exclusions
   c. out-of-pocket services
   d. expensive services

6. A statement summarizing how the insurance carrier determined reimbursement for services received by the patient is called a(n):
   a. explanation of benefits (EOB)
   b. remittance advice (RA)
   c. day sheet
   d. personal financial statement

7. The medical insurance that covers medical care for certain qualifying low-income individuals is:
   a. Medicare
   b. CHAMPUS
   c. TRICARE
   d. Medicaid

8. To ensure that there is a successful flow of adequate income in the clinic or office, the medical assistant should:
   a. bill the insurance carrier or patient as needed
   b. complete forms properly
   c. keep track of aging accounts
   d. all of the above

9. Improper billing practices are considered:
   a. fraud
   b. nonproductive
   c. abuse
   d. risky

10. Which of the following is a problem with work-related health insurance coverage?
    a. Part-time employees are usually not eligible.
    b. Medical benefits may not transfer equally.
    c. Insurance companies often refuse to provide coverage for some procedures, including experimental treatments.
    d. All of the above

11. The person covered under the terms of an insurance policy is called the:
    a. primary
    b. secondary
    c. beneficiary
    d. elector

12. When more than one policy covers the individual, the _____ determines which of the policies will pay first.
    a. deductible
    b. exclusion
    c. coinsurance
    d. coordination of benefits

13. Where does one find the address to which insurance claims are to be sent?
    a. The telephone book
    b. On the back of the insurance card
    c. In the insurance provider manual
    d. None of the above

14. Blue Cross and Blue Shield are examples of:
    a. managed care organizations
    b. health maintenance organizations
    c. preferred provider organizations
    d. traditional insurance organizations

LEARNING APPLICATION

Critical Thinking

1. When children of married parents are covered under both parents' policies, how is the birthday rule used to determine which policy is primary?

   _____

   _____

   _____

2. You are the medical assistant working the front desk and one of your responsibilities is to screen patients for insurance. What questions will you ask when collecting these data, and how will you word each question so that accurate information is received from the patient?

   _____

   _____

   _____

   _____

   _____

   _____

   _____

   _____

   _____

3. An established patient is seen today by the provider, who determines that a liver scan is necessary to determine a diagnosis. You must ascertain if this procedure is a covered benefit, determine what the payment rate will be by the carrier, and secure preapproval if necessary. How will you go about collecting this information?

   _____

   _____

   _____

4. You must establish proof of eligibility for a patient. How will you go about doing this?

   _____

   _____

   _____

Case Studies

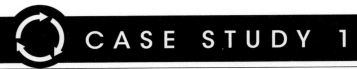

CASE STUDY 1

Lourdes Austen, a 1-year survivor of breast cancer, is covered by an HMO. Lourdes's primary care provider, Dr. King, recommends that Lourdes receive a colonoscopy because she has a family history that is positive for colon cancer, and medical studies have demonstrated a link between colon and breast cancers in families. Lourdes's HMO requires preauthorization before a specialist's care can be provided. Dr. King supplies the referral to a gastroenterologist who will perform the colon screening test and gives Lourdes the necessary completed referral form to take with her to her scheduled appointment. During the colonoscopy procedure, one benign polyp is removed, and the gastroenterologist requests that Lourdes return for a follow-up examination in 1 week.

Lourdes makes an appointment with the specialist's administrative medical assistant. When she returns 1 week later, the medical assistant informs Lourdes that she must have a new referral form for the clinic visit or the HMO will not approve payment; Lourdes will have to pay for the examination herself. "But we drove 40 minutes to get here, and no one ever told me I'd need another form for this. I thought it was all covered under the colonoscopy," Lourdes says.

CASE STUDY REVIEW QUESTIONS

1. Lourdes's HMO policy requires preauthorization. Is there anything that can be done to secure a proper referral without having to schedule another appointment for the patient or force the patient to pay for the clinic visit?

   _____

   _____

   _____

   _____

2. What is the role of the specialist's administrative medical assistant in this situation? Could the situation have been prevented?

   _____

   _____

   _____

   _____

Hands-On Activities

1. **Obtaining a Referral for a Patient:** Arrange the students into pairs. One will assume the role of the medical assistant, while the other assumes the role of the representative at the insurance company. The medical assistant will ask the insurance representative the following questions to portray the important duty of obtaining a referral for a patient:

   a. Is the service/procedure covered by the insurance? (If so, the medical assistant must provide the DOS at this time to indicate when the initial service will potentially take place.)

   b. Referral/authorization number

   c. Co-payment amount and deductible information

   d. How many visits are authorized?

   e. What is the expiration date?

   f. Name and telephone number of the contact person (or the person with whom you spoke)

2. **Calculating Allowed Charges and Determining Patient Responsibility:** A new patient, Carol Cooper, age 67, has just received services at the family practice clinic where you work. Her charges for the day come to $200.00. She is a Medicare beneficiary with no secondary coverage. Your practice is a participating provider with Medicare and accepts assignment. You have already contacted Medicare and verified that her Medicare deductible responsibility has already been met, and that her services are covered. It is now time to calculate what Medicare will potentially pay for her services. Fill in the appropriate amounts.

   a. New patient clinic visit charge:

   b. Allowed amount for the service according to Medicare's fee schedule:

      1. 80% to be paid by Medicare:

      2. Amount to be written off by the provider:

      3. Patient responsibility:

Web Activities

Mr. Jones is in reasonably good health and incurs drug expenses less than $1,000 per year. Review the Medicare drug plans for your area and select the optimum plan for Mr. Jones. If his prescription drug costs increased to $1,800 per year, how would this change the plan selection? (Visit http://www.medicare.gov on the Internet and select "Compare" under Prescription Drug Plans.")

CHAPTER POST-TEST

Perform this test without looking at your book.

1. An MCO will contract with an insurance carrier to take care of the medical needs of an enrolled group for a fixed fee per enrollee for a fixed period. This payment system is called:

   a. capitation

   b. adjustment

   c. remittance

   d. coinsurance

2. The amount of money that the insured must incur for medical services before the policy begins to pay:

   a. coinsurance

   b. deductible

   c. co-payment

   d. exclusion

3. Most policies have a specific _____ before coverage is extended to help cover for preexisting conditions.

   a. time frame

   b. donut hole

   c. benefit period

   d. waiting period

4. The _____ helps to determine which insurance is primary and which is secondary when there are dependents covered under two insurance policies.

   a. remittance advice

   b. birthday rule

   c. benefit period

   d. coordination of benefits

5. The amount the insurance will cost the patient's employer each month is the:
   a. co-payment
   b. deductible
   c. premium
   d. coinsurance

SELF–ASSESSMENT

1. Take a close look at your insurance coverage. If you do not have medical insurance coverage, take a look at the coverage of a close friend or relative or choose a policy you would like to have.
   a. Does it require a co-payment?
   b. How much is the co-payment for a provider's visit?
   c. How much is the co-payment for a hospital stay? Surgery?
   d. How much is the co-payment for medication?
   e. Does prescribed medicine have to be from a formulary list?
   f. How much is the total amount you would have to pay for any given year?

2. Some people advocate doing away with health insurance for clinic visits and medications and just having insurance for big expenses such as catastrophic coverage. Discuss this idea with a group of at least three people. These people may be your classmates or friends/family. Write up a list of advantages and disadvantages.

3. Some people advocate a "socialistic" method of health insurance such as Canada has. Look online for information about Canada's health care system and make a list of the advantages and disadvantages. Which way would you vote if you had a choice?

C H A P T E R **18**

Medical Insurance Coding

CHAPTER PRE-TEST

Perform this test without looking at your book.

1. HCPCS stands for:
   a. Health Common Procedure Code System
   b. Healthcare Common Procedure Coding System
   c. Health Care Classification Procedural Coding System
   d. Healthcare Common Permanent Code Solution

2. CPT stands for:
   a. Comprehensive Patient Treatments
   b. Current Procedural Terminology
   c. Curative Procedures Tried
   d. Curative Patient Treatments

3. ICD stands for:
   a. Incidental Codes of Diagnosis
   b. Internal Codes for Decisions
   c. International Codes for Diagnosis
   d. International Classification of Diseases

4. An individual who receives Medicare is referred to as:
   a. Beneficiary
   b. Claimant
   c. Policy owner
   d. Individual

5. The type of code from ICD-9-CM that explains the external cause of an injury or poisoning is called a(n):
   a. V code
   b. M code
   c. E code
   d. J code

VOCABULARY BUILDER

Misspelled Words

Find the words below that are misspelled; circle them, and then correctly spell them in the spaces provided.

bundeled codes

claim register

Current Procedural Terminoligy

E codes

encounter form

explanation of benifts

Healthcare Common Procedure Coding System

International Classification of Deseases

modifyers

point-of-service device

Uniform Bill (UB-04)

V codes

_____

_____

_____

_____

_____

Definitions

Write the definitions of the following terms or phrases.

1. Bundled codes

   _____

2. Claim register

   _____

   _____

3. Current Procedural Terminology

   _____

   _____

4. E codes

   _____

   _____

5. Encounter form

   _____

   _____

   _____

6. Explanation of benefits

_____

_____

_____

7. Healthcare Common Procedure Coding System

_____

_____

8. *International Classification of Diseases*, 9th Revision, Clinical Modifications (ICD-9-CM)

_____

_____

9. Point-of-service device

_____

_____

10. Uniform Bill (UB-04)

_____

_____

11. V codes

_____

_____

12. Modifiers

_____

_____

LEARNING REVIEW

Short Answer

1. CPT is updated annually and published by the American Medical Association. It is divided into six main sections. List them in the order in which they appear in the CPT codebook.

_____

_____

_____

_____

_____

_____

2. Codes for diagnoses are found in the ICD-9-CM. The ICD-9-CM is divided into three volumes. Specify what information each volume contains.

   A. Volume I:

   _____

   _____

   B. Volume II:

   _____

   _____

   C. Volume III:

   _____

3. In which volume of the ICD would a medical assistant first look to find the diagnosis code for osteomyelitis? What is the diagnosis code for unspecified osteomyelitis of the ankle or foot?

   _____

4. Injury codes cannot stand alone but must be accompanied by E codes. What does the "E" stand for?

   _____

5. Errors in coding insurance claims can have far-reaching effects for both the patient and the provider. Name three effects.

   _____

   _____

   _____

   _____

   _____

   _____

6. Differentiate between bundled and unbundled codes.

   _____

   _____

   _____

7. List five common errors that may occur when completing insurance claim forms.

   _____

   _____

   _____

   _____

8. Identify seven basic elements necessary to have documented in a compliance program.

   _____

   _____

   _____

   _____

   _____

Diagnosis and Procedure Identification

For each entry in the following table, insert a "D" for diagnosis or a "P" for procedure on the first line. Then, enter the appropriate diagnosis or procedure code, referencing the textbook, the current revision of the ICD, or the current edition of the CPT.

Diagnosis/Procedure	Entry	Code
	1. Supplies and materials provided by the physician over and above those usually included with the office visit	
	2. Medicine given or taken in error	
	3. Anorexia nervosa	
	4. Pneumonocentesis, puncture of lung for aspiration	
	5. Diabetic ketoacidosis	
	6. Urinalysis; qualitative or semiqualitative, except immunoassays, micro-scopic only	
	7. Bruxism	
	8. *Pneumocystis carinii* pneumonia	
	9. Amniocentesis	
	10. Epstein-Barr virus infection	
	11. Gait training (includes stair climbing)	
	12. Medical testimony	
	13. Therapeutic or diagnostic injection (specify material injected); subcuta-neous or intramuscular	
	14. Narcotics affecting fetus or newborn via placenta or breast milk	

CERTIFICATION REVIEW

These questions are designed to mimic the certification examination. Select the best response.

1. What is the name of the coding system that includes codes for services provided to Medicare or Medicaid patients?
   a. HCFA
   b. CPT
   c. ICD-9
   d. HCPCS
   e. WHO

2. A diagnosis code of 670.51 has been entered on the claim form. What system is used to assign that code?
   a. CPT
   b. ICD-9-CM
   c. ICD-10-CM
   d. HCPCS
   e. RVS

3. In the CPT manual, the description of the level of E&M codes includes which of the following?
   a. Complexity of the medical decision making
   b. Level of history taken
   c. New versus established patient
   d. All of the above

4. Which of the following is a description of Volume II of the ICD-9?

    a. Known as the Tabular Index, lists all diagnostic codes in numeric order

    b. An alphabetic listing of all known diagnoses, including symptoms and accidents and their causes

    c. Lists procedures in tabular form

    d. All of the above

5. Deliberately billing a higher rate than what was performed to obtain greater reimbursement is called:

    a. encoding

    b. down-coding

    c. up-coding

    d. exploding

6. One way to prevent a breach of confidentiality when processing insurance claim forms is to:

    a. ask the patient, parent, or guardian to sign an Authorization to Release Medical Information form before the claim is completed

    b. ask the patient for verbal approval before sending in the claim

    c. have the patient write a letter requesting that the information be forwarded

    d. have the insurance carrier contact the patient

7. When coding, it is imperative:

    a. to be as precise as possible

    b. not to guess

    c. not to code what is not there

    d. all of the above

8. Submitting claims electronically:

    a. can improve cash flow

    b. ensures consistency

    c. will reduce the amount of supplies required

    d. all of the above

9. Using an electronic device for direct communication between medical offices and a health care plan's computer is called:

    a. subrogation

    b. point of service

    c. diagnosis-related groups

    d. prospective payment

10. The most common claim form for the ambulatory setting is the:

    a. CMS-1450

    b. HCFA-1000

    c. CMS-1500

    d. CPT-1500

11. The codes showing that a patient has been seen for reasons other than sickness or injury are:

    a. S codes

    b. D codes

    c. V codes

    d. X codes

12. The insurance claims processor will confirm that:
    a. there are no exclusions or restrictions for payment of that diagnosis
    b. the claim was received within seven days of the appointment
    c. the procedure relating to the diagnosis is medically necessary
    d. a and c

13. A provider's fee profile is:
    a. based on an average of all the practice's fees
    b. a continuous record of usual charges made for specific services
    c. an average of fees charged over a period of 3 months
    d. the amount paid by insurance carriers

LEARNING APPLICATION

Critical Thinking

1. Electronic claims filing is mandatory for Medicare. Karen recently graduated from an accredited medical assisting program and is employed in the insurance department of a busy medical practice. She has asked her supervisor how she can gain more knowledge in coding and electronic billing procedures and how she might decrease the number of rejected claims. How would you respond to her if you were the supervisor?

_____
_____
_____
_____
_____
_____
_____

2. The supervisor has given Karen a number of rejected claims and asks her to determine why the claims were denied and to maintain a log of these reasons to be discussed at the next staff meeting. How should Karen proceed with this assignment?

_____
_____

3. Karen finds that many claim forms were rejected because important information was omitted. How might Karen suggest corrections for these omissions?

_____
_____

Case Studies

CASE STUDY

Lourdes's colonoscopy required the following diagnoses and procedures. Give the correct coding for processing the insurance claim for this patient.

CASE STUDY REVIEW QUESTION

Colonoscopy with biopsy, single or multiple   _____

Benign neoplasm of the colon   _____

Family history of malignant neoplasm of the gastrointestinal tract   _____

Personal history of malignant neoplasm of the breast   _____

Low-complexity office visit   _____

CPT Review

For each procedure listed, give the correct procedure code and name the CPT section in which the code can be found.

Chemotherapy administration, intravenous infusion technique,
up to 1 hour   _____   _____

Hepatitis B surface antibody (HBsAb)   _____   _____

Simple repair of superficial wounds of scalp, neck, axillae, external
genitalia, trunk, or extremities (including hands and feet) 7.6 to 12.5 cm _____   _____

Electrocardiogram, routine ECG with 12 leads; with interpretation
and reports   _____   _____

Hepatic venography, wedged or free, with hemodynamic evaluation,
radiologic supervision, and interpretation   _____   _____

Hepatitis Be antigen (HBeAg)   _____   _____

Anesthesia for arthroscopic procedures of hip joint   _____   _____

Web Activities

Go onto your favorite search engine and key in "ICD-10-CM Implementation." Many websites will appear. What should a medical facility do to properly prepare for this change in diagnosis coding? Why has the United States postponed the implementation to 2014?

CHAPTER POST-TEST

Perform this test without looking at your book.

1. International Classification of Diseases is released every year in what month?

   a. November

   b. September

   c. October

   d. January

2. OCR stands for:
   a. Office of Coding Review
   b. Optical Character Recognition
   c. Optical Character Relations
   d. Office of Clinical Review

3. The CPT code of 58150 would be found in which section of the CPT codebook?
   a. Surgery
   b. Radiology
   c. Evaluation and Management
   d. Medicine

4. To separate the components of a procedure and bill them individually is known as:
   a. down-coding
   b. up-coding
   c. overbilling
   d. unbundling

5. The CMS-1500 (08-05) claim form permits a maximum of how many procedure codes to be listed?
   a. Five
   b. Six
   c. Seven
   d. Four

6. Block 32 of the CMS-1500 (08-05) claim form contains what type of information?
   a. The name and address of the service facility
   b. The name and address of the insurance company
   c. The name and address of the referring physician
   d. The name and address of the policyholder

7. Codes that represent durable medical equipment may be found in:
   a. CPT
   b. ICD-9-CM
   c. HCPCS
   d. ICD-10-CM

8. Select the piece of information that an explanation of benefits does not include.
   a. Date of service
   b. Diagnosis code
   c. Patient ID number
   d. Procedure code

9. CPT modifier 22 is used to describe services that are:
   a. bilateral
   b. multiple
   c. reduced
   d. unusual

10. An electronic device that provides immediate and direct access to patient eligibility information is known as a (an):
    a. point-of-service machine
    b. scanner
    c. electronic health system
    d. optical character reader

SELF-ASSESSMENT

1. Have you considered whether you would like to be an insurance coder and biller? Think about the following questions.
   a. What qualities do you possess that would make you a good candidate for a career in medical billing and coding?

   _____

   _____

   b. What qualities do you not possess but could obtain?

   _____

   _____

   c. What do you think you would like best about a position in medical billing and coding?

   _____

   _____

   d. What would be your least favorite part of the job?

   _____

2. Explore the profession of medical coding. Look on the Internet for coding organizations offering certification examinations. Differentiate among the various credentials available to coders. Which one(s) appeal to you the most and why?

   _____

   _____

   • _____

   _____

   • _____

   _____

   • _____

   _____

   • _____

   _____

   _____

   • _____

   _____

C H A P T E R **19**

Daily Financial Practices

CHAPTER PRE-TEST

Perform this test without looking at your book.

1. The management of the business details of a practice usually becomes the responsibility of:
   a. The medical assisting staff
   b. The practice administrator
   c. The physician
   d. The office accountant

2. For Medicare patients, a form officially known as _____ is the only legal means a clinic has to collect payment on charges not allowed by Medicare.
   a. Advanced Patient Notice
   b. Advanced Charge Notice
   c. Advanced Beneficiary Notice
   d. Advanced Payment Notice

3. The one advantage to the ambulatory care setting that accepts credit/debit cards is that monies for fees charged usually are:
   a. Of minimal amounts
   b. Available within 24 hours
   c. Available within 48 hours
   d. Instantaneous

4. On a patient account or ledger, the credit column is:
   a. On the right and is used for entering charges
   b. On the left and shows the amount due
   c. On the right and is used for entering payments
   d. None of the above

5. The amount of cash on hand for the purpose of petty cash is usually within the range of:
   a. $75 to $100
   b. $85 to $125
   c. $50 to $150
   d. $50 to $100

VOCABULARY BUILDER

Misspelled Words

*Find the words below that are misspelled; circle them, and correctly spell them in the spaces provided. **Then insert correct vocabulary terms from the list that best fit into the descriptive sentence below.***

accounts payible	day sheat	notary
accounts recievable	debit	payee
adjustments	encounter form	pegboard system
balance	guaranter	petty cash
cashier's check	leadger	poasting
certified check	money market account	traveler's check
credit	National Provider Identifier	voucher check

_____   _____   _____

_____   _____   _____

1. _____ A record of daily patient transactions used in conjunction with pegboard systems

2. _____ Small cash sum kept on hand in the office for minor or unexpected expenses

3. _____ Decreases the balance due

4. _____ Replaces all other identifiers used by providers for reimbursement and other transactions with private payers and the government

5. _____ As a noun, this term denotes "the amount owed"; as a verb, the term means "to verify posting accuracy"

6. _____ Accounting function that describes the act of recording financial transactions into bookkeeping or accounting systems

7. _____ Increases or decreases to a patient account not due to charges incurred or payments received

8. _____ Sum owed by a business for services or goods received

9. _____ Sum owed to a business for services or goods supplied

LEARNING REVIEW

Short Answer

1. Identify six habits essential to creating and maintaining accurate paper financial records.

2. Identify seven of the nine features that may be a part of the checking account.

3. What are five rules to ensure that checks are properly written and recorded?

4. Give three reasons why it is important to ensure that proper control is utilized when purchasing supplies and equipment.

5. When office supplies arrive, what should be done to verify that the correct items and quantities have been received? What should be done to prepare the invoice for payment?

6. Describe the following types of checks, which are different from checks issued from a standard business checking account.

   (a) Cashier's check:

   (b) Certified check:

   (c) Money order:

(d) Voucher check:

_____

_____

(e) Traveler's checks:

_____

_____

7. Adjustments are entries made to a patient's account that do not represent charges or payments. Name three reasons why adjustments may sometimes be made to a patient's account.

_____

_____

8. Deposits are generally made daily. All checks to be deposited must be endorsed. Define endorsement. Identify the best method of endorsing checks in the ambulatory care setting and describe the benefits of using this method.

_____

_____

_____

_____

_____

9. If a check is returned to the ambulatory care setting for insufficient funds, what procedures should be followed?

_____

_____

10. It is crucial to balance all financial information for each day and for the month's end. Month-end figures on the day sheet must agree with the patient ledgers. Why is it important to go through this time-consuming accounting process?

_____

_____

_____

_____

11. Differentiate between bookkeeping and accounting.

_____

_____

12. How should a medical office establish and maintain a petty cash system?

_____

_____

_____

_____

_____

_____

CERTIFICATION REVIEW

These questions are designed to mimic the certification examination. Select the best response.

1. The pegboard system of bookkeeping is sometimes called the:
   a. write-it-once system
   b. ledger system
   c. double-entry system
   d. duplicated page system

2. NSF stands for:
   a. nonsufficient funds
   b. not sufficient funds
   c. not satisfactory funding
   d. negligent status of funding

3. A restrictive endorsement stamp is used to:
   a. stamp on the ledger to signify that payment has been made
   b. stamp the doctor's signature on insurance forms and other documents
   c. stamp on the statement to signify that you have sent a check
   d. stamp on the back of a check to signify "for deposit only"

4. When reconciling a bank statement:
   a. the reconciling should be done every month
   b. the checkbook entries should be checked against the bank statement
   c. the reconciling should be done daily by computer
   d. all reconciling should be done in ink to avoid any unauthorized entries
   e. a and b

5. If a check has been deposited and is now returned because of insufficient funds, it will be necessary to:
   a. redeposit the check
   b. call the bank that returned it and verify availability of funds so the check can then be redeposited
   c. call the patient who wrote the check
   d. discard the check and credit the amount back to the patient's account

6. The most common method(s) of tracking a patient's balance is (are):
   a. the pegboard system
   b. computerized financial systems
   c. the ledger card
   d. a and b

7. The pegboard system consists of:
   a. day sheets
   b. ledger cards
   c. encounter forms
   d. receipt forms
   e. all of the above

8. In cases of divorced parents where one parent has physical custody of the child and is considered the one responsible for payment if the child is not insured with a contracted insurance carrier, the parent is called:

    a. the payee

    b. the guarantor

    c. the subscriber

    d. none of the above

9. The number required by the Centers for Medicare & Medicaid Services (CMS) on claims for clinical diagnosis services is called the:

    a. insurance registration number

    b. client number

    c. National Provider Identifier

    d. contract number

10. The Advanced Beneficiary Notification form is used primarily for:

    a. Medicaid patients

    b. HMO patients

    c. Medicare patients

    d. CHAMPUS patients

11. A patient encounter form:

    a. is also called a charge slip

    b. is also called a superbill

    c. is also called a pegboard form

    d. both a and b

12. In most practices there is a need to have cash available on a daily basis to:

    a. make change for a patient paying cash for services

    b. make funds available for all office personnel

    c. pay for minor and incidental expenses

    d. provide funds for weekly lunches for all employees

13. When a check must be guaranteed for the amount in which it is written, a _____ is issued.

    a. cashier's check

    b. certified check

    c. voucher check

    d. traveler's check

14. Restricting the use of a check should it be lost or stolen may be done through:

    a. reconciling

    b. balancing

    c. special endorsement

    d. blank endorsement

15. The ledger is placed under the charge slip or encounter form in a pegboard system and:

    a. verified before posting

    b. aligned before posting

    c. entered before posting

    d. reconciled before posting

LEARNING APPLICATION

Critical Thinking

1. Discuss the types of checks identified in the text. Give an example of how each might be used or seen in the ambulatory care medical setting.

_____

_____

_____

_____

_____

_____

2. Check with a local bank or two to determine how after-hours deposits are made. Are any special supplies necessary? What is the bank's responsibility? What is the responsibility of the office staff?

_____

_____

_____

_____

_____

_____

_____

_____

3. When you reconcile the practice bank statement, you see that a check written almost 30 days ago to one of your suppliers has not been deposited. What course of action do you take, if any?

_____

_____

_____

_____

4. Even when a computer software system is used for the management of the practice's finances, discuss why following the bookkeeping guidelines for a manual system still has merit.

_____

_____

_____

_____

Hands-on Activities

1. Administrative medical assistant Karen Ritter is responsible for assisting the office manager and accountant in performing accounts payable activities for Inner City Health Care. On September 4, she receives a $323.45 bill from RJ Medical Supply Company for blood pressure equipment the office received on August 30. Noting that the company demands payment within 30 days of billing, Karen writes a check disbursing funds to the company on September 15. The balance in the office's checking account before this check is written is $26,100.00. Using this information, write out the check and stub below. Karen will submit the check to Susan Rice, M.D., for her signature.

BALANCE FORWARD				
2417				**2417**

DATE _____ 20 ____

TO _____

FOR _____

	TOTAL	
	THIS PAYMENT	
	BALANCE	

TAX DEDUCTIBLE ✓

Inner City Heatlth Care
222 S. First Avenue
Carlton, MI 11666
(814) 555-7155

_____ 20 ____

PAY TO THE
ORDER OF _____ $ _____

_____ DOLLARS

First Bank
5411 Brown Rd.
Carlton, MI 11666

FOR _____ ⑈⑈2⑈0⑈⑈4⑈9⑈3⑈2   _____

© Cengage Learning 2014

2. Office manager Walter Seals, CMA (AAMA), is responsible for purchasing office supplies for Inner City Health Care. On September 10, Walter completes purchase order #1742 to Mayflower Supply, requested by administrative medical assistant Karen Ritter. The items are taxed at 8%, and the shipping fee is prepaid. The items are billed and shipped to Inner City Health Care; the terms are net due 30 days. Complete the purchase order form below.

PURCHASE ORDER   NO. 1742

Bill To:

Ship To:

Vendor:

REQ BY	BUYER	TERMS

QTY	ITEM	UNITS	DESCRIPTION	UNIT PR	TOTAL

	SUBTOTAL	
	TAX	
	FREIGHT	
	BAL DUE	

© Cengage Learning 2014

Inner City Health Care
8600 Main Street, Suite 201
River City, NY 01234
(123) 555-0326

Mayflower Supply, Inc.
642 East 65th Street
River City, NY 01234
(123) 555-9999

2 boxes of fax paper, #62145, at $8.99 a box

5 day-view desk calendars, #24598, at $4.25 each

4 cases of copier paper, #72148, at $20.00 a case

5 boxes of highlighter pens, 12 to a box, #26773, at $3.98 a box

4 computer printer cartridges, #96187, at $49.99 each

Web Activities

Using your favorite Internet search engine, determine how many medical or ambulatory care computerized book-keeping systems might be available. One popular computerized system is called Medisoft. What does your research tell you about their prescription processing? Discuss the advantage or disadvantage of such a process.

CHAPTER POST-TEST

Perform this test without looking at your book.

1. The encounter form is also known as the:
   a. charge slip
   b. multipurpose billing form
   c. superbill
   d. none of the above
   e. all of the above

2. A refund on a patient's account will usually occur when:
   a. there has been a mathematical error in bookkeeping
   b. the insurance carrier pays more than anticipated
   c. any time there is a payment from Medicare
   d. the write-it-once system was not used properly

3. Which of the following is NOT usually a piece of information that is included on an encounter form?
   a. Requested return visit
   b. Patient account number
   c. Previous balance
   d. Coverage effective date

4. Which of the following is true about petty cash procedures?
   a. Petty cash is used to make change for patients when they pay their co-payment.
   b. The amount of petty cash on hand is usually between $50 and $150.
   c. Petty cash should be balanced each day before closing.
   d. The amount on hand should be enough to cover several weeks of incidental expenses.

5. On a patient account or ledger, the credit column is:
   a. on the right and is used for entering charges
   b. on the left and shows the amount due
   c. on the right and is used for entering payments
   d. none of the above

SELF-ASSESSMENT

1. In your personal checkbook or banking system at home, how often do you reconcile?

2. When you do reconcile, do you balance? How much time will you spend on the reconciliation to balance? If you reconcile your bank statements on a regular basis and balance each month, congratulations! If you do not reconcile on a regular basis, start today. Gather your last bank statement. If you do not have one, call the bank and have them send you one or download one from the Internet if your bank offers Internet banking. Accept the beginning balance on the bank statement. Gather the check stubs/copies that you have written within the bank statement's beginning and end dates. Check off all the checks that have gone through the bank and are listed on the statement.

   Add up the outstanding checks (i.e., the ones that have not gone through yet). Subtract them from the ending balance. Add in any interest you have earned for the month. Subtract any fees you have been charged. Does your amount match the bank statement? If not, go back over your math to make sure you added and subtracted correctly and fix any errors. If you still cannot balance, call the bank and ask to sit down with a representative/clerk so they can help you balance. After you balance once, the next month will be much easier. If your bank offers Internet or online banking, and you are not using that option, consider it. Why are you not using it? Talk to a representative to be sure the online service is secure and your information is protected. If you are satisfied that it is a safe and secure service, consider taking advantage of the online option. Reconciling the monthly statements online is easy to do because the math is done for you by the computer! If you are using online banking, do you think it saves you time? Does it save you money? Is it easier than reconciling manually?

C H A P T E R **20**

Billing and Collections

CHAPTER PRE-TEST

Perform this test without looking at your book.

1. The Truth-in-Lending Act states:
   a. Providers cannot charge more than 10% interest on their patient accounts.
   b. Providers must charge interest if the account is more than four months past due.
   c. Providers must notify patients in writing if interest is to be charged on their accounts.
   d. If the provider and patient agree to an installment plan of more than four payments, the installment charge must be stated in writing.

2. The best opportunity for collection is:
   a. One month after the time of service
   b. At the time of service
   c. When cycle billing is performed for the month
   d. When the account is sent to a collection agency

3. In a cycle billing system, all accounts usually are:
   a. Divided into groups according to balance owed
   b. Sent on Friday at the end of every week
   c. Divided alphabetically with each group billed at a different time
   d. Sorted by insurance company

4. Management consultants recommend collecting at least a portion of the fees at the time of service and a collection ratio of:
   a. 90%
   b. 95%
   c. 80%
   d. 85%

5. In most states, a debtor may be contacted only between:
   a. 9 AM and 9 PM
   b. 8 AM and 9 PM
   c. 8 AM and 8 PM
   d. 9 AM and 10 PM

VOCABULARY BUILDER

Misspelled Words

Find the words below that are misspelled; circle them, and correctly spell them in the spaces provided. Then match the correct vocabulary term to its definition below.

accounts recievable ratio   collection ratio   statute of limatations
collection agency   probate court   Truth-in-Lending Act

_____   _____

1. _____ Also known as the Consumer Protection Act of 1967; an act requiring providers of installment credit to state the charges in writing and to express the interest as an annual rate

2. _____ An outside establishment that collects outstanding debt

3. _____ Defines the period of time in which legal action can take place

4. _____ Shows the status of collections and the possible losses in a medical facility

5. _____ A measure of how effective collections are and an indication of how quickly outstanding accounts are paid

LEARNING REVIEW

Short Answer

1. A billing efficiency report allows for careful monitoring of follow-up bills; that is, whether they were paid, if the insurance has paid, and an assessment of the patient's responsibility for payment. What five pieces of data are included in these reports from which production efficiency is calculated?

_____

_____

2. Describe the importance of the Truth-in-Lending Act as it relates to a medical clinic.

_____

_____

_____

_____

3. Identify and explain the five most common reasons some patient accounts become past due.

_____

_____

_____

_____

_____

4. In the pegboard system, what method is used to identify the age of accounts?

_____

_____

_____

5. Name five criteria according to which computer programs can age accounts.

_____

_____

6. The computer can also generate accounts receivable reports. Name three pieces of information included on a computer-generated accounts receivable report.

_____

7. Collection agencies generally provide two services to an ambulatory care facility. Name and describe each type of service.

_____

_____

_____

_____

8. Collection of fees when a patient has died is directed to the executor of the estate. Place an X next to each action below that represents a responsible action in collecting past due accounts from deceased patients' estates.

__ If there is no known administrator, address the statement to "Estate of [insert patient's name]" and mail to the patient's last known address.

__ Send an invoice via certified mail with a complete breakdown of all monies owed to the deceased patient's spouse or closest relative, noting that the survivor is responsible for making payment in full.

__ Mail the account information via certified mail, return receipt, to the administrator of the estate, whose name can be obtained from the probate department of superior court.

__ If unsure how to proceed, contact the clinic's attorney or the probate court for advice.

9. With regard to collections, the statute of limitations is usually defined by the class of the overdue account. Name the three classes of accounts.

_____

_____

10. There are certain legal rules and ethical guidelines to follow when placing collection calls. Circle all that apply.

a. _____

b. Threaten to turn the account over to a collection agency.

c. _____

d. _____

CERTIFICATION REVIEW

These questions are designed to mimic the certification examination. Select the best response.

1. Patients who owe money but have moved and left no forwarding address are referred to as:
   a. deadbeats
   b. skips
   c. nonpayers
   d. dead accounts

2. Statutes of limitations vary from state to state but should be investigated if an unpaid account is more than:
   a. 3 years old
   b. 5 years old
   c. 10 years old
   d. without a time limit if the account is more than a certain amount

3. Lack of payment from a patient may not be considered serious until after:
   a. 30 days
   b. 60 days
   c. 90 days
   d. 120 days

4. For an insurance claim pending more than 45 days, the medical assistant should:
   a. call the carrier and find out if the claim was received
   b. rebill the insurance company
   c. check on the processing status of the claim with the carrier
   d. a and c

5. The most appropriate time to discuss fees and the patient's financial concerns is:
   a. when services are rendered
   b. when scheduling an appointment
   c. by mail after services are rendered
   d. when the insurance company does not pay the fee

6. The Truth-in-Lending Act is also known as the:
   a. Consumer Protection Act of 1967
   b. Fair Debt Collection Practice Act
   c. Patient Bankruptcy Protection Act
   d. Accurate Billing and Collection Act

7. The charge slip is also known as the:
   a. ledger
   b. encounter form
   c. day sheet
   d. CMS-1500

8. When a patient files for bankruptcy:
   a. there is little likelihood that the debt can be collected
   b. it is best to close the account and identify the loss
   c. file a proof-of-claim form and provide a copy of the patient's outstanding account to the bankruptcy court
   d. take the account to small claims court

9. In determining how aggressive to be in debt collections, you should consider:
   a. the previous month's billing backlog
   b. production efficiency
   c. the terms of the insured's policy
   d. the value of the dollar owed

10. Chapter 13 Bankruptcy is otherwise known as:
    a. Wage Earner's Bankruptcy
    b. Farmer's Bankruptcy
    c. Fair Lending Bankruptcy
    d. Allowable Debt Bankruptcy

LEARNING APPLICATION

Critical Thinking

1. An elderly widow covered only by Medicare Parts A and B is a patient in your clinic. You know her resources are limited. She receives a very small pension and Social Security benefits. She is facing hip replacement that will involve surgery, hospital care, rehabilitation care prior to her return to her apartment, and outpatient physical therapy. Describe what steps your clinic might take to ease her financial burden for this much needed care.

   _____

   _____

   _____

   _____

2. You are making a collections call. You follow all the rules and you are gracious in your approach. Before you realize what is happening, however, you have listened to a tale of woe, the patient is in tears, and you want to write your own check for the balance due. What happened? What will you do now?

   _____

   _____

   _____

   _____

3. Collections are an activity that many medical assistants shy away from and prefer not to do. What factors contribute to that feeling?

   _____

   _____

   _____

   _____

4. When the office manager calls a patient regarding a past-due account, she is told by the patient, "I'm not about to pay that bill. The treatment made my pain worse, not better." What steps might be taken now?

   _____

   _____

   _____

   _____

_____

_____

_____

_____

Hands-On Activity

Complete the charge slip for Charles Williams's clinic visit, based on the information below.

Charles Williams, 62 years old, is a new patient of Dr. Winston Lewis at the clinic of Drs. Lewis and King. On July 1, 20XX, five days before the patient's birthday, Charles comes to see Dr. Lewis for an appointment with a chief complaint of intermittent, irregular heartbeats or palpitations, dizziness, and chest pain. Dr. Lewis performs a comprehensive physical examination and orders several tests, including an ECG, complete blood count (CBC), and urinalysis with microscopy. The total fee for the clinic visit and tests is $345—$200 for the physical examination, $75 for the ECG, $25 for the urinalysis, $25 for venipuncture, and $20 for the CBC, which Charles pays for by check at the time of service. Charles is insured by a private carrier, All-American Insurance Company, group #333210, ID number 112-45-9980, which he receives through his employer, High Tech Computer Group. Dr. Lewis asks Ellen Armstrong, CMA (AAMA), to schedule a return appointment in exactly one week to go over the results of Charles's tests. Ellen schedules the appointment and prepares a charge slip for Charles's visit. She refers to his patient information sheet for the correct personal information. Charles Williams lives at 123 Greenside Street, Northborough, OH 12346.

Role-Play Activity

In pairs, role-play a collection call using the information in Figure 20-6 in your text. One student should role play the medical assistant, and one should be Patient O'Keefe. At the conclusion of the role-play, the "medical assistant" and "patient" should each discuss how it felt to be the person in that role. Then have the students switch places and perform the scenario again, with the same type of discussion afterward.

Web Activities

1. Research the Internet for information on debt collections. Consider key words such as "credit law," "collections," and "debt recovery." What sources of information are found that might be helpful to an ambulatory care facility?

2. Research the statute of limitations in your state. How much time is allowed for legal action to take place in collecting a past-due account?

CHAPTER POST-TEST

Perform this test without looking at your book.

1. The Truth-in-Lending Act states:
   a. Providers can charge more than 10% interest on their patient accounts.
   b. Providers can charge interest only if the account is more than four months overdue.
   c. Providers must notify patients in person if interest is to be charged on their accounts.
   d. If the provider and patient agree to an installment plan of more than four payments, the installment charge must be stated in writing.

2. Someone who leaves with an outstanding bill and no forwarding address is known as a(n):
   a. debtor
   b. indigent
   c. skip
   d. collector

3. This defines the period in which legal action may take place:
   a. statute of limitations
   b. Fair Debt Reporting Act
   c. Truth in Lending Act
   d. Anti-Kickback Statute

4. This measures the speed in which outstanding accounts are paid:
   a. collection ratio
   b. accounts receivable ratio
   c. accounts payable ratio
   d. debt collection ratio

5. A method used to gauge the effectiveness of the ambulatory care setting's billing practices:
   a. accounts payable ratio
   b. debt collection ratio
   c. collection ratio
   d. delinquency ratio

SELF-ASSESSMENT

Think about a time or times when you paid a bill late or did not paid it until the following month. Without disclosing too much personal information, answer the following:

1. What was your reason(s)?

2. Did you receive an overdue notice or a phone call?

3. Which do you think would be more difficult to receive, the notice or the phone call?

4. Are you likely to become defensive if the caller or notice has a threatening tone or a more understanding tone? Justify your response.

5. Could the tone of the notice/call leave you feeling good/bad about the event? Explain.

6. Identify ways the situation could have been handled better.

7. Will your experience affect the way you treat people who owe your clinic money?

_____

_____

_____

C H A P T E R **21**

Accounting Practices

CHAPTER PRE-TEST

Perform this test without looking at your book.

1. Properties owned by the business such as supplies and equipment are known as:
   a. Liabilities
   b. Assets
   c. Owner's equity
   d. Accounts

2. The purpose of cost analysis is to determine the:
   a. Costs of each service
   b. Fixed costs
   c. Variable costs
   d. Total of all of the above

3. Financial records should provide:
   a. Amount collected in a given period
   b. Amount earned in a given period
   c. Where the expenses were incurred in a given period
   d. All of the above

4. An unwritten promise to pay a supplier for property or merchandise purchased is:
   a. Accounts receivable
   b. Trial balance
   c. Accounts payable
   d. Cost accounting

5. An itemized statement of the assets, liabilities, and owner's equity of a medical facility as of a specified date:
   a. Cost analysis
   b. Accrual basis
   c. Accounting ledger
   d. Balance sheet

VOCABULARY BUILDER

Misspelled Words

Find the words below that are misspelled; circle them, and correctly spell them in the spaces provided. Then match the vocabulary words to the appropriate definition below.

accounting	cash bases	income statement
accounts payible	check register	libilities
accounts recievable ratio	collection ratio	owner's equity
accrual basis	cost analisys	trial balance
assets	cost ratio	utilazation review
balance sheet	fixed costs	varieble costs

_____   _____   _____

_____   _____

_____   _____

1. _____ Financial statement showing net profit or loss

2. _____ Costs that vary in direct proportion to patient volume

3. _____ Categorizes and records all checks written

4. _____ Formula that measures the speed in which outstanding accounts are paid

5. _____ The purpose of this is to determine the cost of each service

6. _____ An itemized statement of assets, liabilities, and owner's equity; also called the statement of financial condition

7. _____ System of reporting income where income is recognized at the time the money is collected

8. _____ Costs that do not vary in total as the number of patients varies

9. _____ System of monitoring the financial status of a facility and the financial results of its activities, providing information for decision making

10. _____ Debts and other financial obligations for which one is responsible

11. _____ Formula that shows the percentage of outstanding debt collected

12. _____ Properties of value that are owned by a business entity

13. _____ Created by totaling debit balances and credit balances to make sure that total debits equal total credits

14. _____ The amount by which a business's assets exceed the business's liabilities

15. _____ Formula that shows the cost of a procedure or service and helps determine the financial value of maintaining certain services

16. _____ System of reporting income where income is reported at the time charges are generated

17. _____ A review of medical services before they can be performed

LEARNING REVIEW

Short Answer

1. There are a variety of methods used for financial management in the ambulatory care setting. Name three of the bookkeeping systems that are appropriate for use in a medical clinic.

_____

_____

2. Medical software packages have the ability to code information obtained in the ambulatory care setting for use in a database. When completing insurance claim forms or generating reports, the software has the capability to include the most common procedural and diagnostic codes. What other kinds of codes can a computerized accounting system generate that will facilitate the billing?

_____

_____

3. The computer can also be used in the preparation of financial documents. Name four financial documents.

_____

4. Name three ways computer service bureaus handle accounts from medical facilities.

_____

_____

_____

_____

5. Identify at least four steps to take to reduce the chance of embezzlement.

_____

_____

_____

_____

6. To protect the practice from financial loss, providers can purchase fidelity bonds. Name and describe the three kinds of bonds. Place an X in front of the one that offers the most assurance.

7. How might the office manager use data from the budget sheet?

_____

_____

8. Why is it important to implement and track budgets for specific categories of income and expense in the ambulatory care setting?

_____

_____

Matching I

Match the appropriate noncomputerized bookkeeping system to the following duties performed by the medical assistant.

A. Single-entry

B. Pegboard

C. Double-entry

_____ 1. Office manager Walter Seals was responsible for implementing a computer system at Inner City Health Care. Before the computerized accounting program was put into effect, the urgent care center relied on a manual system of checks and balances that allowed the provider-employers to keep a firm hold on the relation between the facility's assets and the sum of liabilities and net worth.

_____ 2. During a temporary one-week down period in the computer system at the clinic of Drs. Lewis and King while a system upgrade is being installed, administrative medical assistant Ellen Armstrong completes each day's financial transactions in a daily journal, then transfers this information to the ledger through the posting process. The information will be entered into the computer once the system is up and running again.

_____ 3. When the patient returns the charge slip to the reception desk after an examination, medical assistant Karen Ritter carefully replaces and lines up the charge slip with the patient's name on the day sheet, then correctly inserts the ledger card under the last page of the charge slip. She proceeds to enter the total charges due and any patient payments.

Fixed and Variable Costs Exercise

Fixed costs are expenses that do not vary in total as the number of patients seen by the medical practice grows or shrinks. Variable costs are expenses that are directly affected by patient volume. From the list below, identify expenses that qualify as fixed costs (FC) and those that are variable costs (VC).

_____ 1. Interpreting laboratory test results

_____ 2. Annual depreciation of the cost of an automatic electrocardiograph (ECG) machine

_____ 3. Medical benefits for the clinic staff

_____ 4. Purchase of reagent test strips for urinalysis

_____ 5. Magazine subscriptions for the facility reception area

_____ 6. Monthly telephone expenses

_____ 7. Medical journal subscriptions for the providers

_____ 8. Purchase of a HemoCue blood glucose system

_____ 9. Printing cost of a patient education brochure

_____ 10. Purchase of open-shelf lateral files

_____ 11. Adding a new position, such as a clinical medical assistant, to the clinic staff

_____ 12. Property taxes on the medical facility building and grounds

_____ 13. The monthly cost of janitorial services

_____ 14. Purchase of disposable needle-syringe units

_____ 15. Disposable paper gowns for patient examinations

CERTIFICATION REVIEW

These questions are designed to mimic the certification examination. Select the best response.

1. The system that is based on the accounting principle that assets equal liabilities plus owner's equity is the:
   a. single-entry system
   b. double-entry system
   c. standard of billing services bureaus
   d. accounts receivable accounting principles

2. Of the following statements, which is false?
   a. Double-entry bookkeeping is expensive.
   b. Double-entry bookkeeping is accurate.
   c. Double-entry bookkeeping is more time consuming.
   d. Double-entry bookkeeping has checks and balances in place.

3. Owner's equity is *not* the same as:
   a. net worth
   b. proprietorship
   c. capital
   d. accounts payable

4. Bonds may be purchased to protect the practice from:
   a. embezzlement
   b. financial loss
   c. malpractice suits
   d. a and b
   e. all of the above

5. A total practice management system has the ability to:
   a. process insurance claims electronically
   b. manage payroll and purchases
   c. generate financial records
   d. all of the above

6. Computerization of medical facilities has increased because of:
   a. emphasis being placed on the accurate documentation of medical records
   b. patient load
   c. increase in managed care plans
   d. a and c

7. The trial balance is created by:
   a. collecting data from the current year and previous year and converting them into a ratio
   b. totaling debit balances and credit balances to confirm that total debits equal total credits
   c. reporting outside revenue sources and overhead expenses
   d. recording two sets of entries, such as increase in assets and increase in liabilities

8. Providers should purchase fidelity bonds because they:
   a. are worth the price
   b. provide a sense of security
   c. lessen the chances of embezzlement
   d. will reimburse the practice for any monetary loss caused by the practice's employees

9. A proper contract should be negotiated and signed with any computer and billing service bureau because it:
   a. is considered a legal document
   b. ensures confidentiality and strict privacy of patient information
   c. is in compliance with HIPAA
   d. b and c

10. Financial records should provide the following at all times:
    a. salaries earned by providers and staff
    b. amount earned, owed, and collected within a given period
    c. where expenses were incurred in a given period
    d. b and c

11. A hospital cost report for Medicare is a part of:
    a. financial accounting
    b. managerial accounting
    c. cost accounting
    d. cost analysis

12. Examples of variable costs include all of the following *except:*
    a. clinical supplies
    b. equipment costs
    c. depreciation
    d. laboratory procedures

13. The accounts receivable trial balance:
    a. tells you how much the practice owes to creditors
    b. shows any problems between the daily journal and the ledger
    c. tracks all disbursements and compares the total with the purchases
    d. uses an NCR transfer strip to copy pertinent information

14. Calculating and reviewing costs provide ambulatory care settings with:
    a. data to set fees
    b. monitoring of the practice's performance
    c. offline batch processing
    d. a and b

15. Salary calculations, withholding taxes, and Social Security calculations are the responsibility of the:
    a. practice administrator
    b. administrative medical assistant
    c. office manager
    d. provider

LEARNING APPLICATION

Critical Thinking

1. Discuss the pros and cons of an on-site complete computer system and a computer service bureau.

   _____

   _____

   _____

   _____

   _____

   _____

   _____

   _____

2. The accounting equation can be reported in more than one formula. It can be stated as:
   a. Assets = Liabilities + Owner's Equity, or
   b. Assets – Liabilities = Owner's Equity
   Is one easier to interpret? Why or why not? Add some totals of your choice to illustrate.

   _____

   _____

   _____

   _____

3. Recall from previous chapters and other studies in which you may be involved some basic guidelines for using computers in the medical facility. Identify these. What is one critical procedure that is done quite regularly, especially at the end of a project or the end of the day?

_____

_____

_____

_____

_____

_____

_____

_____

_____

_____

4. Where and how are financial records and reports kept? Who is responsible for their storage? Is there a length of period that the records should be kept?

_____

_____

_____

_____

_____

Case Studies

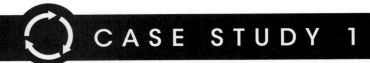

CASE STUDY 1

When the clinic of Drs. Lewis and King agreed to accept individuals covered by a large managed care organization, the decision of the provider-owners was based on a complete financial analysis and projection of the expected effects the new patient load would have on the medical practice. As a result, the group practice added a second office manager and a new clinical medical assistant to the existing staff.

CASE STUDY REVIEW QUESTIONS

1. As Drs. Lewis and King absorb the new managed care patients into the practice, what can the provider-owners do to determine whether their financial analysis and projection were accurate?

_____

_____

2. Once the practice has assembled financial data on the effects of the new patient load, how will these data be used?

_____

_____

_____

_____

_____

3. What beneficial effects might the addition of a clinical medical assistant have on the medical practice?

_____

_____

_____

_____

⟳ CASE STUDY 2

A group practice of radiologists charges $225 for a routine mammogram. Total expenses related to the mammogram procedure equal $30,000 per month, and the practice performs a monthly average of 200 mammograms.

CASE STUDY REVIEW QUESTIONS

1. What is the average cost ratio for the mammogram procedure? (Show your calculations in the space provided).

_____

2. Given the cost to patients for mammograms, is the group practice making a profit or loss on performing mammograms? What amount is the profit or loss per mammogram? What amount is the profit or loss for the entire month?

_____

_____

Hands-on Activities

1. At the clinic of Drs. Lewis and King, the total accounts receivable at the end of May is $100,000 and the monthly receipts total is $75,000; the total accounts receivable at the end of June is $82,000 and the monthly receipts total is $31,000; the total accounts receivable at the end of July is $86,000 and the monthly receipts total is $20,000; the total accounts receivable at the end of August is $93,000 and the monthly receipts total is $45,000. What is the accounts receivable ratio for each month? Show your calculations in the space provided. Which month has the healthiest accounts receivable ratio? Why?

May:	July:
June:	August:

_____

_____

2. For the month of September, receipts at the clinic of Drs. Lewis and King totaled $35,000. The Medicare/Medicaid adjustment for the month was $1,750, and the managed care adjustment was $4,500. Total charges for the month of September equaled $53,000. What is the collection ratio for the month of September? (Show your calculation in the space provided).

_____

3. For the month of October, receipts at the clinic of Drs. Lewis and King totaled $41,000. The Medicare/ Medicaid adjustment for the month was $2,000, the Worker's Compensation adjustment was $750, and the managed care adjustment was $4,700. Total charges for October equaled $55,000. What is the collection ratio for the month of October? (Show your calculation in the space provided).

_____

4. Income statements reveal the cumulative profit and total expenses for each month. Monthly income and expenses are then added to arrive at year-to-date totals, which are compared with the annual budget for particular income and expense categories. Use the following information to complete the expense analysis table for the first quarter office expense costs of the clinic of Drs. Lewis and King. The total office expense budget for the year is $20,000 divided evenly per quarter.

Telephone expenses	January $323.46
	February $425.93
	March $393.87
Postage and mail expenses	January $725.45
	February $550.90
	March $601.33
Office supply expenses	January $1,200.62
	February $325.45
	March $446.26
Yearly budget	Telephone expenses $4,000
	Postage and mail expenses $8,000
	Office supply expenses $8,000

Office Expenses	January	February	March	Year to Date	Budget for Year
Telephone	_____	_____	_____	_____	_____
Postage	_____	_____	_____	_____	_____
Office supplies	_____	_____	_____	_____	_____
TOTALS	_____	_____	_____	_____	_____

Web Activities

1. If you have trouble comprehending the accounting equation, research "The Accounting Equation" on the Internet. What helpful sites did you find? Are there any examples that show how the equation relates to a medical practice? Give an example of what you find.

2. Research "Medical Practice Management" for software packages that include the accounting reports described in this chapter. Identify at least two that seem to have the broadest coverage of how computers are used in a medical practice. Identify the pieces in the package and what they cover.

CHAPTER POST-TEST

Perform this test without looking at your book.

1. Accounts _____ is the amount the provider is owed by patients.
   a. receivable
   b. payable
   c. expendable
   d. profitable

2. The purpose of cost analysis is to:
   a. determine the costs of each service
   b. determine the fixed costs
   c. determine the variable costs
   d. determine the total of all of the above

3. A review of the patient service required before it may be actually performed is known as:
   a. procedure review
   b. management review
   c. utilization review
   d. authorization review

4. The _____ formula shows the cost of a procedure or service.
   a. care ratio
   b. cost ratio
   c. collection ratio
   d. accounting ratio

5. This is designed to cover specific individuals by name and generally requires a personal background investigation:
   a. personal bond
   b. position-schedule bond
   c. blanket-position bond
   d. accountability bond

SELF-ASSESSMENT

Personal finances, as well as the finances of businesses such as ambulatory care settings, require careful planning, management, and budgeting. You can use the systems of business financial management to gain insights into your personal spending patterns and to help develop and fine-tune smart financial habits and attitudes. For each statement, circle the response that best describes you.

1. I think saving money is:
   A. important; I make every effort to put away a sum of money as savings on a regular basis.
   B. great if you can find a way; I would like to save, but I have trouble finding ways to do it.
   C. not important right now; I have too many expenses—what I really need is a loan!

2. When planning a large purchase, such as a computer or a car, I:

   A. set a limit for spending and affordable installment payments and stick to it.

   B. have a rough idea of what I can afford, but do not do any advance planning.

   C. try to buy what I want and think about paying for it later.

3. When considering monthly personal income and expenses, I:

   A. know exactly how much money is coming in and how much is going out to pay bills.

   B. know I can cover my bills but do not keep track of exactly how much I make or spend.

   C. hope for the best, and if I fall short—charge it!

4. When I have extra money, I:

   A. save one-third, use one-third to pay off debts, and use the last third on a special purchase.

   B. save half or use it to pay off debts and spend the other half on a special purchase.

   C. spend it all on a special purchase.

5. My checkbook is:

   A. always balanced.

   B. sometimes balanced.

   C. rarely balanced.

6. When choosing a bank for my savings or checking, I:

   A. research interest rates, features, funds, and services carefully to find the best deal.

   B. choose the bank that pays the highest interest rate.

   C. just pick whatever is most convenient; banks are all the same.

7. I think planning for retirement is:

   A. a priority now; the sooner you start saving, the more your money grows!

   B. important but not the most essential financial responsibility I have right now.

   C. not something I think about now—that is too far away; besides, who can predict the future?

8. People think of me as someone who:

   A. pays attention to detail and is neat and organized.

   B. always manages to get the job done at the last minute.

   C. struggles to keep up with routine or repetitive tasks.

9. I think analyzing financial data is:

   A. a smart way to assess current spending patterns and guide future spending.

   B. a great thing to do if you have enough time and willpower.

   C. a waste of time; besides, I just do not want to know.

10. I am the kind of person who:

    A. sets short- and long-term financial goals for income and spending and works toward implementing them in a responsible way.

    B. has short- and long-term financial goals but cannot get around to planning for them.

    C. makes financial decisions on a day-to-day basis; it is enough to deal with one day at a time.

Scoring

If your answers were mostly A's, congratulations! You have developed a financially responsible outlook and good record-keeping habits. If your responses were mostly B's, you are thinking about financial realities and recognize the importance of a strong financial awareness. Focus on specifics where you can improve your financial skills. If your responses were mostly C's, you need to work on achieving good personal financial habits. Start working on your record-keeping skills by taking the plunge and keeping a weekly journal of expenses to see where your money goes!

C H A P T E R **22**

Infection Control and Medical Asepsis

CHAPTER PRE-TEST

Perform this test without looking at your book.

1. There are necessary steps that must be followed to allow the spread of infectious disease. This is referred to as:
   a. Bacteria
   b. Chain of infection
   c. Infection control
   d. Disinfection

2. Influenza is a disease that results from exposure to:
   a. Bacteria
   b. Virus
   c. Fungus
   d. Protozoa

3. The governmental agency that is responsible for disease prevention and control is the:
   a. CIA
   b. FBI
   c. CDC
   d. IRS

4. An example of an infectious body fluid is:
   a. Blood
   b. Vaginal secretions
   c. Cerebrospinal fluid
   d. All of the above

5. What is the most important aspect of all infection control procedures?
   a. Personal protective equipment
   b. Antibiotics
   c. Handwashing
   d. Sterilization

6. If an employee has suffered an occupational exposure, how long must that medical record be kept?

   a. The length of employment plus 10 years

   b. The length of employment plus 20 years

   c. The length of employment plus 30 years

   d. The length of employment only

7. What is the body's first line of defense?

   a. Handwashing

   b. Intact skin

   c. Immune system

   d. Antibiotics

8. Medications, known as immunomodulators, are prescribed to treat which of the following diseases?

   a. Hepatitis

   b. HIV

   c. Influenza

   d. None of the above

9. The antigen-antibody reaction is also known as:

   a. Immunization

   b. Prodromal stage

   c. Resistance

   d. Sepsis

VOCABULARY BUILDER

Misspelled Words

Find the words below that are misspelled; underline them, and then correctly spell them in the space provided. Then insert one of the correct vocabulary terms into the sentences below. Each word will be used once.

bloodborne pathogin	microorganisms	vector
communicable	nosecomial	
immunoglobulins	palyative	

_____   _____   _____

1. Antibodies are called _____.

2. Infections that are acquired from the hands of health care professionals are known as _____ infections.

3. Diseases that are carried by animals or insects are spread by _____ transmission.

4. Viral infections are difficult to treat. Most of the care provided is designed to relieve symptoms and is known as _____ treatment.

5. Diseases that are easily spread by contact with an infected person are known as _____ diseases.

6. Contact with blood should be avoided because _____ are common causes of disease processes.

7. _____ are microscopic living organisms that are capable of causing illness and disease.

LEARNING REVIEW

Short Answer

1. Describe the scoop technique for recapping needles.

_____

_____

_____

_____

2. List two types of immune responses and describe the process of each.

_____

_____

_____

_____

3. Describe the handling of infectious waste.

_____

_____

_____

4. What are the five stages of infectious disease? Describe each.

_____

_____

_____

_____

_____

_____

_____

5. What are the four items that are considered personal protective equipment? Describe each one.

_____

_____

_____

_____

_____

6. What are the factors that influence the susceptibility of the host?

_____

_____

_____

_____

_____

_____

Matching I

Identify the causative agent of each of the following diseases. Place a (B) beside those that are caused by bacteria or a (V) beside those that are caused by a viral agent.

_____   A. Lyme disease

_____   B. Avian flu

_____   C. AIDS

_____   D. Pertussis

_____   E. Rubella

_____   F. Chicken pox

_____   G. Toxic shock syndrome

_____   H. SARS

_____   I. VRE

_____   J. MRSA

Matching II

Match each of the following types of transmission with the correct definition.

Contact transmission

Droplet transmission

Airborne transmission

Vector transmission

Fomite transmission

Bloodborne transmission

_____   1. Involves animals and insects that are capable of transmitting diseases

_____   2. Microorganisms are transferred from an inanimate object such as a door-knob, table, or medical equipment

_____   3. Occurs when respiratory droplets are generated by a patient who is coughing, sneezing, or talking

_____   4. Occurs when microorganisms are suspended in the air for long periods of time

_____ 5. Physical contact between an infected person, or their body fluids, and a susceptible person that results in a transfer of microorganisms

_____ 6. Infected blood enters a susceptible host through exposure to blood or body fluids

CERTIFICATION REVIEW

These questions are designed to mimic the certification examination. Select the best response.

1. The body's way of responding to an invasion of a pathogen is known as:
   a. immune response
   b. inflammatory response
   c. fight or flight response
   d. all of the above

2. A common way to accidentally come in contact with blood and body fluids is:
   a. phlebotomy
   b. administering an injection
   c. performing or assisting with suturing or removal of sutures
   d. all of the above

3. Eyelashes, eyebrows, skin, and mucous membranes are considered:
   a. physical/mechanical barriers to infection
   b. chemical barriers to infection
   c. cellular factors
   d. all of the above

4. Common infectious agents are:
   a. bacteria
   b. viruses
   c. parasites
   d. all of the above

5. Pus-filled boils, pimples, and rashes are symptoms of:
   a. Avian flu
   b. Chicken pox
   c. MRSA
   d. meningitis

6. The most important aspect of infection control is:
   a. immune response
   b. sterilization
   c. handwashing
   d. mode of transmission

7. The portal of exit is a part of the chain of infection. The best description of the portal of exit is:

   a. the method by which an infectious agent leaves the reservoir

   b. people, equipment, supplies, water, food, and animals or insects

   c. microorganisms that are the causative agents of disease

   d. specific ways in which microorganisms travel from one place to another

8. A disease that must be reported to the CDC is:

   a. rabies

   b. encephalitis

   c. influenza

   d. a and b

9. Methods of disinfection include:

   a. boiling

   b. steam autoclave

   c. gas sterilization

   d. ultrasonic cleaning

10. Microorganisms that can cause infectious disease are:

   a. normal flora

   b. immunosuppressants

   c. pathogens

   d. all of the above

LEARNING APPLICATION

Critical Thinking

1. Analyze the importance of infection control and give five examples of how a medical assistant would practice infection control in the ambulatory care setting.

_____

_____

_____

_____

_____

_____

_____

_____

_____

_____

_____

_____

2. Your patient has a draining wound. After you change the dressing, explain how to prevent the transmission of microorganisms from the wound and dressing to you or to another patient.

_____

_____

_____

3. Give an example of how the proper disposal of contaminated objects can break a link in the chain of infection.

_____

_____

_____

_____

_____

4. You notice a coworker sanitizing surgical instruments in preparation for sterilization. He or she did not scrub the serrations on the instruments well. What will be the result of his or her improper sanitization technique? Explain your answer.

_____

_____

_____

_____

5. Describe eight procedures/techniques that you could be performing on a patient that could expose you to bloodborne pathogens.

_____

_____

_____

_____

_____

_____

6. What alternative do you have if you do not have access to soap and water after performing a procedure on a patient?

_____

7. Explain the differences between sanitation and disinfection.

_____

_____

_____

_____

8. Considering the growth requirements for pathogens, describe how to discourage bacterial growth in the patient examination room.

_____

_____

_____

_____

Case Studies

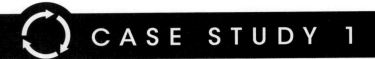

Your provider–employer asks you to help develop an exposure control plan. Include the measures the employer must take to eliminate or lessen an employee's risk for exposure to blood or other potentially infectious materials.

CASE STUDY REVIEW QUESTIONS

1. What should be included in an exposure control plan?

_____

_____

_____

_____

_____

_____

_____

_____

_____

_____

CASE STUDY 2

Veronica Hernandez, a medical assisting intern at the Northborough Family Medical Group of Drs. Winston Lewis and Elizabeth King, attends to patient procedures and examinations under the supervision of office manager Jacquie Cavanaugh, CMA (AAMA). Although Veronica is careful to follow all infection control methods during patient care, severe dermatitis has developed on her hands. She is concerned that this condition, which has not responded to creams and lotions, is related to the latex gloves she wears during procedures.

CASE STUDY REVIEW QUESTIONS

1. Discuss the possible causes of Veronica's symptoms.

_____

_____

_____

_____

2. Suggest a course of action that both addresses Veronica's condition and maintains the proper degree of asepsis.

_____

_____

_____

Hands-on Activities

Complete the following forms with the indicated information.

1. You tested the eyewash station on the first of this month. Complete the Eyewash Testing Log below in the next space.

Tested by:	Date	Assessment Action taken
Janie Carter, RN	August 14, 20xx	Flushed until clear, working appropriately.
B. Abbott, RMA (AMT)	September 16, 20xx	Flushed until clear, working properly.
Joe Guerrero, CMA (AAMA)	October 10, 20xx	Flushed until clear, working appropriately.

© Cengage Learning 2014

2. You checked the emergency cleanup spill kits in all your exam rooms and in the clinical laboratory. You made sure they were complete, had not expired, were intact without tears, and were ready to use when needed. Make notation of your checks on the following form.

Location	Checked by	Date	Assessment Action taken
Exam Room #1			
Exam Room #2			
Exam Room #3			
Lab Station #1			
Lab Kit #2			

© Cengage Learning 2014

3. You were exposed to a patient's blood through an accidental needlestick. Fill out the following form.

OSHA's Form 301

Injury and Illness Incident Report

U.S. Department of Labor
Occupational Safety and Health Administration

Form approved OMB no. 1218-0176

Attention: This form contains information relating to employee health and must be used in a manner that protects the confidentiality of employees to the extent possible while the information is being used for occupational safety and health purposes.

This *Injury and Illness Incident Report* is one of the first forms you must fill out when a recordable work-related injury or illness has occurred. Together with the *Log of Work-Related Injuries and Illnesses* and the accompanying *Summary*, these forms help the employer and OSHA develop a picture of the extent and severity of work-related incidents.

Within 7 calendar days after you receive information that a recordable work-related injury or illness has occurred, you must fill out this form or an equivalent. Some state workers' compensation, insurance, or other reports may be acceptable substitutes. To be considered an equivalent form, any substitute must contain all the information asked for on this form.

According to Public Law 91-596 and 29 CFR 1904, OSHA's recordkeeping rule, you must keep this form on file for 5 years following the year to which it pertains.

If you need additional copies of this form, you may photocopy and use as many as you need.

Information about the employee

1) Full name _____

2) Street _____

City _____ State _____ ZIP _____

3) Date of birth ___/___/___

4) Date hired ___/___/___

5) ☐ Male
   ☐ Female

Information about the physician or other health care professional

6) Name of physician or other health care professional _____

7) If treatment was given away from the worksite, where was it given?

Facility _____

Street _____

City _____ State _____ ZIP _____

8) Was employee treated in an emergency room?
   ☐ Yes
   ☐ No

9) Was employee hospitalized overnight as an in-patient?
   ☐ Yes
   ☐ No

Information about the case

10) Case number from the *Log* _____ (Transfer the case number from the Log after you record the case.)

11) Date of injury or illness ___/___/___

12) Time employee began work _____ AM / PM

13) Time of event _____ AM / PM ☐ Check if time cannot be determined

14) *What was the employee doing just before the incident occurred?* Describe the activity, as well as the tools, equipment, or material the employee was using. Be specific. *Examples:* "climbing a ladder while carrying roofing materials"; "spraying chlorine from hand sprayer"; "daily computer key-entry."

15) *What happened?* Tell us how the injury occurred. *Examples:* "When ladder slipped on wet floor, worker fell 20 feet"; "Worker was sprayed with chlorine when gasket broke during replacement"; "Worker developed soreness in wrist over time."

16) *What was the injury or illness?* Tell us the part of the body that was affected and how it was affected; be more specific than "hurt," "pain," or sore." *Examples:* "strained back"; "chemical burn, hand"; "carpal tunnel syndrome."

17) *What object or substance directly harmed the employee?* *Examples:* "concrete floor"; "chlorine"; "radial arm saw." *If this question does not apply to the incident, leave it blank.*

18) *If the employee died, when did death occur?* Date of death ___/___/___

Completed by _____

Title _____

Phone (____) ____ - ____ Date ___/___/___

Web Activities

1. The U.S. Department of Labor Occupational Safety and Health Administration (OSHA) Web site (http://www.osha.gov) provides you with significant amounts of information about the federal agency that seeks to protect health care workers from bloodborne pathogens. Visit the site to determine when the most recent changes have been made to *The Bloodborne Pathogen Standard*. What are the most recent changes?

2. The Centers for Disease Control and Prevention National Center for Infectious Diseases Web site (http://www.cdc.gov) provides a tremendous amount of information regarding infectious diseases and hepatitis in particular. Information is also available regarding HIV and AIDS. Are there other hepatitis viruses in addition to A, B, and C? Look on this site for the treatment of choice for all hepatitis viruses you find and describe the most common side effects of treatment.

CHAPTER POST-TEST

Perform this test without looking at your book.

1. Barriers that protect our bodies from infection are:
   a. skin and mucous membranes
   b. body excretions and secretions
   c. immune system
   d. all of the above

2. When a disease cannot be cured and the only treatment is for relief of symptoms, it is referred to as:
   a. palliative
   b. intervention
   c. curative
   d. none of the above

3. Influenza is transmitted by which route?
   a. bloodborne transmission
   b. vector transmission
   c. droplet transmission
   d. fomite transmission

4. The stage of infectious disease between the exposure to a pathogenic microorganism and the first appearance of signs and symptoms is the:
   a. incubation stage
   b. prodromal stage
   c. acute stage
   d. declining stage

5. Antibodies are also known as:
   a. erythrocytes
   b. immunoglobulins
   c. antigens
   d. all of the above

6. Most health care employers provide immunization for hepatitis B. If an employee does not wish to receive the vaccine, they must sign what form?
    a. Statement of understanding
    b. Employment contract
    c. Declination form
    d. All of the above

7. Diseases that are caused by parasites are:
    a. malaria
    b. amoebic dysentery
    c. trichomoniasis
    d. all of the above

8. People, equipment, supplies, and food and water are considered which part of the chain of infection?
    a. Portal of entry
    b. Susceptible host
    c. Reservoir
    d. Portal of exit

9. The use of biologic agents such as pathogenic microorganisms is considered?
    a. chain of infection
    b. disinfection
    c. bioterrorism
    d. sterilization

10. A person that is capable of contracting a pathogenic organism is called a:
    a. means of transmission
    b. portal of exit
    c. reservoir
    d. susceptible host

SELF-ASSESSMENT

1. Review your childhood history. What infectious diseases did you contract? Research the agent, mode of transmission, symptoms, diagnosis, and treatment. Record your findings below.

Disease	Agent	Transmission	Symptoms	Diagnosis	Treatment

2. In the course of caring for patients as a medical assistant, it is likely that you will be exposed to patients who have life-threatening infectious diseases. What professional skills might you utilize to protect your health and maintain a respectful manner when providing care? Evaluate your belief systems and record methods of demonstrating empathy in this situation.

_____

_____

_____

C H A P T E R **23**

The Patient History and Documentation

CHAPTER PRE-TEST

Perform this test without looking at your book.

1. Which is *not* a component of SOAP charting?
   a. Subjective information
   b. Assessment of symptoms
   c. Symptoms
   d. Plan for treatment

2. POMR stands for:
   a. Privacy of medical records
   b. Problem-oriented medical record
   c. Payment of medical resources
   d. Parts of medical records

3. The medical history form includes the social history, medical history, family history, review of systems, and:
   a. Insurance information
   b. Chief complaint
   c. Provider's history
   d. Diagnosis and prognosis

4. Primary administrative information includes the patient's full name, telephone numbers, insurance information, and:
   a. Addresses
   b. Date of birth
   c. Vital signs
   d. a and b

5. The Continuity of Care Record (CCR):
   a. Ensures that a minimum standard of information is to be shared with other providers
   b. Will have no effect on the entries made in the patient's chart
   c. Is being established by the American Academy of Gerontologists

   d. Can be completed only by providers
   e. All of the above

6. The most commonly accepted order of chart organization is:
   a. Alphabetic
   b. By diagnosis
   c. Chronologic
   d. Numeric

7. TPMS is an acronym for:
   a. Total Patient Management System
   b. Total Practice Management System
   c. Total Patient Medical Solutions
   d. Traditional Patient Management Systems

8. Displaying cultural awareness includes:
   a. Arranging for an interpreter
   b. Scheduling a female patient with a female provider
   c. Learning to speak Spanish
   d. a and b

9. A release of information form allows for:
   a. Obtaining past medical records
   b. Disclosing medical history to family members
   c. Collecting medical debts
   d. None of the above

10. The purpose of the medical record is:
   a. To plan treatment
   b. To review past treatment
   c. To maintain a legal record
   d. All of the above

VOCABULARY BUILDER

Misspelled Words

Find the words below that are misspelled; underline them, and correctly spell them in the spaces provided. Then, insert one of the correct vocabulary terms into the sentences below. Each word will be used once.

allergy's	objective	soarce–oriented medical record (SOMR)
CHEDDAR	problem-oriented medical record (POMR)	subjective
cheif complaint		
clinical diagnosis	SOAP	

_____ _____ _____

1. The _____ is the main reason the patient has come to the doctor.

2. Mary O'Keefe calls Dr. King's clinic to schedule an emergency appointment and tells Ellen Armstrong, CMA (AAMA), that her 3-year-old son Chris awakened during the night with extreme pain in his right ear. This is a _____ complaint, as it is known by the patient but cannot be seen or measured by the provider.

3. Dr. King examines 3-year-old Chris O'Keefe's right ear with an otoscope and observes that the ear is inflamed; the ear is also draining. Since these conditions can be visualized, they are called _____ signs.

4. Dr. Whitney confirms a _____ of acute appendicitis for the female emergency patient, based on subjective and objective information from the patient's history, the findings of the physical examination, and the results of the laboratory tests ordered.

5. _____ is a traditional form of charting that consists of a chronological set of notes for each visit, beginning with the patient's first visit.

6. The charting method that lists patient data in the following order: subjective, objective, assessment, and plan, is referred to as _____ charting.

7. Acquired abnormal immune responses to substances (allergens) that do not normally cause reactions are called _____.

8. The most efficient way of recording chart notes, especially in multiprovider clinics or practices, is _____.

9. _____ is another more comprehensive approach to charting, which encourages greater detail to SOAP/SOAPER.

LEARNING REVIEW

Short Answer

1. Every provider/patient interview is a cross-cultural one. List four questions a medical assistant might ask while taking a medical history that would help bridge social and cultural beliefs to obtain accurate information about a patient's condition that the provider will need to give proper care and treatment.

_____

_____

2. List eight possible characteristics of chief complaints.

_____

_____

3. After the history is taken by the medical assistant, the provider will perform a review of systems (ROS). In addition to the patient's general state of health, list 10 body systems the provider will assess during the ROS.

_____

_____

_____

_____

4. List five charting rules for Electronic Medical Records.

_____

_____

_____

_____

_____

_____

5. List at least ten components of a medical record.

_____

_____

_____

_____

Reading Chart Notes

1/10/XX CC: NVD × 4 days. T: 100°F for 2 days. Loss of appetite.

1. Write what this chart note means.

_____

_____

2. A mistake has been made in the chart note above: three days should be listed instead of four. Using proper procedure for correcting a paper chart, correct the note.

_____

_____

3. To practice charting, translate the following statements (A through H) into medical terms as you would document it in a patient's medical record. Use the lines provided.

A. The patient was examined on January 12, 20XX at ten fifteen in the morning.

_____

_____

B. The patient says she has had lower abdominal pain on the left side for a week and has been feeling more and more tired.

_____

_____

C. Weight is 135 pounds. Height is 5 feet 4 inches. Temperature is 99.8°F, slightly elevated above normal. Respiration is 19 breaths per minute and is clear. Pulse is 78 beats per minute and is regular. Blood pressure reading is 134 (systolic)/82 (diastolic).

_____

_____

D. The patient describes an increasing urge to urinate with a burning sensation upon urination; pressure in abdomen; and lack of energy.

_____

_____

E. The patient has a medical history that is positive for frequent urinary tract infections. The patient was diagnosed with type II diabetes mellitus in 1987 and takes a prescribed dosage of 3 mg of Glynase orally daily in tablet form. The patient quit smoking 20 years ago and has lost 10 pounds in the last 2 years.

_____

_____

F. The patient has no known allergies.

_____

_____

G. There is no change in family history.

_____

_____

H. The patient has less than two glasses of wine per week, does not smoke, and exercises regularly.

_____

_____

CERTIFICATION REVIEW

These questions are designed to mimic the certification examination. Select the best response.

1. The abbreviation ER stands for:
   a. electronic record
   b. electrophysiology review
   c. emergency resuscitation
   d. emergency room

2. Which type of medical record was developed by the American Academy of Family Physicians and the American Academy of Pediatrics to make it easier to share medication information between providers?
   a. Problem-Oriented Medical Record
   b. Source-Oriented Medical Record
   c. Continuity of Care Record
   d. Electronic Medical Record

3. Social and cultural beliefs are reflected as:
   a. background
   b. belief system
   c. family orientation
   d. all of the above

4. Which of the following is important when taking a patient's history?
   a. Allow the conversation to wander and the patient to tell anecdotes; it helps the patient to relax.
   b. Remind the patient that all information will be treated with confidentiality.
   c. Employ passive listening skills.
   d. Use medical jargon.

5. Some topics are sensitive but must be covered during a medical history. Which of the following will assist the medical assistant to obtain the needed information in these areas?

   a. Ask the questions at the beginning of the history to get them out of the way.

   b. Use casual or slang language and don't look directly at the patient.

   c. Laugh if you find the questions funny. Humor can diffuse a tense situation.

   d. Adopt a non-judgmental manner.

6. Which of the following is an objective statement?

   a. My toe hurts. It feels like a brick fell on it.

   b. When I walk to the mailbox, I get very short of breath.

   c. The right eye shows signs of edema and exudates.

   d. None of the above.

7. Which of the following are considered parts of a social history?

   a. Age at the onset of menstruation

   b. Use of alcohol and tobacco

   c. Sexual habits

   d. b and c

8. When the examination includes hoarseness, change in voice, frequent sore throats, and difficulty swallowing, which system is being reviewed?

   a. Nose, throat, and sinuses

   b. Mouth

   c. Throat/neck

   d. Respiratory

9. A demographic data form contains which of the following?

   a. Name

   b. Birth date

   c. Address

   d. All of the above

10. The medical history form includes which of the following?

    a. Release of information

    b. Physical exam

    c. Insurance information

    d. All of the above

LEARNING APPLICATION

Critical Thinking

1. Recall your last visit to your personal medical provider. How well was your medical history recorded? Was it recorded on a paper chart or in EHR? Recalling those circumstances, how would you make a patient feel comfortable in discussing his or her medical history?

   _____

   _____

   _____

   _____

   _____

2. Compare and contrast the patient's chief concern with the provider's chief concern in the cross-cultural model. How can those concerns be brought together with one focus?

_____

_____

_____

_____

_____

3. A male patient you are interviewing denies that he smokes, but his fingers are stained yellow from nicotine and he smells of tobacco smoke. What questions might you ask to clarify his response?

_____

_____

_____

_____

4. The health and well-being of family members contributes what kind of information to a patient's medical history? When that information is essentially unknown for some reason, such as adoption, how is that information addressed in the patient's record?

_____

_____

_____

_____

Case Studies

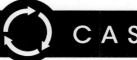 **CASE STUDY**

Yvonne Black is a new patient of Dr. Esposito at Inner City Health Care. Yvonne is an 88-year-old Italian-born woman who comes to the doctor at the urging of her granddaughter, Kristine, who accompanies her to the clinic. Yvonne's primary care provider has just retired after being her family doctor for over 35 years, and she requested Dr. Esposito because he is of Italian descent. Yvonne has many health problems and wants to describe each of them in great detail, making the intake interview complicated and difficult to perform. To add to the challenge, she is a poor historian when relating dates and events and does not always agree with the records obtained from her former doctor. This upsets Kristine, who wants to correct her, and they end up arguing.

CASE STUDY REVIEW QUESTIONS

1. What communication skills will Liz, the CMA (AAMA), need to get the most accurate information from Yvonne?

_____

_____

_____

_____

_____

_____

(continued)

2. What does the manner in which the patient relates information reveal about her?

_____

_____

_____

_____

3. What effect does Kristine have on the process of getting intake information from the patient? Is Kristine helpful or disruptive? What can you do and say to direct the conversation most effectively and efficiently?

_____

_____

_____

_____

_____

Hands-on Activities

1. Interview students from your school's English-as-a-Second-Language program or someone for whom English is not the primary language. Have them describe diseases or conditions that have bothered them in the past or are bothering them now. Discuss the following questions with classmates:

   a. Was there a problem with communication because of the language differences?

   _____

   _____

   _____

   b. What types of creative communication methods did you use?

   _____

   _____

   _____

   c. Did you find that some people can read another language better than they can "hear" it (or vice-versa)?

   _____

   _____

   _____

2. On a separate piece of paper, decode each component of Figure 23-8 in your textbook. Put all the information in lay terms and write out all the abbreviations.

3. Pretend you are a patient and complete the following Health History Questionnaire. You should use "made up" information to protect your privacy, but be sure to put your real name on it for clarification. With another student, take turns role-playing as medical assistant and patient using the forms you have filled out.

CONFIDENTIAL HEALTH HISTORY

Name:_____ Date: _____

Birthdate:_____ Age:_____ Date of last physical examination:_____

Occupation: _____

Reason for visit today: _____

MEDICATIONS List all medications you are currently taking	**ALLERGIES** List all allergies

SYMPTOMS Check (✓) symptoms you currently have or have had in the past year.

GENERAL
- ☐ Chills
- ☐ Depression
- ☐ Dizziness
- ☐ Fainting
- ☐ Fever
- ☐ Forgetfulness
- ☐ Headache
- ☐ Loss of sleep
- ☐ Loss of weight
- ☐ Nervousness
- ☐ Numbness
- ☐ Sweats

MUSCLE/JOINT/BONE
Pain, weakness, numbness in:
- ☐ Arms
- ☐ Hips
- ☐ Back
- ☐ Legs
- ☐ Feet
- ☐ Neck
- ☐ Hands
- ☐ Shoulders

GENITO-URINARY
- ☐ Blood in urine
- ☐ Frequent urination
- ☐ Lack of bladder control
- ☐ Painful urination

GASTROINTESTINAL
- ☐ Appetite poor
- ☐ Bloating
- ☐ Bowel changes
- ☐ Constipation
- ☐ Diarrhea
- ☐ Excessive hunger
- ☐ Excessive thirst
- ☐ Gas
- ☐ Hemorrhoids
- ☐ Indigestion
- ☐ Nausea
- ☐ Rectal bleeding
- ☐ Stomach pain
- ☐ Vomiting
- ☐ Vomiting blood

CARDIOVASCULAR
- ☐ Chest pain
- ☐ High blood pressure
- ☐ Irregular heart beat
- ☐ Low blood pressure
- ☐ Poor circulation
- ☐ Rapid heart beat
- ☐ Swelling of ankles
- ☐ Varicose veins

EYE, EAR, NOSE, THROAT
- ☐ Bleeding gums
- ☐ Blurred vision
- ☐ Crossed eyes
- ☐ Difficulty swallowing
- ☐ Double vision
- ☐ Earache
- ☐ Ear discharge
- ☐ Hay fever
- ☐ Hoarseness
- ☐ Loss of hearing
- ☐ Nosebleeds
- ☐ Persistent cough
- ☐ Ringing in ears
- ☐ Sinus problems
- ☐ Vision - Flashes
- ☐ Vision - Halos

SKIN
- ☐ Bruise easily
- ☐ Hives
- ☐ Itching
- ☐ Change in moles
- ☐ Rash
- ☐ Scars
- ☐ Sores that won't heal

MEN only
- ☐ Breast lump
- ☐ Erection difficulties
- ☐ Lump in testicles
- ☐ Penis discharge
- ☐ Sore on penis
- ☐ Other

WOMEN only
- ☐ Abnormal Pap Smear
- ☐ Bleeding between periods
- ☐ Breast lump
- ☐ Extreme menstrual pain
- ☐ Hot flashes
- ☐ Nipple discharge
- ☐ Painful intercourse
- ☐ Vaginal discharge
- ☐ Other

Date of last
menstrual period_____

Date of last
Pap Smear_____

Have you had
a mammogram? _____

Are you pregnant? _____

Number of children _____

MEDICAL HISTORY Check (✓) the medical conditions you have or have had in the past.

- ☐ AIDS
- ☐ Alcoholism
- ☐ Anemia
- ☐ Anorexia
- ☐ Appendicitis
- ☐ Arthritis
- ☐ Asthma
- ☐ Bleeding Disorders
- ☐ Breast Lump
- ☐ Bronchitis
- ☐ Bulimia
- ☐ Cancer
- ☐ Cataracts

- ☐ Chemical Dependency
- ☐ Chicken Pox
- ☐ Diabetes
- ☐ Emphysema
- ☐ Epilepsy
- ☐ Gall Bladder Disease
- ☐ Glaucoma
- ☐ Goiter
- ☐ Gonorrhea
- ☐ Gout
- ☐ Heart Disease
- ☐ Hepatitis
- ☐ Hernia

- ☐ Herpes
- ☐ High Cholesterol
- ☐ HIV Positive
- ☐ Kidney Disease
- ☐ Liver Disease
- ☐ Measles
- ☐ Migraine Headaches
- ☐ Miscarriage
- ☐ Mononucleosis
- ☐ Multiple Sclerosis
- ☐ Mumps
- ☐ Pacemaker
- ☐ Pneumonia

- ☐ Polio
- ☐ Prostate Problem
- ☐ Psychiatric Care
- ☐ Rheumatic Fever
- ☐ Scarlet Fever
- ☐ Stroke
- ☐ Suicide Attempt
- ☐ Thyroid Problems
- ☐ Tonsillitis
- ☐ Tuberculosis
- ☐ Typhoid Fever
- ☐ Ulcers
- ☐ Vaginal Infections
- ☐ Venereal Disease

CONFIDENTIAL HEALTH HISTORY

HOSPITALIZATIONS

Year	Hospital	Reason for Hospitalization and Outcome

Have you ever had a blood transfusion? ☐ Yes ☐ No

If yes, please give approximate dates: _____

OCCUPATIONAL CONCERNS Check (✓) if your work exposes you to the following:	**HEALTH HABITS** Check (✓) which substances you use and indicate how much you use per day/week.	**PREGNANCY HISTORY**		
		Year of Birth	Sex of Birth	Complications if any
☐ Stress	☐ Caffeine			
☐ Hazardous Substances	☐ Tobacco			
☐ Heavy Lifting	☐ Drugs			
☐ Other	☐ Alcohol			

SERIOUS ILLNESS/INJURIES	DATE	OUTCOME

FAMILY HISTORY Fill in health information about your family.

Relation	Age	State of Health	Age at Death	Cause of Death	Check (✓) if your blood relatives had any of the following Disease	Relationship to you
Father					☐ Arthritis, Gout	
Mother					☐ Asthma, Hay Fever	
Brothers					☐ Cancer	
					☐ Chemical Dependency	
					☐ Diabetes	
					☐ Heart Disease, Strokes	
Sisters					☐ High Blood Pressure	
					☐ Kidney Disease	
					☐ Tuberculosis	
					☐ Other	

I certify that the above information is correct to the best of my knowledge. I will not hold my doctor or any members of his/her staff responsible for any errors or ommisions that I may have made in the completion of this form.

_____   _____
Signature   Date

_____   _____
Reviewed By   Date

Web Activities

1. Electronic medical records or EMR are required for submission of claims for payment to Medicare or Medicaid. The date has been moved several times. Currently, there is a goal of 2014 for complete implementation by providers. In order to assist providers, there is an EMR incentive program in place. Go to http://www.cms.gov and read about the guidelines to participate in the incentive program.

2. Search the Internet for information on the electronic POMR. Are you able to see examples? Discuss the advantages and disadvantages of the electronic record and the POMR.

CHAPTER POST-TEST

Perform this test without looking at your book.

1. When a patient "denies" something, he or she is:
   a. just whining
   b. not being truthful
   c. explaining his or her symptoms
   d. trying to blame someone else

2. The correct abbreviation for physical therapy is:
   a. PT
   b. pt
   c. PhTx
   d. ptx

3. The Joint Commission's prohibited abbreviation list is aimed at:
   a. controlling the use and creation of new abbreviations
   b. enhancing the goal of patient safety
   c. allowing the provider to accurately prescribe medications
   d. all of the above

4. Some benefits of EMR are:
   a. ease of storage
   b. access 24 hours a day
   c. multiple, simultaneous viewers
   d. all of the above

5. When reviewing a note in the patient's record, you see notations regarding the assessment of joint stiffness, muscle pain, back pain, and arthritis. This would be an ROS of which system?
   a. Cardiovascular
   b. Musculoskeletal
   c. Neurological
   d. Endocrine

6. The history of present illness includes:
   a. medications
   b. allergies
   c. other providers or alternative therapy practitioners being seen
   d. all of the above

7. The abbreviation CBC indicates:

   a. Complete Body Chemicals

   b. Complex Biochemicals

   c. Complete Blood Count

   d. none of the above

8. The purpose of a privacy notice is to:

   a. describe patient rights

   b. describe the facility's privacy practices

   c. describe how to file a complaint if a patient feels his or her rights are violated

   d. all of the above

9. The use of abbreviations in charting serves several purposes including:

   a. saving time and space

   b. giving exact meaning to a finding

   c. making legal action confusing

   d. a and b

SELF-ASSESSMENT

Think about your own personal experiences when answering the following questions. Be as self-reflective as you can.

1. When you are asked to complete a medical history form, what are some of the emotions that you experience? Do you dread the effort involved (especially if you aren't feeling well)? Are you concerned that you will not know all the answers, won't have all the dates and numbers, and so on? Are you frustrated because you have filled out so many forms already? Are you ever embarrassed by some of the questions? Do you feel guilty that you will not answer some of the questions honestly? Do you feel stupid if you do not understand all the questions? Do you feel hindered because you did not bring your glasses or you have a sprained wrist or are too sick to fill out the form? Think of other feelings you have that are not listed here.

   _____

   _____

2. Whenever a patient sees a new doctor or has not been in to the doctor for a while, or even on a periodic basis, a new medical history form needs to be filled out. There is always paperwork to complete. Can you think of a better/easier/more efficient way to update patient information? Could computers make the job easier? What do you think will happen in the future?

   _____

   _____

3. Remember your feelings when you ask your patients to fill out the medical history forms, and be sensitive to their needs. How might you assist them, without dedicating time away from your other duties?

   _____

   _____

   _____

C H A P T E R   **24**

Vital Signs and Measurements

CHAPTER PRE-TEST

Perform this test without looking at your book.

1. Elevated blood pressure above the normal range is called:
   a. Hypotension
   b. Hypertension
   c. Normotension
   d. None of the above

2. The definition of afebrile is:
   a. Absence of body temperature
   b. Normal body temperature
   c. Elevated body temperature
   d. Low body temperature

3. The process of losing body heat from the surface of the skin into a cooler environment is known as:
   a. Convection
   b. Conduction
   c. Radiation
   d. Evaporation

4. Airflow during respiration that stops for more than 10 seconds is considered:
   a. Eupnea
   b. Apnea
   c. Tachypnea
   d. All of the above

5. Blood pressure less than 90/60 is referred to as:
   a. Hypotension
   b. Hypertension
   c. Normotension
   d. All of the above

6. Bradycardia is defined as:
   a. Rapid pulse rate
   b. Slow pulse rate
   c. Absent pulse rate
   d. Normal pulse rate

7. Measuring chest circumference in an adult assesses which disease?
   a. Heart disease
   b. Edema
   c. Emphysema
   d. Fractured ribs

8. The normal pulse rate for a newborn is:
   a. 80–140 bpm
   b. 120–160 bpm
   c. 100–150 bpm
   d. 120–170 bpm

9. Tympanic thermometers are used to measure body temperature at what part of the body?
   a. Axillary area
   b. Sublingual
   c. Eardrum
   d. Rectum

10. The most common location an artery is palpated to calculate pulse rate is:
    a. Radial
    b. Carotid
    c. Temporal
    d. Femoral

VOCABULARY BUILDER

Misspelled Words

Find the key vocabulary words below that are misspelled; underline them, and correctly spell them in the space provided. Then, fill in the blanks below with the appropriate terms from the list. Not all words will be used.

arhythmia	hyperpnea	pyrexia
bradycardia	hypertension	strider
bradypnea	hyperventilation	tachycardia
Cheyne-Stokes	hypotention	wheese
dispnea	orthopnia	
frenulum	peripheral	

_____   _____   _____

_____   _____   _____

1. Tachycardia is a common cardiac _____.

2. The fold of mucous membrane under the tongue is known as the _____.

3. In medical directional terms, away from the center of the body is referred to as _____.

4. When a patient' heart rate is above 100 bmp, it is called _____.

5. A pattern of breathing that starts with a long period of apnea followed by increasing depth and rate of respirations is called _____ respiration.

6. Another term used when describing an elevated body temperature is _____.

7. It is common for children who have aspirated a foreign body to have _____ on inspiration.

Matching

Match the following terms listed in Column A with the corresponding descriptions in Column B

Column A	Column B
____ 1. Atherosclerosis	A. Initial measurement against which future measurements are compared.
____ 2. Apical	B. Having a fever.
____ 3. Rales	C. A form of arteriosclerosis marked by calcium deposits in the arterial lining.
____ 4. Baseline	D. One component of blood pressure measurement that represents the lowest amount of pressure exerted upon the arteries during the cardiac cycle.
____ 5. Diastole	E. Deviation from the normal pattern or rhythm of the heartbeat.
____ 6. Febrile	F. Pertaining to the apex of the heart.
____ 7. Arrhythmia	G. Difficulty breathing in any other position than upright.
____ 8. Orthopnea	H. Abnormal bubbling or crackling sounds heard by auscultation during inspiration.

LEARNING REVIEW

Short Answer

1. Temperature, pulse, respirations, and blood pressure are collective referred to as:

   _____

2. How is heat produced within the body? What part of the brain maintains the balance between heat production and heat loss? What are ways the body cools itself in hot weather?

   _____

   _____

   _____

   _____

3. List the five ways in which the body loses heat next to each example below.
   a. Casey climbs into a cold bed. _____
   b. Sarah enjoys her aerobic workout, which causes her to sweat. _____
   c. In the surgical suite, Dr. Beahm likes to keep the temperature at a cool 62 degrees. _____
   d. Phillip uses a portable fan when sleeping to maintain comfort. _____
   e. Bryan performs daily yoga breathing exercises. _____

4. Explain the different pattern of fevers listed below:

    a. Remittent _____

    b. Intermittent _____

    c. Continuous _____

5. Circle the correct words to complete the sentences: A(n) (increase/decrease) in temperature may be caused by several factors, such as eating, medications that increase metabolism, exercise, bacterial infections, and exposure to heat, pregnancy, stress, and age. A(n) (increase/decrease) in body temperature may result from fasting, inactivity, medications that decrease metabolism, exposure to cold, and age.

6. An aural temperature is taken where?

_____

_____

7. Write the normal ranges of blood pressure for the following ages:

Child, aged 10   _____

Adolescent, aged 16   _____

Adult   _____

     _____

8. Define the following terms and explain how each factor affects blood pressure.

Blood volume: _____

_____

Elasticity of artery walls: _____

_____

Peripheral resistance: _____

_____

Strength of the heart muscle: _____

_____

_____

Viscosity of the blood: _____

_____

_____

9. Name and describe the various sounds heard during blood pressure measurement.

Phase I: _____

Phase II: _____

Phase III: _____

Phase IV: _____

Phase V: _____

10. List five types of hypertension and explain each type, whether it is curable, and what the treatment(s) and cause(s) are. Then give an example of each.

Type	Description and Example

Type	Description and Example

11. List three possible causes of hypotension.

_____

_____

12. The medical term for a very rapid pulse is _____.

13. The medical term for a slower pulse rate is _____.

14. The medical term meaning difficulty and/or painful breathing is _____.

15. Write the normal respiratory rates for the following age groups:

Newborns _____

Infants _____

Children (1–7 years) _____

Adults _____

16. Name the common pulse sites described below and then match the site to its proper location on the body in the figure below by placing the correct letter in the space provided.

a. The site most commonly used for blood pressure measurement: _____

b. The site for blood pressure measurement in the leg: _____

c. The site commonly used for infant pulse rate measurement: _____

d. The site used in emergencies and when performing cardiopulmonary resuscitation (CPR): _____

e. The site used to check for circulation in the lower limbs: _____

f. The most commonly used site to measure pulse rate in an adult: _____

g. The site used in an emergency to control bleeding in the leg: _____

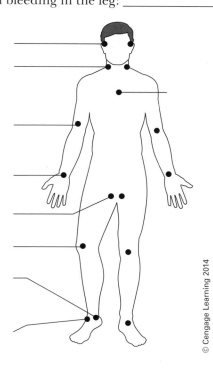

© Cengage Learning 2014

CERTIFICATION REVIEW

These questions are designed to mimic the certification examination. Select the best response.

1. Which of the following is *not* a routine body measurement?

    a. Chest circumference

    b. Head circumference

    c. Ankle circumference

    d. Height

2. In converting inches to feet, which of the following is true?

    a. 62 inches is 5 feet, 2 inches

    b. 62 inches is 6 feet, 2 inches

    c. 62 inches is 6 feet exactly

    d. 62 inches is 5 feet, 6 inches

3. What is considered a normal pulse and respiration rate for an adult?

    a. Pulse of 76 bpm, respiration of 20/min.

    b. Pulse of 80 bpm, respiration of 18/min.

    c. Pulse of 56 bpm, respiration of 16/min.

    d. Pulse of 20 bpm, respiration of 60/min.

    e. Both a and b.

4. Which of the following is *not* a requirement in order to obtain accurate blood pressure?

    a. The cuff should be the proper size.

    b. The cuff should be placed correctly over the radial artery.

    c. The arm should be above the heart level.

    d. The deflation should not be faster than 2–4 mm Hg per heartbeat.

    e. The patient should be seated with feet on the floor and back supported.

5. A pulse obtained at the intersection of the fifth intercostals space at the midclavicular line on the left chest is called the:

    a. femoral pulse

    b. temporal pulse

    c. brachial pulse

    d. apical pulse

6. Malignant hypertension:

    a. is a borderline elevation of the blood pressure

    b. is a blood pressure reading that is below normal

    c. is life threatening

    d. is the same as postural hypertension

7. Heat lost through the normal functioning of the intestinal, urinary, and respiratory tracts is known as:

    a. convection

    b. conduction

    c. radiation

    d. elimination

8. Glass mercury thermometers are being phased out because they contain a hazardous material. Which of the following are applicable during cleanup after breakage?

   a. Use a broom to pick up any spilled mercury.

   b. Use a vacuum to clean up the spilled mercury.

   c. Use an eyedropper or scoop up the mercury with a piece of heavy paper.

   d. All of the above.

9. Respiration that is increased in both rate and depth is called:

   a. hyperpnea

   b. hypoventilation

   c. tachypnea

   d. orthopnea

10. A disorder that causes patient to have daytime sleeping while driving, eating, or participating in other usual activities is known as:

   a. insomnia

   b. narcolepsy

   c. epilepsy

   d. sleep apnea

LEARNING APPLICATION

Critical Thinking

1. Discuss the responsibilities of the medical assistant when measuring vital signs.

   _____

   _____

   _____

2. Describe the care and use for each of the various types of thermometers.

   _____

   _____

   _____

   _____

   _____

   _____

   _____

   _____

   _____

   _____

   _____

   _____

   _____

   _____

3. Discuss the reasons why a professional must be aware that mercury thermometers and other mercury-containing equipment are being phased out of use.

_____

_____

_____

_____

4. Discuss the rationale for not using the thumb for taking the pulse rate of a patient.

_____

_____

5. Discuss the reasons for taking the respiratory rate of a patient without the patient's knowledge.

_____

_____

Case Studies

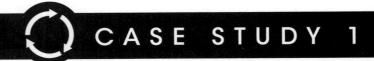

CASE STUDY 1

Wayne lives near Inner City Health Care in a group home for developmentally delayed adults. Wayne has a history of frequent colds and ear infections. He visits the clinic one morning with pain in both ears. He is also drinking a cup of hot coffee.

CASE STUDY REVIEW QUESTIONS

1. What method would Sarah, the CMA (AAMA), use to take Wayne's temperature?

_____

_____

2. How might Sarah explain to Wayne why she is using an alternate method?

_____

_____

CASE STUDY 2

Sam, who is 4 years old, is rushed to Heartland Pediatrics. He is bleeding profusely from a cut on his head. "He fell down the stairs," sobs his mother, Julie. Sam does not seem to be fully conscious and appears confused. Dr. Tony Tyler attends to Sam's laceration, applying direct pressure on the cut to stop the bleeding. He directs clinical assistant Linda Ludemann to call 911 for emergency services. Then Linda takes Sam's pulse. "What are you doing?" Julie asks Linda.

CASE STUDY REVIEW QUESTIONS

1. What site would Linda use to take Sam's pulse?

   _____

2. How might Linda answer Julie's questions about what she is doing as she assesses Sam's vital signs?

   _____

   _____

   _____

   _____

CASE STUDY 3

Abigail, who suffers from many problems related to her advanced age, also has type II diabetes. She is very friendly and has a good rapport with everyone in the clinic—all of whom she says are "just like family"—and she is very eager to please the staff. One winter day she comes to the clinic complaining of flu symptoms. When clinical assistant Audrey asks Abigail to step onto the scale to get her weight, Abigail says, "Oh, do we have to? I just don't feel up to it right now."

CASE STUDY REVIEW QUESTION

1. How might Audrey explain to Abigail about why her weight is important at every visit?

   _____

   _____

   _____

   _____

   _____

Web Activities

1. Using a search engine, access information on the Internet from the American Heart Association regarding essential hypertension and answer the following:

   a. What population of people in the United States is at greatest risk for essential hypertension?

   _____

   _____

   b. List four patient education tips for reducing blood pressure without the aid of medication.

   _____

   _____

   _____

   _____

CHAPTER POST-TEST

1. Which of the following is an essential activity to ensure accurate weight measurement?
   a. Calibration of the scale
   b. Heavy outwear must be removed
   c. Shoes should be removed
   d. All of the above

2. The first sound heard when deflating the blood pressure cuff is the _____ sound:
   a. Phase I
   b. Phase II
   c. Phase III
   d. Phase IV

3. An apical pulse is measured:
   a. in the groin area
   b. on the top of the foot, slightly to the side of midline
   c. at the back of the knee
   d. at the apex of the heart

4. The medical term for a normal respiratory rate is:
   a. apnea
   b. bradypnea
   c. eupnea
   d. tachypnea

5. A pulse oximeter measures:
   a. respiratory rate
   b. amount of oxygen present in arterial blood
   c. amount of oxygen present in venous blood
   d. none of the above

6. Measuring chest circumference is done correctly by:
   a. measuring at the nipple line
   b. measure during deepest inspiration
   c. measure during deepest expiration
   d. all of the above

7. Which age group routinely has height and weight measured at every clinic visit?

   a. Pediatrics

   b. Geriatrics

   c. Adults

   d. All of the above

8. You measure your 50-year-old patient's blood pressure and find that it is 102/50. This is considered:

   a. normotensive

   b. hypotensive

   c. hypertensive

   d. none of the above

9. Pulse pressure is considered:

   a. the difference between the diastolic reading and the pulse

   b. the difference between the systolic reading and the pulse

   c. the difference between the systolic and diastolic readings

   d. the calculation of one third the systolic reading

10. Which of the following may cause an error in a blood pressure reading?

    a. Correct cuff size

    b. Deflation of the cuff is more rapid than 2 to 4 mm Hg per heartbeat

    c. Patient is relaxed and comfortable

    d. Cuff placed appropriately

SELF-ASSESSMENT

As you respond to the following questions, think of how your experiences will affect how you treat your patients.

1. Think of the last time you had your height and weight measured. Did you have enough privacy to make you comfortable?

_____

_____

_____

_____

_____

_____

_____

_____

_____

_____

2. When you had your blood pressure taken, did the medical assistant share your measurements with you? Did you feel comfortable asking questions?

_____

_____

_____

_____

3. Has any health care provider ever discussed any of your vital signs or body measurements with you? Have you been informed of the health factors related to your vital signs or body measurements?

_____

_____

_____

_____

4. Do you still have mercury thermometers in your home? If so, call the health department to find out where you can take them for disposal and then obtain an electronic or digital thermometer for future use at home. How do you think your patients will feel when you encourage them to do the same? Write out exactly what you will say to them to convince them of the importance of replacing all mercury thermometers with a safer alternative. Explain mercury poisoning to them.

_____

_____

_____

_____

_____

_____

_____

_____

_____

C H A P T E R **25**

The Physical Examination

CHAPTER PRE-TEST

Perform this test without looking at your book.

1. Which of the following is *not* a method used during a physical examination?
   a. Percussion
   b. Menstruation
   c. Manipulation
   d. Auscultation

2. Which is a component of a routine physical examination?
   a. What the patient looks like
   b. How the patient walks
   c. Whether the patient has bad breath
   d. All of the above

3. Which of the following is *not* a position used in physical examinations of patients?
   a. Lithotomy
   b. Supine
   c. Dorsal recumbent
   d. Reverse Trendelenburg

4. Choose the correct spelling of the instrument used to examine the inside of the eyeball.
   a. Ophthalmoscope
   b. Optomescope
   c. Opthalmoscope
   d. Otoscope

5. An uncoordinated, wide-based walk is considered:
   a. Gait
   b. Balance
   c. Ataxia
   d. Spastic

6. PERRLA is an abbreviation for:
   a. Pupils equal to light and accommodation
   b. Pupils equal, round, and reactive to light and accommodation
   c. Pupils equal, reactive, radiant, to light and accommodation
   d. Pupils equal, round, rightly aligned

7. Excessive accumulation of fluids that impact a patient's weight is referred to as:
   a. Swelling
   b. Cyanosis
   c. Edema
   d. Scleroderma

8. When the provider assesses stature, which of the following is included?
   a. Height, trunk, and limb proportion
   b. Height, weight, and age
   c. Arm, leg, and trunk proportion
   d. Height, weight, and limb proportion

9. Correspondence in shape and size of body parts located on opposite sides of the body is known as:
   a. Stature
   b. Posture
   c. Symmetry
   d. Reflexes

10. The medical term for loss of voice is:
    a. Laryngitis
    b. Aphasia
    c. Dysphagia
    d. Aphonia

VOCABULARY REVIEW

Misspelled Words

Find the words below that are misspelled, underline them, and then correctly spell them in the space provided. Then identify the correct vocabulary terms most appropriate for each example below from a patient's physical examination.

ataxia	labirynthitis	symmetry
bruits	paller	tinnitus
cianosis	piorrhea	vertigo
jaundice	schleroderma	vertiligo

_____   _____   _____

_____   _____   _____

1. During a physical examination of Louise Kipperley, a 48-year-old woman, Dr. Esposito notices that Louise's facial skin has become tight and atrophied, suggesting possible _____.

2. Leo McKay comes to Inner City Health Care with mouth pain. Dr. Reynolds examines Leo's mouth and discovers _____, which is discharge of pus from the gums around the teeth.

3. Medical assistant Liz Corbin, CMA (AAMA), observes the gait of Geraldine Potter, a 36-year-old woman diagnosed with multiple sclerosis. Geraldine's gait is lurching and unsteady, with her feet widely placed. Liz charts this as _____.

4. Annette Samuels is diagnosed with hepatitis B virus (HBV) by Dr. John Pettit. Among Annette's symptoms, noted by Dr. Pettit during the physical examination, was _____, a distinct yellowing of Annette's skin and the whites of her eyes.

5. Lenny Taylor, an older adult male with Alzheimer's disease, is brought to Inner City Health Care by his son George. Apparently, Lenny has had problems breathing. Dr. Whitney observes _____, a bluish color in Lenny's skin.

6. After performing a routine venipuncture procedure on patient Rhonda Campbell, Sam Huckaby, CMA (AAMA), notices that all color has drained from Rhonda's face. He assumes that her _____ is due to a psychological reaction to the venipuncture, so he has her lie down on the examination table for a few minutes until her color improves.

7. Abigail Johnson's 28-year-old granddaughter Lucy comes in for an examination with Dr. King after observing white patches of depigmentation, or _____, on her hand. "Is this what Michael Jackson had?" she asks Dr. King.

8. While performing a complete physical examination on patient Ann Cook, Dr. King listens for abnormal sounds, or _____, from vital organs while auscultating her abdomen.

9. During a routine physical examination of Joanna Rowe, a young woman confined to a wheelchair, Dr. Lewis checks for balance or _____ of size, shape, and position of body parts on opposite sides of her body.

10. Addi Mountjoy comes in to see Dr. King for ringing in her ears. Dr. King asks her if she is taking large doses of aspirin, which can cause _____.

11. Ashley White's 6-year-old daughter, Brittney, diagnosed with a case of the mumps, returns with her mother for a reexamination with Dr. Lewis when the child experiences a sensation that the room is spinning, caused by inflammation of the labyrinth, called _____.

12. While her blood was being taken, Susan O'Donnell described the room as spinning and felt light-headed. _____ is a common reaction to a stress-induced drop in blood pressure.

LEARNING REVIEW

Matching

Column A	Column B
____ 1. Auscultation	A. On his physical examination of Charles Williams, Dr. Winston Lewis looks at the patient to assess his general health, posture, body movements, skin, mannerisms, and care in grooming while verbally reviewing Charles's medical history with him.
____ 2. Observation or inspection	B. Dr. Mark Woo uses a stethoscope to listen to the bowel sounds that accompany peristalsis.
____ 3. Manipulation	C. Dr. King performs range of motion exercises on patient Margaret Thomas, who is suspected of having Parkinson's disease.
____ 4. Mensuration	D. Dr. Rice taps Edith Leonard's chest to feel and hear the hollow quality expected from clear lungs.
____ 5. Percussion	E. During Marissa O'Keefe's well-baby visit, chest and head circumference measurements are recorded in the patient's medical record.

Short Answer

1. Identify each entry below as a piece of medical equipment (ME), a laboratory procedure (LP), a body part (BP), or a patient illness or condition (PI). Then identify the correct component or sequence of the physical examination to which the entry relates. The first two entries have been completed for you as an example.

   A. Sphygmomanometer   ME   Vital signs

   B. Aphonia   PI   Speech

   C. Lymph nodes   _____   _____

   D. Edema   _____   _____

   E. Anal fissures   _____   _____

   F. Emphysema   _____   _____

   G. Pharyngeal mirrors   _____   _____

   H. Scrotum   _____   _____

   I. Areola   _____   _____

   J. Electrocardiography   _____   _____

   K. Kyphosis   _____   _____

   L. Dysphasia   _____   _____

   M. Urinalysis   _____   _____

   N. Achilles tendon   _____   _____

   O. Tympanic membrane   _____   _____

2. Symmetry would be noted by using what method of assessment?

   _____

3. What is another term for the supine position or the position assumed when lying face up?

   _____

4. *(Circle the correct answer)* Orthostatic hypotension occurs as blood pressure decreases/increases/normalizes.

5. What is the preferred position for administration of an enema or rectal suppositories?

   _____

6. Determining the amount of flexion and extension of a patient's extremities would be which form of assessment?

   _____

Image Identification

Identify each of the positions shown in the photos below.

A.

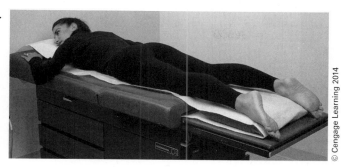

_____

B.

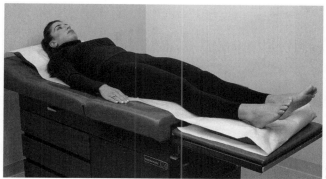

_____

C.

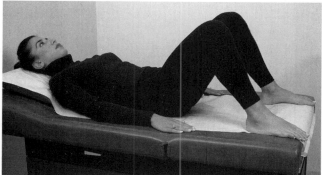

_____

D.

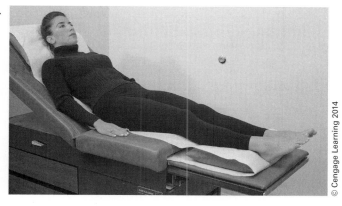

_____

E.

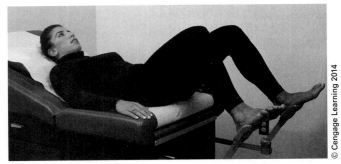

_____

F.

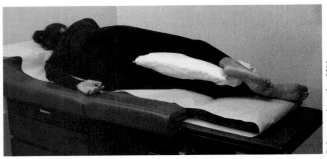

_____

G.

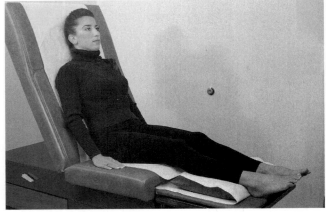

_____

CERTIFICATON REVIEW

1. A patient having an examination of the abdomen should be placed in which position?
   a. Supine
   b. Prone
   c. Lithotomy
   d. Sims'

2. Listening to the patient's chest as he or she breathes is called:
   a. auscultation
   b. percussion
   c. inspection
   d. palpation

3. The process of inspection is also called:
   a. percussion
   b. mensuration
   c. observation
   d. palpitations

4. Movements that are intended to be made by the patient are called:
   a. involuntary movements
   b. gait
   c. palsy
   d. voluntary movements

5. Which of the following is *not* a word used to describe skin color?
   a. Jaundice
   b. Cyanosis
   c. Bruits
   d. Pallor

6. Examination of the ears is an important aspect of a physical exam. Which of the following is *not* utilized when examining the ear?
   a. Ophthalmoscope
   b. Tuning fork
   c. Otoscope
   d. Audiometer

7. Eliciting sounds from the body by tapping is the examination technique referred to as:
   a. observation
   b. inspection
   c. percussion
   d. palpation

8. The most comfortable position for patients with back or abdominal problems when lying on an exam table is:
   a. semi-Fowler's
   b. supine
   c. lithotomy
   d. dorsal recumbent

9. The technique that includes height, weight, length of limbs, and degrees of flexion or extension is:
   a. auscultation
   b. mensuration
   c. manipulation
   d. none of the above

10. Which of the following are instructions that might be given to a patient during a breast exam?
   a. "Place your hand behind your head."
   b. "Take a deep breath."
   c. "Please swallow."
   d. "Close your right eye."

LEARNING APPLICATION

Critical Thinking

1. Discuss the responsibilities of the medical assistant when preparing the patient for a physical examination.

   _____

   _____

   _____

   _____

   _____

   _____

2. Review the six methods used in the physical examination.

   _____

   _____

   _____

   _____

3. Explain the sequence of a physical examination.

   (1) _____

   _____

   (2) _____

   _____

4. Describe the cleaning process that the following instruments will need after their use in an examination:
   a. Nasal speculum _____

   _____

   b. Tuning fork _____

   c. Percussion hammer _____

   d. Reusable otoscope speculum _____

   _____

5. List and describe the three sources of information the provider uses to aid in making a diagnosis.

   (1) _____

   _____

   (2) _____

   (3) _____

   _____

6. List two procedures or tests the medical assistant might perform as part of the patient's physical examination.

   _____

   _____

   _____

Case Studies

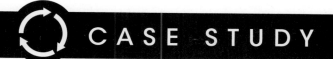

CASE STUDY

Holly Carmona brings her young daughter, Wren, to Charlotte Pediatrics with a suspected case of mumps, which her older sister is just recovering from. As Sarah Thomas, CMA (AAMA), helps the child remove her shirt for the examination, Wren becomes increasingly fearful and begins to cry. It is obvious the child is feverish and not feeling well.

CASE STUDY REVIEW QUESTIONS

1. What aspects of the physical exam will be important to make a diagnosis of mumps?

_____

_____

_____

_____

_____

2. How can Sarah be the most helpful to the provider to allow ease of examination?

_____

_____

_____

_____

_____

Role-Play Exercises

Using the list of patient positions from the textbook, practice placing your classmates into the various positions for examination. Pay special attention to knee and back problems and any physical limitations patients may have.

Web Activities

Explore the Web for information about the following conditions and their possible causes:

a. Changes in retinal blood vessels

b. Enlarged liver

c. Ascites

d. Varicose veins

e. Vertigo

CHAPTER POST-TEST

1. If a rectal exam is to be performed by the provider, which position would be best for this exam?
   a. Lithotomy
   b. Prone
   c. Sims'
   d. None of the above

2. Which examination tool is utilized to check a patient's reflexes?
   a. Tuning fork
   b. Pen light
   c. Tape measure
   d. Percussion hammer

3. To assess the health of a joint, which examination technique is utilized?
   a. Manipulation
   b. Percussion
   c. Palpation
   d. Inspection

5. The order of physical examination proceeds in which manner?
   a. Anterior to posterior
   b. Medial to lateral
   c. Superior to inferior
   d. Proximal to distal

6. Cyanosis is an indicator of diseases of which systems?
   a. Gastrointestinal
   b. Respiratory
   c. Cardiovascular
   d. b and c

7. When a penlight is directed into the eye, the pupil is expected to:
   a. dilate
   b. equalize
   c. constrict
   d. deviate

8. To examine the mouth and throat, the provider will require which of the following instruments?
   a. Flashlight or pen light
   b. Cotton swab
   c. Tongue depressor
   d. a and c

9. Auscultation, palpation, and mensuration are utilized to examine what area of the body?
   a. Abdomen
   b. Breast
   c. Heart
   d. Chest

10. Which examination includes internal genitalia, external genitalia, and rectal exam?
    a. Female genital
    b. Male genital
    c. a and b
    d. None of the above

SELF-ASSESSMENT

Think about the last time you went to the doctor. As you answer the following questions and remember your personal experience(s), think about how your experience(s) will affect the way you treat your patients in the future. If you have no personal experiences, try to imagine how you would feel and react.

1. Did you have to undress at all? How did that feel? Did you get cold or feel a bit awkward?

   _____

   _____

   _____

2. When you had your blood pressure taken, did the cuff cause pain or discomfort as it got tighter? Did you say something to the medical assistant? Do you think most people speak up when they are uncomfortable?

   _____

   _____

   _____

   _____

3. Have you ever noticed a sick patient in a public place? What were the clues that told you the patient was sick? Do you think your skills of observation will be enhanced after you complete this chapter?

   _____

   _____

   _____

   _____

   _____

CHAPTER **26**

Obstetrics and Gynecology

CHAPTER PRE-TEST

Perform this test without looking at your book.

1. Which of the following are addressed during the initial prenatal visit and examination?
   a. Genetic diseases/conditions in the family
   b. Kidney and heart diseases/conditions and diabetes
   c. Nutritional deficiencies
   d. All of the above

2. The Pap smear is designed to detect which type of cancer?
   a. Cervical
   b. Vaginal
   c. Ovarian
   d. All of the above
   e. a and b

3. The contraceptive patch prevents pregnancy by:
   a. Preventing ovulation
   b. Destroying sperm cells
   c. Providing a barrier between sperm and the opening of the cervix
   d. Causing thickening of cervical mucous

4. Gynecologic exams are recommended for women who:
   a. Are sexually active
   b. Have begun menstruation
   c. Have reached the age of 21
   d. a and c

5. A cervical punch biopsy must be preserved by placing it in:
   a. Alcohol
   b. A sterile cup
   c. Formalin
   d. All of the above

6. Complementary therapy for the OB patient may include:
   a. Stress reduction
   b. Acupuncture
   c. Massage therapy
   d. All of the above

7. Ovarian masses, fibroids, and endometriosis may be diagnosed using a(n):
   a. Pelvic exam
   b. Pap smear
   c. Ultrasonography
   d. Dilation and curettage

8. Which of the following might be included in post–IUD insertion patient education?
   a. It is possible to become pregnant with an IUD in place.
   b. No bleeding is expected other than regular menstruation.
   c. The IUD is excellent protection against STDs.
   d. An IUD must be replaced every year.

9. Barrier methods for contraception include which of the following?
   a. Diaphragm
   b. Condoms
   c. Cervical cap
   d. All of the above

10. The medical term for pregnancy-induced hypertension is:
    a. Hyperemesis gravidarum
    b. Placenta previa
    c. Eclampsia
    d. Hypoxia

VOCABULARY REVIEW

Misspelled Words

Find the words below that are misspelled; underline them, and then correctly spell them in the space provided. Then fill in the blanks in the following sentences with the correct vocabulary terms from the list.

abortion	delation	hipoxia
amniotomy	dismenorrhea	hystersalpingogram
Bartholyn Gland	dyspareunia	hyperemesis gravidarum
colposcopy	ektopic	lokia
coupling agent	effacement	meconium
cryosurgery	guestation	multigravida

nullypara   placenta previa   Tay-Sachs

parturation   sickle cell anemia   trichomoniasis

pelvic inflammatory disease

_____   _____   _____

_____   _____   _____

_____   _____   _____

1. _____ is the medical term for abnormal tissue development.

2. The provider instructs you to prepare the room for a _____ in order to examine the patient's vagina and cervix using a lighted instrument that has magnification capabilities.

3. The diagnosis of _____ results when the *Trichomonas* parasite is identified.

4. In order to enhance the penetration of sound waves through the tissue, especially when listening to the fetal heartbeat, a _____ is applied to the mother's abdomen.

5. Ms. Eubanks is pregnant for the first time. For this reason _____ is recorded in her medical record to reflect this fact.

6. An _____ may be performed if fetal membranes do not spontaneously rupture.

7. The first stool of the newborn, _____, may indicate fetal distress.

8. Ms. Ann Boyles is seen in the clinic today and reports that intercourse is painful. The medical term for this condition is _____.

9. Due to _____, pregnant women vomit excessively and may become dehydrated and fail to gain weight appropriately.

10. Abnormal cells found on the cervix are commonly treated with a freezing technique known as _____.

LEARNING REVIEW

Short Answer

1. The obstetric history includes the total number of pregnancies and the number of live births. For each history, give the number of pregnancies and the number of live births.

Obstetric History	Pregnancies	Live Births	Abortions
A. Gravida 2 Para 1 Abortion 1			
B. Gravida 6 Para 4 Abortion 2			
C. Gravida 3 Para 1 Abortion 2			

2. What branch of medicine treats the mother and fetus through all stages of labor, delivery, and postpartum?

_____

3. List at least two signs/symptoms of preeclampsia.

_____

_____

_____

4. Describe the dilation and curettage procedure and the indications for this procedure.

_____

_____

_____

5. List some of the benefits of breastfeeding for the mother and the baby.

_____

_____

_____

6. List and describe the six types of abortion.

_____

_____

_____

_____

_____

7. Describe the emergency condition of placenta previa.

_____

_____

_____

8. Describe Rh incompatibility and treatment options.

_____

_____

_____

_____

9. List and describe the three stages of labor.

_____

_____

_____

10. Recall the screenings that are a usual part of an annual gynecologic exam.

_____

Matching

Match the term in Column I to its description in Column II.

Column I

_____ 1. PID

_____ 2. Menopause

_____ 3. Endometriosis

_____ 4. Ovarian cancer

_____ 5. Ovarian cysts

_____ 6. Dysmenorrhea

Column II

A. Technique consisting of breathing exercises to ease and facilitate labor and delivery

B. Painful menstruation

C. The period from the end of the third stage of labor until involution of the uterus is complete

D. Inflammatory disease of the pelvis involving some or all of the reproductive organs

E. Sudden separation of the placenta from the uterine wall

F. Cysts located on the ovaries

_____ 7. Lamaze

_____ 8. Puerperium

_____ 9. Placenta abruptio

_____ 10. Oxytocin

G. A pituitary hormone that stimulates the muscles of the uterus to contract

H. Painful condition characterized by endometrial cells adhering to tissues and organs outside of the uterus

I. Malignant cells found in the ovaries

J. The end of menstruation

Image Labeling

Identify each part of the female reproductive system below. Describe each part and its function in the spaces provided. Use your medical dictionary if needed.

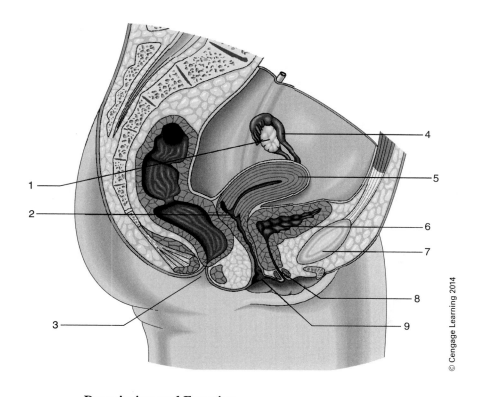

© Cengage Learning 2014

Part	Description and Function
1. _____	_____
2. _____	_____
3. _____	_____
4. _____	_____
5. _____	_____
6. _____	_____
7. _____	_____
8. _____	_____
9. _____	_____

CERTIFICATION REVIEW

These questions are designed to mimic the certification examination. Select the best response.

1. Discharge of blood, mucus, and tissue from the uterus during the period after childbirth is called:
   a. meconium
   b. lochia
   c. menorrhea
   d. papule

2. Which of the following is the medical term for the period of development from conception to birth?
   a. Parturition
   b. Postcoital
   c. Prenatal
   d. Puerperium

3. If there is implantation of a fertilized ovum outside of the uterus it is considered a(n):
   a. placenta abruption
   b. coupling agent
   c. ectopic pregnancy
   d. gestational diabetes

4. When cells are destroyed by an electrical current, it is referred to as:
   a. fulguration
   b. cryosurgery
   c. colposcopy
   d. dysplasia

5. A term that means "painful menses" is:
   a. dyspareunia
   b. dysmenorrhea
   c. dysplasia
   d. none of the above

6. Symptoms of an ectopic pregnancy may include:
   a. one-sided abdominal or pelvic pain
   b. fever
   c. infertility
   d. blood-tinged mucous vaginal discharge

7. Which of the following is the term given to a woman who has not carried a pregnancy to birth?
   a. Nullipara
   b. Primigravida
   c. Multigravida
   d. Gravidity

8. The medical term for giving birth is:
   a. effacement
   b. gestation
   c. parturition
   d. prenatal

9. The small flexible ring that is inserted in the vagina and slowly releases hormones is:

   a. a diaphragm

   b. a cervical cap

   c. spermicide

   d. a vaginal ring

10. During a prenatal visit, the urine is tested for which two substances?

    a. Drugs, including alcohol, and glucose

    b. Infection and glucose

    c. Glucose and protein

    d. Bilirubin and protein

LEARNING APPLICATION

Critical Thinking

1. A pregnant woman, who has had no prenatal care, has not had a period for 6 months. She has called the OB/GYN clinic to schedule an appointment because she is experiencing vaginal bleeding. She continues to feel fetal movement.

   a. What laboratory tests or procedures will the provider order?

   _____

   _____

   b. What might you say to the patient to reassure her during this stressful time?

   _____

   _____

2. Lower abdominal pain and back pain that increases just before and during menses may be caused by what condition?

   _____

   _____

   _____

   _____

   _____

3. Emily Harris is scheduled to have a cervical punch biopsy. What is the primary reason for a cervical punch biopsy? Explain the post-biopsy instructions she will need.

   _____

   _____

   _____

   _____

   _____

   _____

   _____

   _____

Case Studies

CASE STUDY

CASE STUDY REVIEW QUESTION

1. In the clinic, the provider instructs you that a Pap smear and pelvic examination will be performed on Ms. Dobson in Room 1. Describe your role in assisting with these procedures.

_____

_____

_____

_____

_____

_____

_____

_____

_____

_____

_____

_____

_____

_____

_____

_____

_____

_____

_____

Web Activities

Obstetrics

1. Access a Web site for expectant parents to locate information about the following:
   - Obtain fact sheets about each trimester.
   - Compile a list of tests, complications, and postpartum recovery suggestions.

2. Visit the National Library of Medicine Web site to find the answers to the following:
   - What are the time frames for each stage of labor?
   - What are the possible breech presentations?

3. Search for a Web site that provides information about the Lamaze method of childbirth. Create a patient education handout describing the benefits of this method.

4. Search the Internet for a Web site that suggests a postpartum exercise regimen. Also, visit http://www.medscape.com for information.

Gynecology

Locate a Web site specific to cancer of the female reproductive tract to complete the following:

1. What treatment options are available for cancer of the endometrium?

2. What tests are available to diagnose cancers of the female reproductive system?

3. Print a list of local support groups for women with ovarian cancer.

4. Visit the American College of Obstetricians and Gynecologists Web site for information about managing pregnant patients with the following conditions:
   - Hypertension
   - Cardiovascular disease
   - Rh factor incompatibility

5. Visit the American Cancer Society's Web site. Find information about diethylstilbestrol (DES) and male offspring malignancies.

6. Research HPV and its prevention. Develop a sample patient teaching brochure that addresses risk factors and immunization.

POST-ASSESSMENT

1. The medical term dysplasia means:
   a. normal tissue
   b. abnormal development of tissue
   c. infection
   d. cancer

2. A procedure in which a lighted scope is inserted via a surgical incision to view the inside of the pelvic cavity is:
   a. laparoscope
   b. D&C
   c. cervical biopsy
   d. cryosurgery

3. Painful intercourse is referred to as:
   a. dysmenorrhea
   b. dysfunction
   c. dyspareunia
   d. dysuria

4. Guardasil® is an immunization to prevent:
   a. syphilis
   b. STDs
   c. HPV
   d. HIV

5. Types of contraception include:
   a. oral contraceptives
   b. vasectomy
   c. tubal ligation
   d. all of the above

6. The examination of the vagina and cervix by means of a lighted instrument that has a three dimensional magnifying lens is:
   a. colonoscopy
   b. culposcopy
   c. endometrial biopsy
   d. cryosurgery

7. A radiographic technique used to visualize the uterus and fallopian tubes is called:
   a. KUB
   b. MRI
   c. CT
   d. hysterosalpingogram

8. Types of abortion include:
   a. induced
   b. complete
   c. missed
   d. all of the above

9. A test that can detect thalassemina, sickle cell anemia, or Tay-Sachs in a fetus is referred to as:
   a. punch biopsy
   b. dilation and curettage
   c. chorionic villus sampling
   d. none of the above

10. The post-partum period is also known as:
    a. pre-natal
    b. puerperium
    c. palliative
    d. pregnancy

SELF-ASSESSMENT

Think about the last time you went to your provider for an examination. As you answer the following questions and remember your personal experiences, think about how your experiences will affect the way you treat your patients in the future. If you have no personal experiences, try to imagine how you would feel and react. All of the following situations may be discussed in small groups with your classmates.

1. Which questions were you asked the last time you or a significant female in your life went to your provider for a pelvic examination? Try to think of five.

   _____

   _____

   _____

2. When the provider came into the room, were you dressed and in the examination room? Were you undressed and sitting on the examination table? Were you undressed and lying down? Were you undressed and lying down in the lithotomy position? Which of the previous scenarios would make you the most comfortable? Which would make you the most uncomfortable?

_____

_____

_____

_____

3. How comfortable are you with discussing private information with your provider? How about with your medical assistant? Are you more comfortable with one or the other? Why do you suppose you would be?

_____

_____

_____

_____

CHAPTER **27**

Pediatrics

CHAPTER PRE-TEST

Perform this test without looking at your book.

1. Toddlers are:
   a. Children from birth to 2 years old
   b. Children from about 1 to about 3 years old
   c. Children from the time they are able to walk until they are in kindergarten
   d. Children from about 2 to 5 years old

2. Normal childhood immunizations include which of the following?
   a. DTaP, MMR, Hib, and HIV
   b. Tetanus, DTaP, MMR, and IPV
   c. IPV, MMR, DTaP, Hib, and HBV
   d. HBV, Hib, pertussis, and HAV
   e. Both c and d

3. The preferred site for injections for a child younger than 2 years is:
   a. The vastus lateralis
   b. The gluteus medius
   c. The deltoid
   d. Any of the above is acceptable

4. Normal pulse and respiration for an 8-year-old child is:
   a. Pulse of 80, respiration of 30
   b. Pulse of 80, respiration of 12
   c. Pulse of 120, respiration of 20
   d. Pulse of 86, respiration of 18
   e. None of the above

5. If drainage from the ear becomes infected, the discharge will be referred to as:

   a. Suppurative otitis media

   b. Cerumen

   c. Febrile illness

   d. None of the above

6. Which disease causes paralysis of skeletal muscles and diaphragm so that breathing is interrupted?

   a. Diphtheria

   b. Hepatitis

   c. Poliomyelitis

   d. Pertussis

7. An axillary temperature is measured where?

   a. Tympanic membrane

   b. Rectally

   c. Under the arm

   d. Temporal artery

8. The treatment of sensorineural hearing loss is:

   a. Cochlear implantation

   b. Hearing aid

   c. Speech therapy

   d. American Sign Language

9. Male circumcision is:

   a. Removal of the testes

   b. Removal of the prepuce of the penis

   c. A religious rite

   d. b and c

10. What is a common illness during childhood that has a primary symptom of a "bark-like" cough?

   a. Tonsillitis

   b. Pediculosis

   c. Croup

   d. Asthma

VOCABULARY BUILDER

Misspelled Words

Find the words below that are misspelled, underline them, and then correctly spell them in the spaces provided.

arosolized	exudate	neyonate
circumcision	fontanele	pedicullosis
cokelear implantation	myringotomy	phynelketonuria

_____   _____   _____

_____   _____   _____

Definitions

Define the following vocabulary terms.

____ 1. Aerosolized

____ 2. Exudate

____ 3. Lyophilized

____ 4. Myringotomy

____ 5. Neonate

____ 6. Organomercurial

____ 7. Phenylketonuria

____ 8. Tympanostomy

____ 9. Fontanel

A. Placement of a tube through the tympanic membrane

B. Soft spot lying between the bones of the skull of a fetus, newborn, or infant

C. A form of medication that requires reconstitution.

D. Incision into the tympanic membrane

E. Newborn child, typically less than a month old

F. An oozing of pus

G. Dispensed by means of a mist

H. Any organic compound containing mercury

I. Hereditary disease that is caused by the body's inability to oxidize the amino acid phenylalanine

LEARNING REVIEW

Short Answer

1. Mary O'Keefe has called for an emergency appointment with Dr. King for her 3-year-old son, Chris, who awakened during the night with a high fever and severe pain in his right ear, which is draining. Ellen Armstrong, CMA (AAMA), must prepare the examination room for the patient. Based on Chris's symptoms, what equipment will Ellen want to assemble for Dr. King's physical examination of Chris? List the equipment in the order it will most likely be used in the examination.

_____

_____

_____

2. When Mary O'Keefe arrives with her son, Ellen takes them to examination room 2 and prepares the patient for Dr. King's physical examination. Ellen takes and records the child's vital signs: T 102.1°F (Ax); P 115 (AP) bounding, sinus arrhythmia; R 28; BP 76/42/0, rt. arm, sitting. Ellen tells Mary that Dr. King will be examining Chris's ear and may want to take some laboratory tests.

A. What method did Ellen use to take Chris's temperature?

_____

B. What method did Ellen use to measure Chris's pulse? Where on the body is this measured?

_____

C. Are Chris's vital signs normal?

_____

_____

_____

_____

_____

D. Chris is fussy and disagreeable, but not uncooperative, while Ellen takes his vital signs. What can a medical assistant do to facilitate the measurement of a fussy child's vital signs?

_____

_____

_____

_____

3. Ellen assists Dr. King with the physical examination of the patient. After assessing the vital sign measurements taken by the medical assistant, Dr. King examines Chris's ear and lungs. A swab of fluid discharge is taken from the patient's ear. What is the role of the medical assistant during the provider's examination of this patient?

_____

_____

_____

_____

4. Dr. King makes a clinical diagnosis of otitis media for this patient and orders laboratory testing to be performed on the patient's specimen. What criteria are necessary for a provider to make a clinical diagnosis?

_____

_____

_____

_____

5. What is otitis media? Why are children more likely at risk for this condition? How is otitis media commonly treated? What patient education can the health care team offer? (Consult a medical reference or encyclopedia for help in answering this question.)

_____

_____

_____

_____

_____

_____

_____

CERTIFICATION REVIEW

These questions are designed to mimic the certification examination. Select the best response.

1. The head circumference of a newborn should range between:
   a. 12.5 and 14.5 inches
   b. 14.5 and 16.5 inches
   c. 16.5 and 18.5 inches
   d. 18.5 and 20.5 inches

2. The respiratory rate of a 1-year-old child should range between _____ breaths per minute.
   a. 20 and 30
   b. 20 and 40
   c. 16 and 20
   d. 12 and 20

3. Otitis media is:
   a. an inflammation of the middle ear
   b. an infestation of parasitic lice
   c. a spasm of the bronchi
   d. an infection of the tonsils

4. When administering a vaccine to a pediatric patient, which of the following would be appropriate needle gauges?
   a. 14 to 16 gauge needle
   b. 18 to 20 gauge needle
   c. 22 to 25 gauge needle
   d. 27 to 29 gauge needle

5. During the toddler years, height growth averages about _____ inches per year.
   a. 1
   b. 2
   c. 3
   d. 4

6. The infant stage of development is from _____.
   a. birth to 1 month
   b. 2 months to 6 months
   c. birth to 3 months
   d. 1 month to 1 year

7. When administering vaccines, which should be taken into consideration to assure optimal response?
   a. Proper needle selection
   b. Reconstitution
   c. Inspecting vaccine
   d. All of the above

8. For most infants requiring an intramuscular injection, which of the following needles is most appropriate?
   a. ¾ inch 27 gauge needle
   b. 1 inch 22 gauge needle
   c. 1½ inch 20 gauge needle
   d. Any of the above

9. Which of the following immunizations should be given subcutaneously?
   a. Varicella
   b. MMR
   c. HPV
   d. a and b

10. Length and weight of an infant are plotted on which document?

    a. Medication record

    b. Demographic record

    c. Growth chart

    d. All of the above

LEARNING APPLICATION

Critical Thinking

1. You notice when you undress a 2-year-old child to prepare for a physical examination that there are bruises on the buttocks and what appear to be burns on the feet. What course of action do you take?

    _____

    _____

    _____

    _____

    _____

2. Explain the importance of growth charts.

    _____

    _____

    _____

3. Describe the appropriate positions in which to place an infant for obtaining a rectal temperature.

    _____

    _____

    _____

4. Describe the appearance of the pediatric urine collector bag. What is the best way to make certain it will adhere to the child's body?

    _____

    _____

    _____

    _____

5. Explain the type of chart used to test visual acuity in young children.

    _____

    _____

    _____

6. What do the curved lines printed across growth charts indicate?

    _____

    _____

    _____

Case Studies

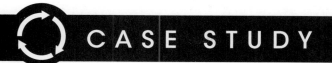

The following is a true story of a young boy (about 8 years of age) who came in to the office with testicular torsion, which occurs when the testicle twists on its cord and often becomes ischemic, resulting in tissue death. The surgeon needs to explore the area to determine if the testicle can be saved or if it needs to be removed. The testicle is usually quite swollen and tender. When the child was told that he needed to go to the surgery center and that the doctor would take care of his problem and make him feel better, he began to cry. He was inconsolable. Why do you think he was so upset? Here are some options to discuss with fellow classmates:

1. He was afraid of the pain.

2. He was afraid of the surgery.

3. He was embarrassed.

4. Other?

CASE STUDY REVIEW QUESTION

1. Discuss what you could do as a medical assistant to help the boy and his parents with all of the above possible scenarios. The reason the child was afraid might surprise you and reminds us all to be careful not to assume we know what a patient is thinking.

_____

_____

_____

Web Activities

1. Search the American Academy of Pediatrics website (http://www.aap.org) and complete the following activities.

   • Select a free online webinar, found under the Professional Resources tab on the home page, to view and prepare a presentation for the class regarding the key points of the educational offering.

   • There is a focus on preventing violence against children through resources found under the Connected Kids tab (also found under Professional Resources). Review the Connected Kids Overview. Print the Clinical Guide and review the counseling suggestions for each age group.

2. Visit the Zero to Three website (http://www.zerotothree.org). Listen to the podcast **Night-Night... or Not: Talking About Babies, Toddlers, and Sleep.** Prepare a parent's education handout for parents of a 3-year-old.

CHAPTER POST-TEST

Perform this test without looking at your book.

1. If two injections must be administered to deliver immunizations, the best manner to handle this is to:

   a. give injections at least 1 inch apart if the same limb is utilized

   b. give injections into two separate limbs

   c. combine the two and give only one injection

   d. a and b

2. The angle of injection for an intramuscular injection on a newborn is:
   a. 15 degrees
   b. 45 degrees
   c. 90 degrees
   d. any of the above

3. If a child does not meet the expected standards of growth, this might lead to a diagnosis of:
   a. failure to thrive
   b. failure to survive
   c. poliomyelitis
   d. none of the above

4. The vaccine schedule for pneumococcal conjugate is:
   a. age 7 years and then every 10 years for life
   b. two doses 3 months apart after age 2 years
   c. 2 months, 4 months, 6 months, and 12 to 15 months
   d. 12 to 18 months or any age without exposure

5. The appropriate IM injection site for children older than 2 years is:
   a. deltoid
   b. dorsal gluteal
   c. vastus lateralis
   d. ventrogluteal

6. Urinary output for a newborn is expected to be:
   a. 1 to 3 mL/hour
   b. 2 to 3 mL/hour
   c. 3 to 4 mL/hour
   d. 4 to 5 mL/hour

7. Females demonstrate evidence of sexual development at what age?
   a. 6 to 10 years
   b. 8 to 13 years
   c. 10 to 15 years
   d. 12 to 16 years

8. Blood pressure measurements should begin for healthy children at what age?
   a. 1 year
   b. 2 years
   c. 3 years
   d. 4 years

9. To provide ongoing drainage of the middle ear, a surgical procedure called _____ is performed for children with chronic otitis media.
   a. cochlear implant
   b. myringotomy
   c. tympanostomy
   d. tympanoplasty

10. If a medication is to be inhaled, the _____ method of delivery is appropriate.
    a. aerosolized
    b. humidified
    c. lyophilized
    d. liquidized

SELF-ASSESSMENT

As you respond to the following questions, think of how your experiences will affect how you treat your patients.

1. Think of your first memory of going to the doctor's office or getting any medical treatment. Think of how you felt from what you can remember. You may have more than one vivid memory, or you may have to think really hard to come up with any memories. Maybe your memories are not from a hospital or doctor's office; that is, maybe you received medical care from your parents, grandparents, or a neighbor. Your memories might not be exactly accurate, but they are a child's perception, and the feelings are real. This awareness can help you interact well with your young patients. Circle all of the words from the following list that come to mind as you take this mental journey back in time (if you have more than one incident to remember, use different colored inks to circle the words). You may even add a couple of your own descriptors if necessary.

helpless	pain	invaded
embarrassed	guilty	angry
alone	afraid of being punished	afraid of what was happening
afraid of pain	happy with the attention	dizzy
relieved	loved	powerless
excited	safe	afraid of the blood
stupid	other: _____	other: _____

Each of our memories will be different, and we will all have different feelings about them. Try to keep this in mind as you treat your young patients. Try to respect what feelings they have and strive to make them comfortable. Reassure them as much as you can.

_____

_____

_____

_____

_____

_____

_____

CHAPTER **28**

Male Reproductive System

CHAPTER PRE-TEST

Perform this test without looking at your book.

1. The most common disease afflicting men older than 50 years is:
   a. Prostate cancer
   b. Benign prostatic hypertrophy (BPH)
   c. Epididymitis
   d. Testicular cancer

2. ED stands for:
   a. Erectile disorder
   b. Erectile dysfunction
   c. Elemental disease
   d. Epididymal disorder

3. Which of the following is *not* a sexually transmitted disease (STD) that afflicts men?
   a. Genital herpes
   b. Chlamydia
   c. Gonorrhea
   d. Epididymis

4. Vasectomy consists of:
   a. Dissection of the seminal vesicles
   b. Dissection of the vas deferens
   c. Dissection of the testicles
   d. Removal of the epididymis

5. A urodynamic study evaluates:
   a. Bladder capacity
   b. Strength of contraction
   c. The ability to retain urine
   d. All of the above

6. A transilluminator is used for:
   a. Evaluation of the penis
   b. Evaluation of the testes
   c. Evaluation of the prostate
   d. All of the above

7. Spread of cancer from the primary site to another site is termed:
   a. Metamorphosis
   b. Metastasis
   c. Menorrhagia
   d. Moxibustion

8. TURP is the abbreviation for what medical procedure?
   a. Transurethral resuscitation of the prostate
   b. Transurethral resection of the prostate
   c. Therapeutic resection of the prostate
   d. Transurethral reattachment of the prostate

9. A normal PSA value is:
   a. <2.5 mg/mL
   b. >2.5 mg/mL
   c. <3.5 mg/mL
   d. >3.5 mg/mL

10. Causes of infertility include:
   a. A history of STDs
   b. Diminished motility of the sperm
   c. Genitourinary tract infection
   d. All of the above

VOCABULARY BUILDER

Misspelled Words

Find the words below that are misspelled, underline them and then correctly spell them in the space provided.

balanitis	lybido	phymosis
criptorchidism	nocturia	retension
intravenous pyelogram	orchidecktomy	spermatogenesis

_____   _____   _____

_____   _____

Matching

Match the term in Column 1 to its description in Column II.

Column I

___ 1. Cryptorchidism

___ 2. Intravenous pyelogram

___ 3. Orchidectomy

___ 4. Retention

___ 5. Transurethral resection

Column II

A. Urine held in the bladder; inability to empty the bladder

B. Undescended testicle

C. X-ray study of the kidneys, ureter, and bladder using a contrast medium

D. Removal of prostate tissue using a device inserted through the urethra

E. Surgical excision of a testicle

LEARNING REVIEW

Short Answer

1. Identify each part of the male reproductive system below. Describe each part and its function in the space provided. Then, using the textbook, a medical dictionary, or the Internet, list at least one common disorder that would adversely affect the part described.

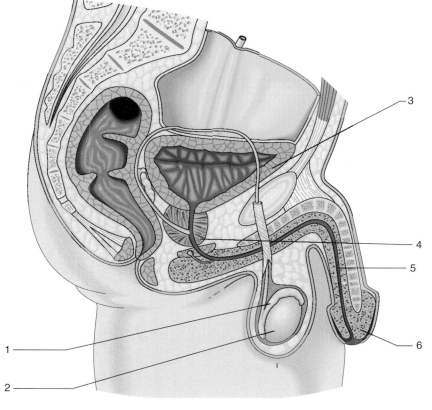

© Cengage Learning 2014

Part	Common Disorder(s)
1. _____	_____
2. _____	_____
3. _____	_____
4. _____	_____
5. _____	_____
6. _____	_____

2. List at least two symptoms of a benign hypertrophic prostate gland.

_____

_____

3. The third leading cause of cancer deaths among men is _____.

4. Name at least two sexually transmitted diseases.

_____

5. PSA tests should be performed _____ beginning at age 40.

CERTIFICATION REVIEW

These questions are designed to mimic the certification examination. Select the best response.

1. Testicular cancer is one of the leading causes of death in men younger than:
   a. 25
   b. 60
   c. 40
   d. 50

2. Male individuals from the onset of puberty should examine their testicles every:
   a. 6 months
   b. year
   c. month
   d. 3 months

3. BPH is a condition of the prostate. It stands for:
   a. benign prostatic hypertrophy
   b. benign prostatic hyperplasia
   c. beginning prostate hyperactivity
   d. benign prostate hyperactivity

4. Balanitis is caused by:
   a. bacteria
   b. fungi
   c. soap
   d. all of the above

5. The best way to determine that a patient has prostate cancer is by a:
   a. biopsy of the prostate
   b. PSA blood test
   c. rectal examination
   d. x-ray examination

6. Which of the following STDs is *not* treated with antibiotics?
   a. *Chlamydia* infection
   b. Gonorrhea
   c. Syphilis
   d. Genital herpes
   e. None of the above

7. Treatment for erectile dysfunction includes:
   a. oral medications
   b. localized injected medications
   c. penile implant
   d. all of the above

8. Gonorrhea is diagnosed by what laboratory test?
   a. Urinalysis
   b. Urethral smear
   c. Culture of lesion
   d. Blood test

9. Predisposing factors for testicular cancer include:
   a. cryptorchidism
   b. STDs
   c. history of mumps
   d. a and c

10. The medical term for inflammation of the prostate is:
    a. prostatitis
    b. epididymitis
    c. balanitis
    d. urethritis

LEARNING APPLICATION

Critical Thinking

1. Describe how a testicular self-examination should be performed.

   _____

   _____

   _____

   _____

2. What is the purpose of severing the vas deferens?

   _____

   _____

   _____

3. List several symptoms of BPH and explain why the symptoms occur.

   _____

   _____

   _____

   _____

   _____

   _____

   _____

   _____

4. Describe the blood test that is helpful to diagnose prostatic cancer.

_____

_____

5. At what PSA level does the provider consider the possibility that the patient may have cancer of the prostate?

_____

_____

_____

6. Explain why BPH is more common in men aged 50 years and older.

_____

_____

_____

7. What age group is afflicted by testicular cancer, and how can the patient take action to detect it?

_____

_____

8. How is a rectal examination on a patient useful to the provider in determining a diagnosis for a patient who has nocturia?

_____

_____

_____

_____

Case Studies

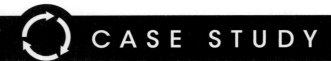

CASE STUDY

CASE STUDY REVIEW QUESTION

1. Mr. Jones, a 75-year-old patient, has just been diagnosed with prostatic cancer. The provider has explained what is to be expected, but Mr. Jones is upset and asks you for your help in understanding the disease and treatment. How will you help him?

_____

_____

_____

_____

_____

_____

Web Activities

Navigate the web to find a trusted medical website, then answer the following questions:

1. Describe two treatment choices for BPH.

2. Search for information regarding an internal radiation technique that involves "seeds" as a treatment for cancer of the prostate. Develop a patient teaching flyer.

3. Discover two other diseases of the male reproductive system. Describe their symptoms, how they are diagnosed, and how they are treated.

4. What contraindications exist for some men whose provider is considering prescribing Viagra to treat erectile dysfunction?

CHAPTER POST-TEST

Perform this test without looking at your book.

1. Which of the following is necessary for an erection to occur?
   a. Intact stimulus from the brain
   b. Adequate circulation and nerve stimulation
   c. Neither of the above
   d. a and b

2. The laboratory test for prostate cancer is:
   a. CBC
   b. IVP
   c. PSA
   d. culture of the lesion

3. When is the best time for a male to perform the monthly testicular self-examination?
   a. After a large meal
   b. After sexual activity
   c. After a warm shower or bath
   d. After a good night's sleep

4. A test to determine male infertility is:
   a. semen analysis
   b. urodynamic studies
   c. urinalysis
   d. PSA

5. A painful viral illness that is dormant and then recurs periodically for which there is no cure is:
   a. *Chlamydia* infection
   b. genital herpes
   c. gonorrhea
   d. syphilis

6. Nocturia is the medical term for:
   a. difficult urination
   b. urinary tract infection
   c. excessive nighttime urination
   d. glucose present in the urine

7. The sexual drive in humans is termed:

   a. erectile dysfunction

   b. ejaculation

   c. libido

   d. all of the above

8. A surgical procedure for treatment of prostatic cancer is:

   a. TURP

   b. cystoscopy

   c. prostatectomy

   d. proctoscopy

9. Treatment for testicular cancer includes:

   a. surgical excision

   b. radiation therapy

   c. chemotherapy

   d. all of the above

10. The surgical sterilization of a male is called:

   a. infertility

   b. vasectomy

   c. prostatectomy

   d. TURP

SELF-ASSESSMENT

How do you think you will feel when assisting with a genitourinary examination or procedure on a male patient? Do you think it will be easier if the patient is much younger or much older than you are? Do you think older medical assistants feel more comfortable assisting with these types of examinations, regardless of their professional experience? Do you think you will become more comfortable with time? Do you think your male patient is also uncomfortable? After giving these questions some thought, answer the following questions. Discuss your ideas with other students. Discuss your ideas with male friends, family members, or classmates to gain more perspectives.

1. Do you think your behavior or attitude will have anything to do with your patients' comfort level?

   _____

   _____

2. What might you do to make yourself more comfortable during a male genitourinary examination/procedure?

   _____

   _____

   _____

   _____

3. What might you do to make your patient more comfortable?

   _____

   _____

   _____

C H A P T E R **29**

Gerontology

CHAPTER PRE-TEST

Perform this test without looking at your book.

1. To assist visually impaired patients, the medical assistant should:
   a. Make his or her presence known prior to approaching
   b. Explain his or her location
   c. Identify others who are present
   d. All of the above

2. Macular degeneration is a common finding in older adults when the _____ is examined.
   a. eye
   b. ear
   c. nose
   d. throat

3. A diseases that is specific to aging is:
   a. Diabetes mellitus
   b. Arthritis
   c. Myocardial infarction
   d. None of the above

4. Hyperthermia occurs in the elderly due to:
   a. Sweat glands decreasing in size
   b. The body becoming less sensitive to heat and cold
   c. More heat being generated when ambulating
   d. a and b

5. The brain shrinks in size as one ages due to:
   a. Less sensory stimulation
   b. Poor nutrition
   c. Cells not continuing to divide
   d. All of the above

6. Dementia affects the following:

   a. Memory, personality, and cognitive functioning

   b. Memory, mobility, and nutrition

   c. Memory, social status, and mobility

   d. None of the above

7. The diminishment of testosterone levels as men age is known as:

   a. Menopause

   b. Andropause

   c. Spermatogenesis

   d. Erectile dysfunction

8. The study of problems associated with aging is known as:

   a. Gerontology

   b. Geriatrics

   c. Gynecology

   d. Geotechnology

9. A common stereotype related to the elderly is that they are:

   a. Sickly

   b. Burdensome

   c. Sexless

   d. All of the above

10. Elder abuse is defined as:

    a. Committing or omitting an act that results in physical injury to an older adult

    b. Committing or omitting an act that results in emotional injury to an older adult

    c. Both of the above

    d. Neither of the above

VOCABULARY BUILDER

Misspelled Words and Definitions

Find the words in Column A below that are misspelled; circle them, and correctly spell them in the space provided. Then match the following correct vocabulary terms listed in Column A with their corresponding definitions listed in Column B.

	Column A	Correct Spelling	Column B
___	1. Arterialsclerosis	_____	A. The branch of medicine that is concerned with the problems of older adults
___	2. Demenetia	_____	B. Disease marked by degeneration of the macular area of the retina of the eye
___	3. Geriatrics	_____	C. Progressive loss of hearing ability caused by the normal aging process
___	4. Incontinance	_____	D. Temporary loss of blood to the brain, causing stroke-like symptoms
___	5. Macular degeneration	_____	E. Urine remaining in the bladder after urination

Column A	Correct Spelling	Column B
____ 6. Pernicous anemia	_____	F. Loss of the ability to retain urine in the bladder
____ 7. Presbycusis	_____	G. Disorder involving the stomach that causes a deficiency of red blood cells
____ 8. Residule urine	_____	H. Decrease in cognitive abilities, especially memory impairment, often associated with Alzheimer's and Parkinson's diseases
____ 9. Transiant ischemic attack	_____	I. Disease that leads to thickening, hardening, and loss of elasticity of the arteries

LEARNING REVIEW

Short answer

1. List at least five ways to improve communication with the geriatric patient who has memory impairment.

_____

_____

_____

_____

_____

_____

_____

_____

2. Why is gerontology becoming more recognized?

_____

_____

_____

3. Why does food become less appealing as one ages, often decreasing the desire to eat and causing weight loss?

_____

_____

_____

4. Fill in the chart below, listing two problems that might occur with each system as people age. The first row has been filled out as an example for you.

A. Vision and hearing _____

B. Taste and smell _____

_____

C. Integumentary system _____

_____

_____

_____

D. Nervous system

_____
_____
_____
_____
_____

E. Musculoskeletal system

_____
_____
_____
_____

F. Respiratory system

_____
_____
_____
_____

G. Cardiovascular system

_____
_____
_____
_____

H. Gastrointestinal system

_____
_____
_____
_____
_____

I. Urinary system

_____
_____
_____
_____

J. Reproductive system

_____
_____
_____
_____

CERTIFICATION REVIEW

These questions are designed to mimic the certification examination. Select the best response.

1. Dementia can include:
    a. memory loss
    b. confusion
    c. depression and agitation
    d. all of the above

2. The nervous system is affected by aging, resulting in all of the following *except*:
   a. insomnia
   b. problems with balance
   c. increased pain sensation
   d. problems with temperature regulation

3. The buildup of plaque in blood vessels is called:
   a. incontinence
   b. heart attack
   c. arteriosclerosis
   d. cardiopulmonary dysfunction

4. The progressive loss of hearing ability caused by the normal aging process is called:
   a. senility
   b. presbycusis
   c. deafness
   d. audio deficiency

5. Poor nutrition and poor absorption of nutrients can result in:
   a. anemia
   b. malnutrition
   c. weight gain
   d. a and b

6. Ways to assure that a hearing impaired adult is able to understand instructions include:
   a. providing written instructions
   b. facing the hearing-impaired person when speaking
   c. assuring that the environment is quiet without distractions
   d. all of the above

7. Loss of a spouse, chronic illness, and financial difficulties can cause _____ in older adults.
   a. dementia
   b. depression
   c. myocardial infarction
   d. arteriosclerosis

8. Changes in an area of the retina that is associated with aging is:
   a. macular degeneration
   b. glaucoma
   c. cataracts
   d. all of the above

9. An unusually high body temperature is termed:
   a. hypothermia
   b. hyperthermia
   c. hyperemesis
   d. hypochondria

10. Being aware of feelings, emotions, and behavior of another is considered:

    a. sympathy

    b. empathy

    c. dystrophy

    d. depression

LEARNING APPLICATION

Critical Thinking

1. What are some ways that older adults can keep bones from becoming brittle?

2. Describe a vision problem that leaves older adults with difficulty seeing color intensity.

3. What are four causes of urinary incontinence?

4. Give three ways to enhance communication with older adults.

5. What is the best way to approach a visually impaired person?

6. How can you encourage older adults to choose a healthy lifestyle?

Case Studies

◯ CASE STUDY 1

CASE STUDY REVIEW QUESTION

1. Sam Jones, 84 years old, has been examined by the provider and is ready to leave the office. Mr. Jones tells you that he is having trouble remembering to take the many medications the doctor has given him. As a medical assistant, what can you do to help him remember to take his medication?

_____

_____

_____

◯ CASE STUDY 2

Adelaide Robinson, 83 years old, has an appointment Thursday morning for a recheck of her most recent complaint. She tells you that she is moving slower than she did just 6 months ago, and she has noticed less flexibility as well.

CASE STUDY REVIEW QUESTIONS

1. What are the possible causes of Mrs. Robinson's complaints?

_____

_____

_____

_____

2. What effect will these problems have on Mrs. Robinson's daily routine?

_____

_____

_____

3. What might Dr. King suggest Mrs. Robinson do to help alleviate symptoms?

_____

_____

_____

CASE STUDY 3

Sally Donovan, 92 years old, is in the gerontology clinic today. Her main concern, problem, and reason for appointment is that she "cannot taste or smell much anymore and food doesn't taste good." She wants suggestions from the provider about how to improve her taste and smell so she can enjoy food more freely.

CASE STUDY REVIEW QUESTIONS

1. What are some reasons that older adults lose their sense of taste and smell?

   _____

   _____

   _____

2. Describe any dangers that can be associated with loss of taste and smell.

   _____

   _____

   _____

   _____

   _____

   _____

   _____

Web Activities

1. The American Psychological Association website (http://www.apa.org) gives information about psychology. Find information that pertains to older adults and their psychological health. What are some resources for metal health issues that can be helpful to older adults?

2. The U.S. government has a website (http://www.aoa.gov) for concerns and information about aging. What government agencies can an older adult contact for help with health insurance questions?

3. The National Osteoporosis Foundation website (http://www.nof.org) provides information about osteoporosis. Retrieve information about osteoporosis that is useful for all older adults.

4. Locate a website for older adults who have arthritis. Find some techniques for these patients to make their activities of daily living less difficult.

CHAPTER POST-TEST

Perform this test without looking at your book.

1. When assisting a patient with visual impairment, you should:

   a. grip the patient firmly by the shoulders and guide them

   b. walk behind the patient

   c. walk at your pace

   d. none of the above

2. Signs of mistreatment or abuse may include which of the following?
   a. Welts
   b. Longing for death
   c. Anxiety
   d. All of the above

3. Factors influencing the increased life expectancy of adults in the United States are:
   a. poor nutrition
   b. stress reduction
   c. today's technology
   d. b and c

4. Unusually low body temperature is known as:
   a. hyperthermia
   b. hypothermia
   c. hypothyroidism
   d. hypertension

5. Some causes for unstable balance in older adults might be:
   a. medication
   b. rapid muscular response
   c. presbycusis
   d. nevus

6. Infection and inflammation of the bladder is medically termed:
   a. cystitis
   b. nephritis
   c. urethritis
   d. appendicitis

7. Research demonstrated that older Americans are generally _____ healthy than the same age group from 100 years ago.
   a. less
   b. more
   c. equally
   d. none of the above

8. A major factor that impacts functional changes in older adults is:
   a. insurance
   b. adult daycare
   c. lifestyle
   d. clothing

9. Patient teaching to encourage healthy living to an older adult might include:
   a. eating a balanced diet
   b. smoking only cigars
   c. exercising regularly
   d. a and c

10. Techniques that might be utilized when speaking to memory-impaired adults might include:
    a. speaking very loudly
    b. giving detailed directions verbally
    c. lowering the tone of your voice
    d. laughing as much as possible

SELF-ASSESSMENT

Without looking in the textbook, list 15 adjectives that describe older adults. Then list 15 adjectives that describe young adults. As you make your list, consider your personal biases toward older adults. Consider the differences in the two lists and think of why you chose those descriptors. When you are finished, discuss your lists with classmates. Share stories about people in your lives who are extraordinarily healthy and happy as they age. Think about the prejudices and assumptions you carry toward aging patients. Try to remember these as you work with those patients. It might be a good idea to create a list of tips to remember about geriatrics and keep it posted by your workstation.

_____

_____

_____

_____

_____

C H A P T E R **30**

Examinations and Procedures of Body Systems

CHAPTER PRE-TEST

Perform this test without looking at your book.

1. An upper GI series (barium swallow) is used to examine the:
   a. Entire large intestine
   b. Stomach and entire small intestine
   c. Esophagus, stomach, and part of the small intestine
   d. Esophagus, stomach, and small and large intestines

2. Nitrogenous waste filtered from the blood by the kidneys includes:
   a. Urea
   b. Protein
   c. Creatinine
   d. a and c

3. The test to discover blood in the stool is called:
   a. CBC
   b. Urinalysis
   c. Fecal occult blood
   d. Culture

4. An important test to diagnose Ménière's disease is:
   a. Opticokinetic drum test
   b. Phacoemulsification
   c. Electrocochleography
   d. Tympanography

5. Color vision is checked using the _____ chart.
   a. Snellen
   b. Ishihara
   c. Landolt C
   d. LEA symbol

6. A simple tool to assess hearing that is commonly used in a provider's office is the:
   a. Audiometer
   b. Phonograph
   c. Tuning fork
   d. Tympanometer

7. A bronchodilator is:
   a. An instrument used to increase lung capacity
   b. A tool to measure lung capacity
   c. A drug that causes the expansion of bronchi and bronchioles
   d. A respirator

8. When using a pulse oximeter, a reading of ≥ 95% indicates:
   a. Hypoxemia
   b. Normal oxygenation
   c. Pyrexia
   d. Cyanosis

9. There are more than _____ muscles in the body.
   a. 200
   b. 400
   c. 600
   d. 800

10. A neurologic examination includes a mental status examination. Components of this examination might include:
    a. Level of consciousness
    b. Reflexes
    c. Muscle tone
    d. Motor function

VOCABULARY BUILDER

Misspelled Words

Find the words below that are misspelled, underline them, and correctly spell them in the spaces provided. Then fill in the blanks in the sentences that follow with the correct vocabulary terms listed below with their proper definitions.

afasia	carbancle	erythemia
auricle	conjunctyvitis	malaise
biopsy	demyelination	strabismus
bullemia	dyslocation	

_____   _____   _____

_____   _____   _____

1. A _____ is an inflammation of the skin and deeper tissues that terminates in slough and suppuration.

2. _____ is a form of macula showing diffused redness of the skin.

3. Infection of the membranes lining the eyelids is called _____.

4. Destruction or removal of the myelin sheath is _____.

5. The provider obtains a representative tissue sample for microscopic examination during a _____.

6. A disease that is characterized by binging on food and then vomiting or using laxatives to prevent weight gain is _____.

7. _____ is the absence or impairment of the ability to communicate through speech.

8. A general feeling of discomfort or unease is known as _____.

9. The _____ is the portion of the external ear that is not connected to the head.

10. Joint trauma that involves the _____ of the head of a bone from its socket is a common injury to the shoulder.

11. _____ is a disorder in which the eyes do not line up in the same direction.

LEARNING REVIEW

Short Answer

1. List five components of a urinalysis.

   _____

   _____

   _____

2. What is the treatment for gastroenteritis?

   _____

   _____

   _____

3. List two causes of erosion of the mucous lining of the stomach.

   _____

   _____

   _____

4. There are many diseases that can be diagnosed by evaluating a patient's blood. List four blood tests that are commonly ordered.

   _____

   _____

5. List at least four endoscopic procedures that require a patient to remain NPO.

   _____

   _____

6. Describe the difference between internal and external respiration.

   _____

   _____

7. Describe treatment of dislocation.

_____

_____

_____

8. List and describe the three kinds of allergy skin testing.

_____

_____

_____

_____

_____

_____

   Patch test: _____

_____

   Intradermal test: _____

_____

Image Labeling

1. Identify the parts of the digestive system.

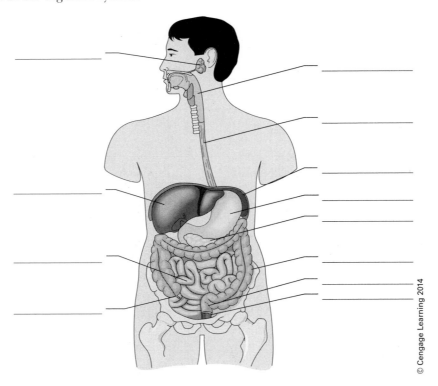

2. Identify the parts of the eye.

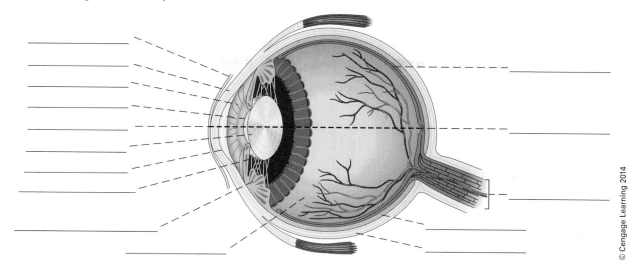

© Cengage Learning 2014

3. Identify the parts of the ear.

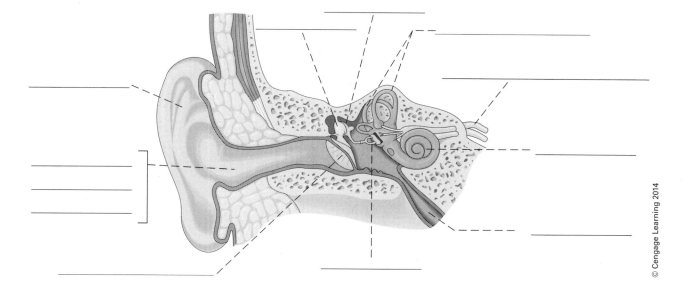

© Cengage Learning 2014

CERTIFICATION REVIEW

These questions are designed to mimic the certification examination. Select the best response.

1. Common symptoms of urinary tract diseases and disorders are:

    a. dysuria, proteinuria, hematuria, and frequency

    b. dysuria, frequency, oliguria, and headache

    c. hematuria, pain, frequency, and headache

    d. frequency, hematuria, vaginal discharge, and dysuria

2. Cystitis is another name for what disorder?
   a. Kidney cysts
   b. Gallbladder disease
   c. Multiple cysts of the breasts or other area
   d. Bladder inflammation

3. UTI means:
   a. urinary tract infection
   b. urinary tract inflammation
   c. urinary tract involvement
   d. urinary treatment initiated

4. The medical term meaning "hidden" is:
   a. cult
   b. occult
   c. crypt
   d. retro

5. Which of the following is an eating disorder?
   a. Bulimia
   b. Anorexia nervosa
   c. Diverticulosis
   d. Crohn's disease
   e. a and b

6. The medical condition of having an increase in intraocular pressure is called:
   a. glaucoma
   b. retinal detachment
   c. cataract
   d. macular degeneration

7. Ear lavage or irrigation is performed for:
   a. impacted sebum
   b. impacted cerumen
   c. impacted lacrimal glands
   d. otitis media

8. The clear tissue covering the pupil and iris is the:
   a. sclera
   b. lens
   c. cornea
   d. retina

9. A cholecystectogram is a test for:
   a. kidney stones
   b. diseases of the gallbladder
   c. diseases of the blood vessels
   d. gastrointestinal disorders

10. Which of the following is not determined by a chest radiograph?
    a. Bronchitis
    b. Pneumonia
    c. Pharyngitis
    d. Tuberculosis

11. Coronary artery bypass surgery might be used to help prevent which of the following cardiovascular conditions?
    a. Myocardial infarction
    b. Pericarditis
    c. Thrombophlebitis
    d. Coronary artery disease

12. Which of the following cardiovascular diseases may be treated with antibiotics?
    a. Thrombophlebitis
    b. Pericarditis
    c. Angina pectoris
    d. Valve stenosis

13. Which of the following diseases is caused by a lack of dopamine?
    a. Epilepsy
    b. Depression
    c. Reye's syndrome
    d. Parkinson's disease

LEARNING APPLICATION

Critical Thinking

1. Is there an advantage to catheterizing a patient for urinalysis and culture and sensitivity? Why or why not?

_____

_____

_____

_____

_____

_____

2. What is the use and purpose of the audiometer? How is the test administered?

_____

_____

_____

_____

_____

_____

_____

_____

3. Explain the rationale for using a solution when doing an eye irrigation solution from the inside canthus to the outer canthus of the eye.

_____

_____

_____

_____

4. Differentiate among bronchitis, emphysema, and asthma.

_____

_____

_____

_____

_____

_____

_____

5. What is the medical assistant's role when assisting with spirometry?

_____

_____

_____

6. What are the cast care guidelines that the medical assistant gives to the patient?

_____

_____

_____

_____

7. When a mental status examination is given, what five areas are being assessed?

_____

_____

_____

8. Explain the medical assistant's role when assisting with a lumbar puncture.

_____

_____

_____

_____

_____

_____

Case Studies

CASE STUDY

CASE STUDY REVIEW QUESTIONS

1. While visiting with family members, your elderly aunt shares with you that she has noticed that her stools are black. This has been happening off and on for several months and now she says her "belly feels swollen" and she is constipated a lot, which is not normal for her. How will you respond?

_____

_____

_____

2. Your aunt becomes alarmed and says she is afraid of what they will do to her; maybe she will need surgery, and she cannot leave her husband alone, and what if it is cancer. She obviously has many concerns and is quite worried. How can you assist her?

_____

_____

_____

_____

_____

_____

_____

_____

Web Activities

Use the Internet to search for information from a trusted medical site to find answers to the following:

1. Using a search engine of your choice, go to Web MD and gather information regarding the following conditions:
   - Kidney stones
   - Polycystic kidneys
   - Describe the etiology and treatment of each

2. Search for possible treatments for sleep apnea. Web addresses that might be of assistance are:

   http://www.mayoclinic.com
   http://www.nhlbi.nih.gov

3. What are some harmful effects of cigarette smoking? Go to http://www.cdc.gov and search for cigarette smoking for information.

4. Go to http://my.clevelandclinic.org and search for pancreatitis. Discover the signs and symptoms of acute pancreatitis. How is the diagnosis made by the provider? What is the most common cause of chronic pancreatitis?

5. Go to http://www.cdc.gov and search for bacterial meningitis. Create a flyer that describes the causes, risk factors, transmission, signs and symptoms, diagnosis, and treatment.

CHAPTER POST-TEST

1. Shingles is a type of:
   a. herpes
   b. psoriasis
   c. dermatitis
   d. acne

2. The type of disease in which the white blood cells become prolific is:
   a. anemia
   b. infectious mononucleosis
   c. leukemia
   d. lymphedema

3. High levels of nitrogenous waste in the blood may result in:
   a. polyuria
   b. oliguria
   c. uremia
   d. pyuria

4. A sigmoidoscopy is a diagnostic examination of:
   a. the inner ear
   b. the bladder
   c. a part of the colon
   d. the eye

5. Guaiac slides are used to detect:
   a. occult blood in the stool
   b. the type of bacteria found in otitis media
   c. thrush of the mucous membranes of the mouth
   d. cholelithiasis

6. A diagnostic test done to determine the presence of stones, duct obstruction, or inflammation of the gallbladder is called a:
   a. barium enema
   b. barium swallow
   c. cholecystogram
   d. gastroscopy

7. The space between the cornea and iris/pupil filled with a clear fluid known as aqueous humor is called:
   a. anterior chamber
   b. posterior chamber
   c. posterior cavity
   d. choroid layer

8. Inflammation of the pleura caused by bacteria or viruses is termed:
   a. pneumonia
   b. influenza
   c. pleurisy
   d. bronchitis

9. Treatment for multiple sclerosis includes:

   a. steroids

   b. physical therapy

   c. muscle relaxants

   d. all of the above

10. _____ is caused by a virus and is transmitted to humans by scratches or bites from animals infected with the virus.

    a. Meningitis

    b. Rabies

    c. Reye's syndrome

    d. Bell's palsy

SELF-ASSESSMENT

Think of a time when you or a close family member had to go to the provider's office and then go through a diagnostic procedure or test for a medical disorder or a disease. Fill in the following outline with as much information as you can remember.

1. What were the patient's symptoms? Try to list two or three.

   _____

   _____

   _____

   _____

   _____

   _____

2. Describe how the disease started. (Suddenly? Gradually? Over time? Related to an injury?)

   _____

   _____

   _____

3. Did the patient go to the emergency department or to the provider's office first?

   _____

   _____

   _____

4. Did the provider, or his or her staff, clearly explain the test or procedure to the patient or the patient's family?

   _____

   _____

   _____

5. What were some of the feelings that you had during the process? List two or three.

   _____

   _____

   _____

6. Could the medical assistant and doctor have reassured you better or kept you better informed, or did they do a good job of answering your questions and meeting your needs and the needs of the patient?

_____

_____

_____

7. How will your experience influence your interaction with your patients when you are assisting with a diagnostic test or procedure? What will you pay special attention to that you might not have if you had not had the experience described above?

_____

_____

_____

C H A P T E R **31**

Assisting with Office/ Ambulatory Surgery

CHAPTER PRE-TEST

Perform this test without looking at your book.

1. The signs of inflammation are:
   a. Redness, drainage, pain, and swelling
   b. Redness, pain, and swelling
   c. Redness, pain, swelling, and tenderness
   d. Redness, pain, swelling, and warmth

2. An item that is free from all microorganisms and their spores is considered:
   a. Contaminated
   b. Sterile
   c. Decontaminated
   d. Clean

3. An informed consent should include what information?
   a. Risks of the procedure
   b. Alternate therapies
   c. Name and description of the procedure
   d. All of the above

4. The locking mechanisms on surgical instruments are known as:
   a. Hinges
   b. Ratchets
   c. Rings
   d. Teeth

5. The definition of anesthesia is:
   a. Loss of feeling or sensation
   b. Loss of consciousness
   c. Loss of control
   d. Loss of function

6. Which statement best describes a dressing?

   a. Supportive material over a wound

   b. Sterile material applied directly over a wound

   c. A rigid material to support a damaged bone

   d. None of the above

7. When setting up for a surgical procedure, it is good to refer to surgery cards. What information can be found there?

   a. The name of the patient

   b. Specific instruments

   c. Supplies for the procedure

   d. b and c

8. Skin must be prepared prior to any invasive procedure. Which of the following is appropriate skin prep?

   a. Betadine®

   b. Hibiclens®

   c. 70% isopropyl alcohol

   d. All of the above

9. A specialized drape that has an opening for the surgical site is:

   a. Pleated

   b. Serrated

   c. Fenestrated

   d. Striated

10. Infected wound drainage is referred to as:

    a. Exudate

    b. Inflammation

    c. Stricture

    d. All of the above

VOCABULARY BUILDER

Misspelled Words

Find the words in Column I that are misspelled; underline them, and correctly spell them in the spaces provided. Then match each of the vocabulary terms below with the correct definition in Column II.

Column I	Correct Spelling	Column II
____ 1. inflamation	_____	A. The trade name for povidone-iodine, a topical anti-infective
____ 2. ephinephrine	_____	B. Partial or complete loss of sensation, with or without loss of consciousness
____ 3. ligature	_____	C. A hormone secreted by the adrenal medulla in response to stimulation of the sympathetic nervous system; used in conjunction with a local anesthetic. It constricts blood vessels to help lessen bleeding during ambulatory surgery.

____ 4. Hibeclens®   _____   D. A condition free from germs, infection, and any form of life

____ 5. anestesia   _____   E. A narrowing or constriction of the lumen of a tube, duct, or hollow organ

____ 6. Betadine®   _____   F. Trade name for chlorhexidine gluconate, a topical antiseptic

____ 7. isopryl alcohol   _____   G. A thread or wire for tying a blood vessel or other structure to constrict or fasten it

____ 8. strictures   _____   H. The nonspecific immune response that occurs in reaction to any type of bodily injury

____ 9. surgical asepsis   _____   I. A clean, flammable liquid used in medical preparations for external use

Definitions

Match the vocabulary words below with their correct definitions.

____ 1. approximate
____ 2. cautery
____ 3. contamination
____ 4. infection
____ 5. informed consent
____ 6. Mayo stand/instrument tray
____ 7. ratchets
____ 8. suture
____ 9. swaged/atraumatic

A. To bring together the edges of a wound

B. A surgical needle is attached to a length of suture material

C. Surgical material or thread; may describe the act of sewing with the surgical material and needle

D. An invasion of pathogens into living tissue

E. A voluntary agreement to have a procedure or surgery after a patient has been informed about the risks and benefits

F. A portable metal tray table used for setting up a sterile field for minor surgery and procedures

G. The locking mechanisms on the handles of many surgical instruments

H. The destruction of tissue by burning

I. To make something unclean, often used to describe a sterile area being made "unsterile" or exposing a clean area to a pathogenic substance

LEARNING REVIEW

Short Answer

1. Identify each entry below as an example that follows strict sterile principles or in which the sterile area, field, or tray is contaminated. Write "sterile" or "contaminated" in the spaces provided. If the entry is "contaminated," write what was done to render it contaminated.

    A. Bruce Goldman, CMA (AAMA), collects used instruments handed to him by Dr. Mark Woo during a minor surgical procedure to excise an infected sebaceous cyst by placing the instruments in a separate container or area out of view of the patient.

    B. Ellen Armstrong, CMA (AAMA), sets up a sterile field for a minor surgical procedure. After setting up the field, she remembers that a sterile solution is required and leaves the room to obtain the solution to be poured into a sterile cup.

    C. Wanda Slawson, CMA (AAMA), removes a dressing from a wound on a patient's arm and then reaches over the sterile field to discard the used dressing in a biohazard waste container that she has placed on the other side of the sterile field that she set up for the procedure.

    D. Patient Edith Leonard will not stop talking and asking questions as Liz Corbin, CMA (AAMA), removes sutures from a small wound on Edith's arm sustained during a recent fall. The medical assistant is careful to time her responses to Edith so that she is not talking when she is working directly over the sterile field.

    E. Anna Preciado, CMA (AAMA), applies sterile gloves in preparation to assist Dr. Lewis with a minor surgical procedure. During the procedure, she comforts the patient and assists the provider as required. When Anna's hands are not in use, she keeps them down at her sides, careful not to touch her gloved hands to her clothing or any other nonsterile item.

2. Living tissue surfaces, such as skin, cannot be sterilized. Name two examples of ways that skin can be rid of as many pathogens as possible before the use of a sterile covering.

3. Identify and describe the most widely used method of sterilization in the ambulatory care setting.

4. List six general rules that ensure proper sterilization when using an autoclave.

_____

_____

_____

_____

_____

5. Identify the recommended requirements for effective sterilization in an autoclave.

Temperature   _____

Time for sterilization of unwrapped items   _____

Time for sterilization of loosely wrapped items   _____

Time for sterilization of tightly wrapped items   _____

Frequency of draining of water and cleaning   _____
of autoclave

MATCHING I

Match the following equipment with the correct aseptic method. For each instrument or item below, identify the method used for proper asepsis: chemical disinfection (CD), chemical sterilization (CS), or steam sterilization (SS) in an autoclave.

_____ 1. Percussion hammer

_____ 2. Wrapped surgical instruments

_____ 3. Stethoscopes

_____ 4. Fiber-optic endoscopes

_____ 5. Countertops

_____ 6. Wheelchairs

_____ 7. Gynecologic instruments

_____ 8. Examination tables

Matching II

Identify each action that follows as an action appropriate to medical aseptic hand washing technique (MAH) or surgical aseptic hand washing technique (SAH).

_____ 1. Do not apply lotion.

_____ 2. Glove for sterility.

_____ 3. 1 minute duration

_____ 4. Hold hands up during washing and rinsing.

_____ 5. Apply lotion.

_____ 6. Wash hands, wrists, and forearms to the elbows.

_____ 7. Hold hands down during rinsing.

_____ 8. 3- to 6-minute duration

CERTIFICATION REVIEW

These questions are designed to mimic the certification examination. Select the best response.

1. Surgical instruments that have opposing cutting edges are classified as:
   a. hemostats
   b. probes
   c. scissors
   d. scalpels

2. Surgical instruments that have ratchets are used for:
   a. cutting
   b. clamping
   c. probing
   d. exploring
   e. opening

3. Thumb forceps may also be called:
   a. pickups
   b. towel clamps
   c. hemostats
   d. Allis forceps

4. The recommended temperature for effective sterilization in an autoclave is:
   a. 212°F
   b. 270°F
   c. 150°F
   d. 220°F

5. An acceptable border between a sterile and a nonsterile area is:
   a. 1 inch
   b. 2 inches
   c. 4 inches
   d. 5 inches

6. The preferred length for suture material, because it is manageable yet long enough to complete most suture procedures, is:
   a. 10 inches
   b. 8 inches
   c. 12 inches
   d. 18 inches

7. Suture material that is used when more time is needed for healing is coated with:
   a. magnesium
   b. chromium
   c. calcium
   d. iodine

8. Application of a caustic chemical or destructive heat that burns tissue is called:

   a. cryotherapy

   b. evisceration

   c. approximation

   d. cauterization

9. The mechanism located between the rings of the handles of surgical instruments that is used for locking the instrument is called the:

   a. serration

   b. box-lock

   c. ratchet

   d. probe

10. Which of the following is considered a sterile principle?

   a. A sterile object may not touch a nonsterile object.

   b. Turning you back on a sterile field is allowable.

   c. Reaching over the sterile field is allowable with gloved hands.

   d. Some sterile objects are still considered sterile when wet.

LEARNING APPLICATION

Critical Thinking

1. What would be the rationale behind leaving a wound open rather than suturing it? On what basis would the provider make the decision?

   _____

   _____

   _____

   _____

   _____

   _____

   _____

   _____

   _____

   _____

   _____

   _____

   _____

2. While you are preparing a patient for surgery, he confides in you that he doesn't have anyone to drive him home, but he only lives three miles away and he can drive himself. How do you respond?

   _____

   _____

   _____

3. You have thoroughly explained the postoperative instructions to the patient and caregiver. Are written instructions also necessary? Why or why not?

_____

_____

_____

_____

_____

4. While pouring a sterile solution into a bowl on the sterile field, you accidentally splash a very tiny amount of the solution onto the field. What is your next step? Explain your actions.

_____

_____

5. During an incision and drainage of a localized infection you notice a large amount of exudates from the side. What precautions should you take?

_____

_____

_____

_____

Case Studies

CASE STUDY 1

Joyanna Evans, CMA (AAMA), is responsible for maintaining and cleaning the autoclave at Inner City Health Care. Because this equipment is used every day to sterilize instruments, Joyanna cleans the inner chamber of the autoclave daily. Once a week she gives the autoclave a thorough cleaning.

CASE STUDY REVIEW QUESTIONS

1. Describe Joyanna's daily cleaning procedure.

_____

_____

_____

2. Describe Joyanna's weekly cleaning procedure.

_____

_____

_____

_____

_____

3. Why is proper maintenance and cleaning of the autoclave important?

_____

_____

_____

CASE STUDY 2

Joyanna works with a variety of instruments and supplies as she assists in ambulatory care surgery. Answer the following questions related to surgical instruments and supplies.

CASE STUDY REVIEW QUESTIONS

1. From the selection that follows, identify each instrument by name. In the spaces provided, give a brief description of each instrument's use.

Instrument	Instrument Name	Uses
© Cengage Learning 2014		
© Cengage Learning 2014		
© Cengage Learning 2014		
© Cengage Learning 2014		
© Cengage Learning 2014		

continues

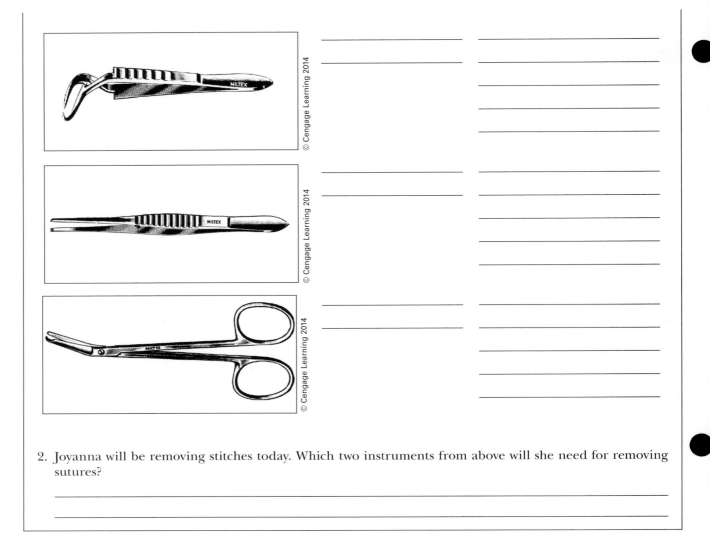

2. Joyanna will be removing stitches today. Which two instruments from above will she need for removing sutures?

_____

_____

Preparing Surgical Packs

Pretend the areas outlined below are labels on surgical packs that you have just wrapped. Label them with the proper information.

a. Iris scissors and 4 × 4 gauze.

b. Needle driver and a #3 scalpel handle.

c. Thumb tissue forceps and a #3 scalpel handle.

Web Activities

Search the Internet to explore the most current ambulatory surgical procedures for varicose veins, cataracts, and cholelithiasis.

1. Using a search engine of your choice, go to a Web site about ambulatory care.
   a. Look for the criteria that the patient must meet to be discharged after surgery.
   b. What are some common complications that can occur in the ambulatory center after any surgical procedure?
   c. Name two other surgeries other than those listed in your book that can be performed in an ambulatory center. Discuss them.
   d. List three to four advantages and disadvantages of ambulatory surgery.

CHAPTER POST-TEST

Perform this test without looking at your book.

1. Which of the following is not a method of sterilization?
   a. Boiling sterilization
   b. Gas sterilization
   c. Steam sterilization
   d. Dry heat sterilization

2. When loading an autoclave, it is important to leave how much space between packages?
   a. 1 to 2 inches
   b. 1 to 3 inches
   c. 2 to 3 inches
   d. 2 to 4 inches

3. Thermolabile is a term that refers to:
   a. a type of dye that changes color when exposed to steam at the proper temperature and pressure and for the proper amount of time
   b. a type of dye that remains the same color when exposed to steam at the proper temperature and pressure and for the proper amount of time
   c. a biological indicator that contains spores to determine an autoclave's efficacy
   d. a culture strip containing heat-resistant spores

4. When an electric current is used to cut or destroy tissue, it is called:
   a. incision
   b. electrosurgery
   c. cryosurgery
   d. laser surgery

5. Select the gauge of the finest suture material:
   a. 0
   b. 2-0
   c. 3-0
   d. 4-0

6. Which of the following is a cutting instrument?

   a. Scissors

   b. Scalpel

   c. Forceps

   d. a and b

7. When cleaning sharp instruments it is good practice to wear:

   a. heavy duty rubber gloves

   b. non-latex gloves

   c. non-sterile disposable gloves

   d. sterile gloves

8. Sterile surgical wicks or wound packing strips are used:

   a. to dress a sutured wound

   b. to close sterile packages

   c. to keep an infected wound open for drainage

   d. all of the above

9. Which of the following is used to create a sterile field over and around the operative site?

   a. Dressing

   b. Sponges

   c. Drapes

   d. Wicks

10. When assisting the provider with a minor surgery, which is the correct order of the activities listed below?

    1. Set up sterile field

    2. Wash hands

    3. Place sterile instruments and supplies on the sterile field

    4. Gather equipment and supplies

       a. 2, 4, 1, 3

       b. 1, 2, 3, 4

       c. 2, 1, 3, 4

       d. 4, 2, 1, 3

SELF-ASSESSMENT

Think of a time when you or a family member experienced a surgical event. If you have not had a personal surgical experience, interview a friend or family member and gather answers to the following questions.

1. Did the doctor or his or her staff explain the procedure clearly?

   _____

   _____

2. Were your questions answered to your satisfaction?

_____

_____

_____

_____

3. What was of greatest concern to you (financial concerns, pain, recovery, results, etc.)?

_____

_____

_____

_____

4. Did the recovery go as expected?

_____

_____

_____

_____

5. Were the results what you expected?

_____

_____

_____

_____

6. What could have made the experience better?

_____

_____

_____

_____

C H A P T E R **32**

Diagnostic Imaging

CHAPTER PRE-TEST

Perform this test without looking at your book.

1. MRI stands for:
   a. Magnetic realistic imaging
   b. Magnetic resonance imaging
   c. Magnetic ray imaging
   d. Magnetic radiologic imagining

2. An X-ray study that measures mineral loss and bone thinning is:
   a. Fluoroscopy
   b. Bone densitometry
   c. Computerized tomography
   d. Magnetic resonance imaging

3. The three main components of an X-ray machine are:
   a. Table, x-ray tube, control panel
   b. X-ray tube, control panel, flat plate
   c. Fluoroscope, x-ray table, x-ray tube
   d. Flat plate, x-ray table, x-ray tube

4. Flat plates are known as "plain" films because:
   a. No contrast medium is used
   b. They require no special technique
   c. They do not require the addition of a patient's name
   d. a and b

5. Radioactive substances that are ingested or injected for nuclear studies are called:
   a. Peptides
   b. Amino acids
   c. Radionuclides
   d. Electrons

6. A common fear for people undergoing an MRI is that of being confined. This is known as:
   a. Hyperventilation
   b. Tachycardia
   c. Claustrophobia
   d. Anxiety

7. A noninvasive test that is utilized to evaluate blood flow through arteries in various areas of the body is called:
   a. PET scan
   b. Doppler ultrasound
   c. Mammography
   d. CAD

8. If X-rays cannot easily penetrate a substance, it is called:
   a. Radiolucent
   b. Radiopaque
   c. Radiology
   d. None of the above

9. Dilated vessels located in the esophagus are called:
   a. Esophageal reflux
   b. Esophageal stricture
   c. Esophageal varices
   d. Esophageal spasm

10. What are the characteristics of a PET scan?
    a. A radioactive substance is injected into the patient's blood
    b. Charged particles are given off that combine with particles in the patient's body
    c. Color images are produced
    d. All of the above

VOCABULARY BUILDER

Misspelled Words

Find the words below that are misspelled; underline them, and correctly spell them in the spaces provided. Then write the following correct vocabulary terms next to their corresponding definitions.

dosimeter

echocardiogram

floroscope

isotope

magnetic resonence imaging

oscilloscope

position emission tomography

radialpaque

radiolusent

transducer

_____

_____

_____

_____

_____

1. _____ Use of fluorescent screen that shows the images of objects inserted between the tube and the screen

2. _____ Sound waves emitted from its head during ultrasound

3. _____ A chemical element

4. _____ A noninvasive procedure where the patient lies inside a cylinder-shaped machine, or an open-bore machine, in which there is an electromagnet

5. _____ A radiographic procedure using a computer and radioactive substance

6. _____ Term a structure is called if X-rays do not penetrate it

7. _____ Noninvasive diagnostic method that uses ultrasound to visualize internal cardiac structure, including valves

8. _____ Small, badgelike device worn above the waist which measures the amount of X-rays a person is exposed to

9. _____ Term a structure is called if X-rays penetrate it easily

10. _____ An electronic device used for recording electrical activity of the heart, brain, and muscular tissues

LEARNING REVIEW

Short Answer

1. Describe the positions used during X-rays and include the direction of the X-rays, if applicable.

Position	Description	Direction of X-rays
Anteroposterior view (AP)		
Posteroanterior view (PA)		
Lateral view		
Right lateral view (RL)		
Left lateral view (LL)		
Oblique view		
Supine view		
Prone view		

2. For each radiologic test listed below, explain the purpose of the test.

Test	Purpose
Angiography	
Barium swallow (upper GI series)	
Barium enema (lower GI series)	
Cholangiography	
Cholecystography	
Cystography	
Hysterosalpingography	
Intravenous pyelography (IVP)	
Mammography	
Retrograde pyelography	

3. Describe the patient preparation needed for each test: before, during, and after. *NOTE*: instructions to the following exams may differ depending on the facility and technology involved.

Test	Patient Preparation
Angiography	
Barium swallow (upper GI series)	
Cholangiography	
Cholecystography	
Cystography	
Hysterosalpingography	
Intravenous pyelography (IVP)	
Mammography	
Retrograde pyelography	

4. Why is exposure to radiation dangerous?

_____

_____

5. What test is performed to study the colon for disease?

_____

CERTIFICATION REVIEW

These questions are designed to mimic the certification examination. Select the best response.

1. If a patient needs to be NPO before a radiologic procedure and the patient drinks a glass of water 3 hours before the appointment, what must you do?
   a. Water is allowed but nothing else.
   b. The provider must be consulted.
   c. The procedure must be canceled.
   d. Three hours is long enough for the water to be through the patient's system.

2. Possible side effects of radiation include:
   a. hair loss, weight loss, nausea, and diarrhea
   b. hair loss, nausea, dizziness, and diarrhea
   c. nausea and vomiting, inflammation of the mouth, and hair loss
   d. all of the above

3. Palliative means:
   a. relieving symptoms, as well as curing
   b. curing but not offering much relief of symptoms
   c. placebo, or an agent that does nothing but the patient thinks it helps
   d. agents, such as pain relievers, used to relieve or alleviate painful or uncomfortable symptoms but do not cure the condition

4. When storing and safeguarding radiographs:
   a. they must be protected from light, heat, and moisture
   b. the environment is of little concern; they are basically plastic and can be wiped clean
   c. they must be kept in a cool, dry place
   d. a and c

5. Which is true about medical assistants and their ability to take X-rays?
   a. With additional training, medical assistants can take films of extremities in some states
   b. If the provider approves, medical assistants can take radiographs as ordered in any state
   c. Medical assistants must have a basic understanding of radiologic studies for the purpose of patient teaching
   d. a and c

6. Diagnostic imaging:
   a. is accessible to all clinics and hospitals
   b. is an inexpensive form of testing
   c. results are easy to read
   d. results can be stored on computer systems

7. In order to obtain an anteroposterior view (AP), which of the following is correct?

   a. The anterior surface of the body faces away from the tube

   b. The anterior surface of the body faces the tube

   c. The posterior surface of the body faces the tube

   d. None of the above

8. MRI and CT scanning are not available for patients with what implantable device?

   a. Metal clips or pins

   b. Pacemaker

   c. Implantable cardioverter-defibrillator

   d. All of the above

9. Stomatitis, bone marrow depression, and nausea and vomiting are side effects of:

   a. mammography

   b. radiation therapy

   c. gastrography

   d. infusion therapy

10. Once radiographic films are taken, they are the property of:

    a. the patient

    b. the provider

    c. the hospital or facility

    d. the insurance

LEARNING APPLICATION

Critical Thinking

1. Describe the purpose of a lead apron and lead-lined walls in the radiology department.

   _____

   _____

   _____

2. In what ways are X-rays utilized to diagnose illness?

   _____

   _____

   _____

3. In what ways are X-rays utilized to treat illness?

   _____

   _____

   _____

4. What is contrast media? How is it used and why?

   _____

   _____

   _____

   _____

   _____

5. To whom do X-ray films belong once they are taken and processed?

_____

6. What special precautions should be taken when a patient is having excretory urography (IVP)?

_____

_____

_____

Case Studies

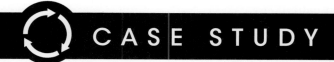

CASE STUDY

You begin working in a clinic where X-ray procedures are done. The provider has informed you that he will teach you the procedure for taking X-rays. In your state, special education and licensure are needed for a medical assistant to perform X-ray procedures. You also notice that no one in the clinic wears a dosimeter, although all are near the X-ray room during the day. Lead aprons are also not used on patients during X-ray procedures.

CASE STUDY REVIEW QUESTIONS

1. How will you handle this situation?

_____

_____

_____

_____

_____

_____

Web Activities

1. Visit the American Society of Radiologic Technicians at http://www.asrt.org. What information can you find that relates to the care of patients undergoing radiologic procedures?

2. Use Google to find a Web site for the "history of MRI." Describe how long it took for the first MRI to produce one image.

3. Using a search engine of your choice, locate information about how CT scans work. What is the fundamental concept of how a CT scan operates?

4. Using the search engine of your choice, discover how nuclear medicine is utilized to diagnose and treat disease.

5. Locate a Web site about medical radiation safety. Find a guide about radiation protection for the patient. What are the risks and benefits of a mammogram? Excretory urogram (IVP)?

6. Go to the World Health Organization's website and explore information on medical radiation exposure.

CHAPTER POST-TEST

Perform this test without looking at your book.

1. Which of the following should be included when educating the patient regarding their upcoming MRI?
    a. Explain that the machine is quiet and calming
    b. They must remove all metal objects such as jewelry
    c. They must lie still and avoid talking
    d. b and c

2. When explaining the excretory urography procedure, what details should be included?
    a. Contrast media will be injected
    b. The kidneys, ureters, and bladder will be visualized
    c. Laxatives are given to improve the visualization of the bladder
    d. All of the above

3. Which is true about positioning of a patient for a supine view?
    a. The anterior surface of the body faces the X-ray tube
    b. The body is lying face down
    c. The body is lying face up
    d. The posterior surface of the body faces the X-ray tube

4. Commonly used contrast media are:
    a. barium sulfate
    b. iodine compounds
    c. air
    d. all of the above

5. X-rays were named when a German physicist discovered them in 1895. What was his name?
    a. Roentgen
    b. Einthoven
    c. Hahn
    d. Pasteur

6. Studies to examine the bile ducts and the gallbladder are:
    a. angiography
    b. cholangiography
    c. cholecystography
    d. b and c

7. Bone densitometry is a study to detect:
    a. osteoarthritis
    b. osteomyelitis
    c. osteopathy
    d. osteoporosis

8. Which of the following is a type of MRI configurations?
   a. Open
   b. Closed
   c. Open-air
   d. All of the above

9. The visual picture that is generated by an ultrasound study is displayed on a(n):
   a. transducer
   b. fluoroscope
   c. oscilloscope
   d. monitor

10. Computer-aided detection is an augmented method to recognize abnormal tissues found on which study?
    a. Ultrasound
    b. MRI
    c. Mammography
    d. CT

SELF-ASSESSMENT

As a clinical medical assistant, if you are taking X-rays or assisting with X-ray procedures, what protective measures would you take? Would the patient take the same precautions? Why would you need more precautions than the patient?

_____

_____

_____

_____

C H A P T E R **33**

Rehabilitation and Therapeutic Modalities

CHAPTER PRE-TEST

Perform this test without looking at your book.

1. The field of medicine that uses physical and mechanical agents to aid in the diagnosis, treatment, and prevention of diseases and bodily injury is called:
   a. Geriatrics
   b. Orthopedics
   c. Rehabilitative medicine
   d. Sports medicine

2. Application of a heating pad or hot pack is _____ therapy.
   a. dry heat
   b. moist heat
   c. paraffin wax
   d. warm soaks

3. Forearm crutches differ from axillary crutches because they are:
   a. Shorter
   b. Less stable
   c. Easier to use
   d. a and b

4. An example of proper body mechanics is:
   a. Always bend over from the hips
   b. Keep the back as straight as possible
   c. Pivot the entire body instead of twisting
   d. b and c

5. The medical term for paralysis on one side is:
   a. Quadriplegia
   b. Paraplegia
   c. Hemiplegia
   d. None of the above

6. When assisting a patient to ambulate, it is important to remember:
   a. The patient should be barefooted to assure stability
   b. To provide the patient with a gait belt for firm hold
   c. To monitor the patent for signs of fatigue
   d. b and c

7. Treatment of disorders with physical and mechanical agents and methods to restore normal function after injury or illness is called:
   a. Physical therapy
   b. Occupational therapy
   c. Speech therapy
   d. Sports medicine

8. Normal daily self-care is termed:
   a. ADLs
   b. ACLS
   c. ACLs
   d. ALS

9. One function of good posture is:
   a. Protecting the patient
   b. Protecting your back
   c. Protecting the entire body
   d. b and c

10. Before beginning a transfer of a patient, you should:
    a. Make sure the equipment is stable and firm
    b. Never allow the patient to put their arms around you
    c. Make sure there are no obstructions in the pathway
    d. All of the above

VOCABULARY BUILDER

Misspelled Words

Find the words below that are misspelled; underline them, and correctly spell them in the spaces provided. Then write the correct vocabulary terms next to the example below that best describes it.

activities of daily living	gait	modality
ambulation	gait belt	range of motion
asistive devices	ghoniometer	thermaltherapy
body mechanics	ghoniometry	ultrasound
contrackures	hemaplegia	vasalconstriction

_____   _____   _____

_____   _____

_____   _____

LEARNING REVIEW

_____ 1. When examining a new patient, a physical therapist must determine which of the physical agents, such as heat, cold, light, water, and electricity, will be most beneficial in treating the patient's condition.

_____ 2. As Margaret Thomas, diagnosed with Parkinson's disease, began to experience balance problems and difficulties in walking, her physical therapist prescribed the use of high-frequency sound waves to generate heat in the deep tissue of her right leg, producing a therapeutic effect.

_____ 3. Cold applications may be used to constrict blood vessels to slow or stop the flow of blood to an area.

_____ 4. Lenny Taylor, suffering the early stages of dementia from Alzheimer's disease, works with an occupational therapist to practice methods of making these everyday tasks easier to perform.

_____ 5. Dr. Winston Lewis recommends this heat modality to help relieve Herb Fowler's chronic lower back pain, which is caused by strain on the back muscles created by the patient's overweight condition.

_____ 6. When patient Linda Maier comes to Inner City Health Care describing a sore back and several recent falls, Dr. Whitney asks clinical medical assistant Bruce Goldman, CMA (AAMA), to secure a gait belt around Linda's waist and have her walk across the room. With Bruce staying a step behind her and slightly to the side, Dr. Whitney carefully observes Linda's progress when performing this task.

_____ 7. As a muscle atrophies, shrinking and losing its strength, joints become stiff and experience development of these deformities. Without constant exercise, the musculoskeletal system deteriorates.

_____ 8. Dr. Susan Rice recommends that patient Linda Maier begin to use a walker at home to prevent further falls. Bruce Goldman secures a gait belt around Linda's waist and positions her inside the walker as he gives her verbal instructions to begin the procedure of learning to ambulate with a walker.

_____ 9. Older adult patient Abigail Johnson is afraid that because she has diabetes mellitus she is at increased risk for stroke. "I don't want to end up a vegetable and a burden to my family," she tells Dr. Elizabeth King, "all paralyzed on one side like that."

_____ 10. Clinical medical assistant Joe Guerrero, CMA (AAMA), applies this practice of using certain key muscle groups together with correct body alignment to avoid injury when assisting patient Lenore McDonell in performing a transfer from her wheelchair to the examination table.

_____ 11. Margaret Thomas's neurologist uses this instrument to measure the angle of her shoulder joint's ROM during a follow-up examination for Parkinson's disease.

_____ 12. Canes, walkers, and crutches are examples of walking aids.

_____ 13. When lying flat with arms at the sides, the average person should be able to move from a 20-degree hyperextension of the elbow joint to a 150-degree flexion.

_____ 14. A physical therapist uses the measurement of joint motion to help evaluate a patient's ROM.

Matching

Match each of the joint movement terminology listed below to its proper definition.

____ 1. Extension

____ 2. Circumduction

____ 3. Plantar flexion

____ 4. Dorsiflexion

____ 5. Eversion

____ 6. Adduction

____ 7. Hyperextension

____ 8. Flexion

____ 9. Inversion

____ 10. Pronation

____ 11. Supination

____ 12. Rotation

____ 13. Abduction

A. Moving the arm so the palm is up

B. Moving a body part outward

C. Straightening of a body part

D. Motion toward the midline of the body

E. Moving a body part inward

F. Turning a body part around its axis

G. A position of maximum extension, or extending a body part beyond its normal limits

H. Motion away from the midline of the body

I. Circular motion of a body part

J. Moving the arm so the palm is down

K. Moving the foot downward at the ankle

L. Moving the foot upward at the ankle joint

M. Bending of a body part

LEARNING REVIEW

Short Answer

1. Name four types of exercise programs that are used for therapeutic or preventative purposes.

   _____

   _____

2. Using the four types of exercise programs identified above, match each one to the example below that best describes it.

   _____   Pat Tidmarsh, who is suffering a sports injury to the muscles surrounding the knee, performs exercises with the help of a rubber exercise band.

   _____   Lourdes Austen performs self-directed exercises at home to improve the ROM and increase strength in her left arm, after lumpectomy and axillary lymph node dissection.

   _____   Lenore McDonell, who is confined to a wheelchair and unable to move her legs voluntarily, works regularly with a physical therapist to avoid atrophy and contractures in the legs and to improve overall circulation.

   _____   Luanne Moore, who is recovering from a shoulder injury, rebuilds upper body strength with a daily regimen of push-ups, first against the wall and then on the floor.

3. Therapeutic exercise is not the only way to treat painful joints or tissues. Many patients respond well to the therapeutic modalities of heat and cold, thermotherapy and cryotherapy. List six precautions that medical assistants must take when applying heat or cold modalities.

   _____

   _____

   _____

   _____

   _____

   _____

_____

_____

_____

_____

4. Identify each modality listed below as either a dry heat therapy (DHT), a moist heat therapy (MHT), a moist cold therapy (MCT), or a dry cold therapy (DCT) by placing the proper letters in the space provided. Then identify whether the modality can be performed at home by the patient, with or without caregiver assistance, or whether the modality must be performed in a clinical setting under the supervision of a health care professional.

_____ A. Ice pack _____

_____ B. Paraffin wax bath _____

_____

_____ C. Cold compress _____

_____ D. Hot water bottle _____

_____

_____

_____ E. Warm compress _____

_____

_____ F. Whirlpool bath _____

_____

_____ G. Heating pad _____

_____

_____

_____ H. Warm soak of one
extremity _____

_____ I. Warm pack _____

_____

_____ J. Total body
immersion in a
Hubbard tank _____

_____

5. For each of the following, identify the proper temperature and correct amount of time the modality should be administered to the patient. The first row has been completed for you as an example.

Modality	Temperature	Time
Aquamatic K-Pad for an older adult patient		
Paraffin wax bath for a patient with rheumatoid arthritis		
An ice pack for a patient with an ankle sprain		
Hot water bottle for an adult patient		
A warm compress to drain pus from a patient's skin infection		
Warm soak of the arm and hand for a patient with osteoarthritis		

6. How do ultrasound waves best travel? What are the special concerns of ultrasound treatment, how long can ultrasound be administered, and who is authorized to perform ultrasound procedures on patients?

_____

_____

_____

_____

_____

_____

Image Labeling

Some patients require assistive devices to ambulate. Name each assistive device shown below, and then name the physical conditions for which each device is best suited to be used as part of a provider's treatment plan. The first row has been completed for you as an example.

	Name	**Uses**

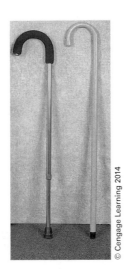

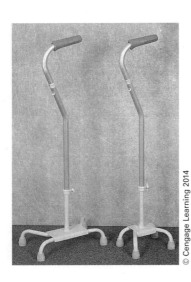

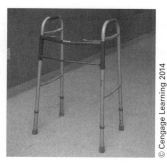

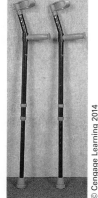

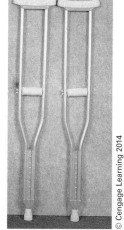

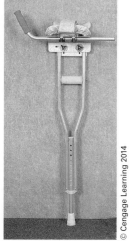

CERTIFICATION REVIEW

These questions are designed to mimic the certification examination. Select the best response.

1. When lifting or carrying heavy objects, you should rely on the following muscle group(s):
   a. abdominal
   b. thoracic
   c. legs and arms
   d. back

2. The type of assistive device that does not require much upper body strength but is not recommended for older adults is:
   a. the walker
   b. the cane
   c. crutches
   d. the wheelchair

3. When a patient is standing with hands on the grip of a walker, the elbow should be bent at a _____ degree angle.
   a. 90
   b. 45
   c. 15
   d. 30

4. The type of crutch that may be used temporarily while a lower extremity heals is:
   a. axillary
   b. forearm
   c. platform
   d. Lofstrand

5. A quad cane is:
   a. two-legged
   b. four-legged
   c. one-legged
   d. three-legged

6. The use of activities to help restore independent functioning after an illness or injury is termed:
   a. physical therapy
   b. occupational therapy
   c. speech therapy
   d. sports medicine

7. Which of the following is key when using lifting techniques?
   a. Use the large muscles of the legs and arms to lift.
   b. Bend from the hips and knees, squat down, and push up with leg muscles.
   c. Get as close as possible to the patient.
   d. All of the above

8. The appropriate way to utilize a gait belt includes:
   a. lifting the patient by grasping the belt from underneath
   b. lifting up
   c. utilizing a firm grip on the patient's arms
   d. a and b

9. Walkers are used for patients who need which of the following?
   a. Maximum assistance
   b. Assistance with poor balance
   c. Stability
   d. All of the above

10. A patient with severe arthritis or poor use of their hands could utilize which of the following assistive devices?
    a. Axillary crutches
    b. Quad cane
    c. Platform crutches
    d. Rolling walker

LEARNING APPLICATION

Critical Thinking

1. Define rehabilitation medicine and explain its importance in patient care.

   _____

   _____

   _____

   _____

2. Describe the procedure for measuring for axillary crutches.

   _____

   _____

   _____

   _____

3. What kind of patient would need a forearm crutch?

   _____

   _____

   _____

4. In crutch-walking gaits, what is a *point*?

   _____

   _____

   _____

5. List the six safety rules for transporting a patient in a wheelchair.

   _____

   _____

   _____

   _____

6. What is joint range of motion, how is it measured, and how is the measurement expressed?

   _____

   _____

7. Describe how ultrasound works and identify the patient conditions for which it is an effective treatment.

_____

_____

_____

8. Explain how to avoid internal damage to the patient when an ultrasound treatment is being performed.

_____

_____

Case Studies

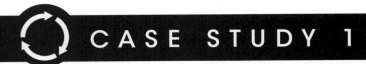

Ellen Armstrong, CMA (AAMA), performs the annual task of assembling and moving inactive patient files into a storage filing area for safekeeping. It is the end of the day and Ellen is tired and eager to finish the job—this task has never been one of Ellen's favorites. When she gets to filling the last of three cartons of files, Ellen moves the carton to a shelf, about shoulder high, in the storage room. She returns and decides to take both of the remaining cartons in one trip. Fatigued, she bends at the waist to pick them up.

CASE STUDY REVIEW QUESTION

1. Describe the proper lifting technique that Ellen should use.

_____

_____

_____

_____

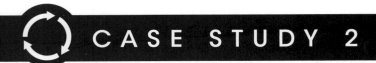

After explaining the procedure to the patient Mary Craig and her son, Wanda Slawson, CMA (AAMA), applies a gait belt and begins the transfer of Mary from a car to a wheelchair in the parking lot of Inner City Health Care. Mary is an older adult blind patient with diabetes mellitus who is suffering from atrophy of the legs. Unfortunately, because of Mary's position in the car, the patient must be transferred with her weaker side closest to the wheelchair. The patient panics during the transfer and throws her arms around Wanda's neck as she is lifting and pivoting Mary to the right to position her in the wheelchair. The patient's son, John, rushes forward to grab onto his mother.

CASE STUDY REVIEW QUESTIONS

1. What is the best action of the medical assistant?

_____

_____

2. What is the best therapeutic response of the medical assistant?

3. Could the situation have been avoided? If so, how? If not, why not?

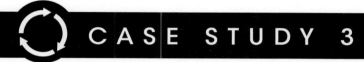

CASE STUDY 3

Dr. Susan Rice asks Bruce Goldman, CMA (AAMA), to instruct patient Dottie Tate in the use of a walker to prevent further falls at home. Dottie is silent as Dr. Rice leaves the examination room and Bruce proceeds to set the walker correctly. However, when Dottie sees that Bruce must once again put Dottie in a gait belt for her protection—the belt was used earlier in the examination to assess Dottie's ability to ambulate—the patient gets feisty. She is visibly tired and ready to go home. "I'll learn to use the walker if I have to, but I won't wear that infernal contraption. It makes me feel like a baby. And it's such a bother. Who wants to go through all that? We just don't need it."

CASE STUDY REVIEW QUESTIONS

1. What is the best action of the medical assistant?

2. What is the best therapeutic response of the medical assistant?

3. Could the situation have been avoided? If so, how? If not, why not?

Web Activities

1. Search the Internet for information online about the Americans with Disabilities Act of 1990.

   a. To what group of people does the act apply?

   b. What does the act provide for these individuals?

   c. Does the act have any influence over access to providers' offices and clinics? Please explain.

   d. What is included in the 2010 Standards for Accessible Design?

2. Visit the American Physical Therapy Association (APTA) web site to find information about the following disorders and the therapies that can be prescribed for each:

   a. Repetitive stress injuries

   b. Spinal cord injuries

   c. Sports injuries

CHAPTER POST-TEST

Perform this test without looking at your book.

1. The term for moving away from the midline is:

   a. abduct

   b. adduct

   c. extension

   d. flexion

2. The instructions to start with crutches at the side, move both crutches forward, transfer the weight and swing through with both feet refer to which crutch-walking gait?

   a. Three-point gait

   b. Four-point alternating gait

   c. Swing-through gait

   d. Two-point gait

3. When measuring for axillary crutches, the medical assistant should adjust the height to _____ below the patient's axillae.

   a. 1 inch

   b. 2 inches

   c. 3 inches

   d. 4 inches

4. Canes are usually made of:

   a. wood

   b. steel

   c. aluminum

   d. a and c

5. Which of the following are safety rules to be followed when moving a patient in a wheelchair?

   a. Always enter an elevator with the patient facing forward.

   b. Proceed forward down ramps.

   c. Make sure the patient's feet are on the footrests prior to moving.

   d. Move down the center of corridors to avoid injuring the patient's elbows.

6. The amount of movement that is present in a joint is referred to as:
   a. goniometry
   b. range of motion
   c. flexion
   d. extension

7. Moving a body part inward is termed:
   a. abduction
   b. eversion
   c. inversion
   d. pronation

8. A licensed massage therapist might use petrissage to assist in reducing muscle tension. This term is defined as:
   a. tapping
   b. rubbing
   c. stroking
   d. kneading

9. A high-frequency acoustic vibration that is used to treat deeper tissue injuries is known as:
   a. ultrasound
   b. radiation
   c. percussion
   d. effleurage

10. A warm bath in which only the hips and buttocks are immersed for relief of pain from conditions such as rectal surgery is called a:
    a. paraffin wax bath
    b. wet compress
    c. sitz bath
    d. warm soak

SELF-ASSESSMENT

1. Have you ever considered the field of physical or occupational therapy as a career?

   _____

   _____

   _____

   _____

2. What makes you think you would do well or not do well in those fields?

   _____

   _____

   _____

   _____

3. What do you think you would not care for in working with rehabilitative medicine? What would you like the most?

_____

_____

_____

_____

4. What are some of the skills, talents, interests, and abilities a person would need to have to do well in rehabilitative medicine? List a dozen or more, and then consider and circle all of those that you possess. Which on the list could you learn in a rehabilitative medicine program (insert an *S* for school), and which would be a natural part of your makeup (insert an *N* for natural)? Is there a direct relation between the skills, talents, interests, and abilities you possess and those that you marked with an *N*? Discuss your results with a small group of fellow students. What conclusion(s) did you reach?

_____

_____

_____

_____

C H A P T E R **34**

Nutrition in Health and Disease

CHAPTER PRE-TEST

Perform this test without looking at your book.

1. The constant internal environment of the body is referred to as:
   a. Hemostasis
   b. Homeostasis
   c. Hemodynamics
   d. Hemoglobin

2. The basic structural unit of a protein is:
   a. Hydrochloric acid
   b. Carbohydrates
   c. Amino acid
   d. Saturated fat

3. Which of the following are fat-soluble vitamins?
   a. A, B, C, and D
   b. C, E, and K
   c. B, C, D, and E
   d. A, D, E, and K

4. Herbal supplements are also known as:
   a. Phytomedicines
   b. Minerals
   c. Botanicals
   d. A and C

5. Development of bones and teeth, transmission of nerve impulses, and blood clotting are valuable functions of which mineral?
   a. Chloride
   b. Potassium
   c. Calcium
   d. Magnesium

6. When reviewing a food label, which of the following is an important piece of information?
   a. Amount of saturated fat
   b. Vitamins and minerals
   c. Amount of fiber
   d. All of the above

7. Childhood obesity and a poor diet can increase the risk of:
   a. Rickets
   b. Cerebral palsy
   c. Type 2 diabetes
   d. Halitosis

8. An infant requires _____ times more calories per kilogram than an adult.
   a. 1 to 2
   b. 2 to 3
   c. 3 to 4
   d. None of the above

9. Severe restriction of caloric intake and excessive exercising is known as:
   a. Bulimia
   b. Malnutrition
   c. Anorexia nervosa
   d. Weight loss

10. The leading cause of death in the United States is:
    a. Cancer
    b. Diabetes
    c. Cardiovascular disease
    d. Obesity

VOCABULARY BUILDER

Misspelled Words

Find the words below that are misspelled; underline them, and then correctly spell them in the spaces provided. Then fill in the blanks below with the correct vocabulary term from the following list.

amino acids	digestion	nutrients
antioxident	electrolytes	nutrition
basal metabolic rate	extracellulare	oxydation
calories	fat-soluble	presearvatives
catalist	glycogen	processed foods
cellulose	homeostasis	saturated fats
coenzyeme	major minerals	trace minerals
diaretics	metabolizm	water-soluable

_____   _____   _____

_____   _____   _____

_____   _____   _____

1. Artificial flavors, colors, and _____ that keep food fresh longer are non-nutritive chemical substances commonly added to processed foods.

2. _____ is the study of the intake of nutrients into the body and how the body processes and uses these nutrients.

3. Toxicity is most likely to occur with _____ vitamins because they are stored in tissues composed of lipids and in the liver and are not carried easily into the bloodstream.

4. The best sources of complete proteins are meats and animal products such as milk and eggs; complete proteins contain all eight of the essential _____.

5. Beverages that contain caffeine and alcohol, which are _____, will cause the body to increase urinary output and lose water. These substances should be avoided when performing activities, such as a good physical workout, as well as when entering environments, such as an airplane passenger cabin, that promote dehydration.

6. A _____ is a nonprotein substance that acts with a catalyst to facilitate chemical reactions in the body.

7. Chlorine (Cl) is a mineral with an important _____ function, one that takes place outside the cells of body tissues in the spaces between layers or groups of cells.

8. The total of all changes, chemical and physical, that take place in the body is called _____.

9. Some minerals are considered _____ in that they become ionized and carry a positive or negative charge; these minerals must be carefully balanced in the body.

10. _____ begins at the mouth with chewing and progresses through the gastrointestinal tract to the small intestine.

11. _____ are ingested substances that help the body maintain a state of homeostasis.

12. The process of _____ maintains a constant internal environment of the human body, including such functions as heartbeat, blood pressure, respiration, and body temperature.

13. A _____ facilitates chemical reactions by speeding up the reaction time without the need for a high-energy output.

14. It is always important to analyze the nutritional labels on _____ purchased in the supermarket.

15. Lard is one example of _____, which have been found to increase the level of fats and cholesterol in the blood and are hydrogenated, or contain hydrogen.

16. The ability to reduce _____ is a characteristic of vitamin E that has led some researchers to suggest that vitamin E may slow the aging process, although its true effectiveness has not yet been demonstrated.

17. The amount of energy a substance is able to supply is measured in _____.

18. Potassium is one of the seven _____ found in the body.

19. Vitamins that are _____ must be constantly ingested to maintain proper blood levels, because these vitamins are not easily stored in the body.

20. Vitamin E is a fat-soluble vitamin that belongs to a group of compounds called _____, which counteract the damaging effects of oxidation. Beta-carotene is another substance in this group.

21. Despite their name, _____ are vital to body functioning and include molybdenum and fluorine.

22. Children, pregnant women, and people with a lean body mass will have a higher _____ because it takes more energy to fuel the muscles than it does to store fat.

23. A type of carbohydrate, _____, is derived from a plant source and supplies fiber in the human diet.

24. Ingested only in small quantities, _____ is an important carbohydrate form for storage of glucose in the body.

LEARNING REVIEW

Short Answer

1. Vitamins are a class of nutrients in which each specific vitamin has a function entirely of its own. These complex molecules are required by the body in minute quantities. What are the two functions of vitamins in the body?

   _____

   _____

2. Identify the correct chemical name for each vitamin listed. Then describe what each vitamin does in the body to promote good health.

   A. One of the B-complex vitamins, also called nicotinic acid:

   _____

   _____

   B. Vitamin B_1:

   _____

   _____

   C. Vitamin E:

   _____

   _____

   D. Vitamin D:

   _____

   _____

   E. One of the B-complex vitamins, also called folacin:

   _____

   _____

   F. Vitamin A:

   _____

   _____

   G. Vitamin B_{12}:

   _____

   _____

   H. Vitamin C:

   _____

   _____

   I. Vitamin B_2:

   _____

   _____

   J. Vitamin B_6:

   _____

   _____

3. Nutrients are divided into two groups: those that provide energy and those that do not. Identify the nutrients listed below as providing energy or not providing energy by placing an X in the appropriate column.

	Energy	**No Energy**
Vitamins		
Carbohydrates		
Fiber		
Minerals		
Lipids (fats)		
Proteins		
Water		

4. What three chemical elements do carbohydrates, fats, and proteins all contain?

_____

_____

5. Name the most important dietary complex carbohydrate. _____

6. Name the only true essential fatty acid in the human diet. _____

7. What additional chemical element does protein alone contain? _____

8. What happens when the body does not have enough carbohydrates or fats in supply as an energy source? What effect does this have on the body?

_____

_____

9. Name two conditions associated with deficiencies in protein.

_____

_____

10. List two distinct ways in which minerals differ from vitamins.

_____

_____

_____

11. For each food source, list the mineral or minerals that each provides.
    (1) Eggs: _____
    (2) Milk: _____
    (3) Cheese: _____
    (4) Salmon: _____
    (5) Bananas: _____
    (6) Green vegetables: _____

12. List six types of fiber that are carbohydrates.

_____

_____

13. What important fiber is *not* a carbohydrate?

_____

_____

14. Americans generally do not consume enough fiber. How much fiber should be consumed each day?

_____

_____

15. Why does brown rice contain more fiber than white rice?

_____

_____

16. What happens when the body takes in more calories than will be expended by the body as energy?

_____

_____

17. What happens when the body uses more energy than the calories it takes in?

_____

_____

18. What is the ideal percentage of total calories for adults that should be consumed as carbohydrates, fats, and proteins?

_____

_____

19. Compare the advantages and disadvantages of the following diets: U.S. Southern, Jewish, and Japanese.

_____

_____

_____

_____

_____

_____

_____

_____

20. Obesity is a major health concern in the United States and often begins in childhood. What can you do as a medical assistant to assist parents to help their children avoid obesity?

_____

_____

Matching

For each of the following in Column A, identify the substance as a water-soluble vitamin (WSV), fat-soluble vitamin (FSV), a major mineral (MM), or a trace mineral (TM) in Column B. Then match the substance to the response in Column C that best fits its character or properties. The first one has been completed for you as an example.

	Column A		Column B	Column C
_____	1. Sulfur	_____		A. This substance works with potassium to maintain proper water balance and proper pH balance; the two also are involved in muscular nerve conduction and excitability.
_____	2. Vitamin B_{12}	_____		B. This substance is part of the pigment rhodopsin found in the eye and is responsible in part for vision, especially night vision.

_____ 3. Iron   _____ C. This substance is vital to life because of its role in the heme molecule, which carries oxygen to every cell in the body.

_____ 4. Vitamin K   _____ D. Rickets and osteomalacia are diseases caused by deficiencies in this substance; when deficiencies occur, usually in childhood, malformation of the skeleton is seen.

_____ 5. Sodium   _____ E. This member of the B-complex, together with pantothenic acid, is generally responsible for energy metabolism.

_____ 6. Pyridoxine   _____ F. Because this substance is found only in foods from animal sources, such as liver, kidney, and dairy products, pernicious anemia, the result of deficiencies, may be a problem for some vegetarians.

_____ 7. Iodine   _____ G. This substance, found in rice, beans, and yeast, is important to protein metabolism.

_____ 8. Biotin   _____ H. This substance is a component of one of the amino acids and is found in protein; it is also involved in energy metabolism.

_____ 9. Retinol   _____ I. About half of the body's requirement for this substance is fulfilled through synthesis by intestinal bacteria; bile is required for its absorption into the bloodstream.

_____ 10. Vitamin D   _____ J. This substance is found only in the thyroid hormones; without it, the thyroid gland would be unable to regulate the overall metabolism of the body.

CERTIFICATION REVIEW

These questions are designed to mimic the certification examination. Select the best response.

1. Carbohydrates, fats, and proteins have one thing in common. What is it?
   a. High calcium content
   b. Their ability to convert into energy
   c. Low sodium content
   d. All of the above

2. An example of a monosaccharide is:
   a. fructose
   b. sucrose
   c. glucose
   d. a and c

3. The compounds composed of carbon, hydrogen, and oxygen that exist as triglycerides in the body are:
   a. fats
   b. fiber
   c. vitamins
   d. minerals

4. The basic structural unit of a protein is:
   a. simple sugar
   b. complex sugar
   c. lipids
   d. amino acids

5. Each gram of a carbohydrate contains how many calories?

    a. Four

    b. Eight

    c. Ten

    d. Twelve

6. Chemical digestion begins with amylase that is secreted by the:

    a. lining of the stomach

    b. pancreas

    c. salivary glands

    d. small intestine

7. Glucose is stored in the form of _____ in the body.

    a. insulin

    b. glycogen

    c. fat

    d. bone

8. Xerophthalmia is a deficiency of Vitamin _____.

    a. A

    b. B

    c. C

    d. D

9. Free radicals are produced when:

    a. amino acids are broken down

    b. the body uses oxygen to burn food for energy

    c. the body fails to excrete nitrogen

    d. DNA breaks down

10. Pyridoxine is the name of which vitamin?

    a. A

    b. B_{12}

    c. B_6

    d. C

LEARNING APPLICATION

Critical Thinking

1. Identify each organ of the digestive system below. Describe the healthy functioning of each organ in the space provided. Then, using a medical dictionary or encyclopedia, look up each organ and list one common disorder that would adversely affect the digestive process.

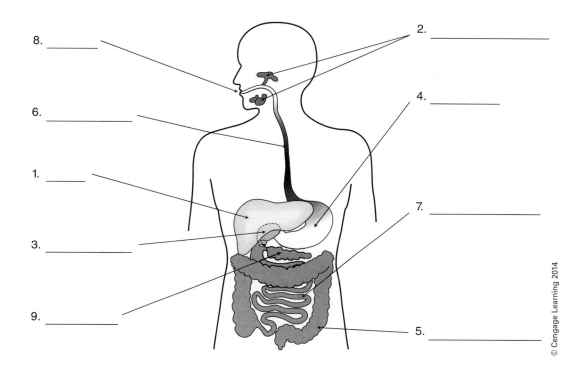

8. _____

6. _____

1. _____

3. _____

9. _____

2. _____

4. _____

7. _____

5. _____

© Cengage Learning 2014

Healthy Function

1. _____
   _____
   _____
   _____

2. _____
   _____
   _____

3. _____
   _____

4. _____
   _____
   _____

5. _____
   _____

6. _____
   _____

Common Disorders

_____
_____
_____
_____

_____
_____
_____

_____
_____

_____
_____
_____

_____
_____

_____
_____

7. _____   _____
   _____   _____
   _____   _____
   _____
   _____

8. _____   _____
   _____   _____

9. _____   _____
   _____   _____
   _____
   _____

2. When helping patients modify their diets, medical assistants need to be knowledgeable about the nutrients in the food we eat. The nutritional analysis label on the back or side of a food package is helpful when figuring out the levels of fat, cholesterol, sodium, carbohydrates, protein, and vitamins contained in a particular food. Obtain a food label and answer the following questions.

   A. The percentage of daily values listed on a food label report the amount of a nutrient obtained by eating how many servings of a product? _____

   B. The percentages are based on a _____-calorie diet.

   C. The listing for total carbohydrates is broken down into what two additional listings? Which type of carbohydrate is more beneficial and why?

   _____

   _____

   D. Why is a high-fiber diet important?

   _____

   _____

   _____

3. Compare the nutrition label from a box of muesli with fruit, nuts, and seeds with the label from a package of pretzel snacks. Which is more nutritious and why? Note that one serving of the muesli, a half cup or 55 grams, is roughly equivalent to 2 servings of pretzels, 14 pretzels or 60 grams.

   _____

   _____

   _____

   _____

   _____

   _____

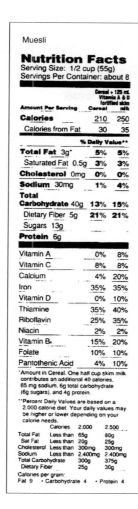

Muesli

Nutrition Facts

Serving Size: 1/2 cup (55g)
Servings Per Container: about 8

Amount Per Serving	Cereal	Cereal + 125 mL Vitamin A & D fortified skim milk
Calories	210	250
Calories from Fat	30	35

	% Daily Value**	
Total Fat 3g*	**5%**	**5%**
Saturated Fat 0.5g	**3%**	**3%**
Cholesterol 0mg	**0%**	**0%**
Sodium 30mg	**1%**	**4%**
Total Carbohydrate 40g	**13%**	**15%**
Dietary Fiber 5g	**21%**	**21%**
Sugars 13g		
Protein 6g		

Vitamin A	0%	8%
Vitamin C	8%	8%
Calcium	4%	20%
Iron	35%	35%
Vitamin D	0%	10%
Thiamine	35%	40%
Riboflavin	25%	35%
Niacin	2%	2%
Vitamin B₆	15%	20%
Folate	10%	10%
Pantothenic Acid	4%	10%

*Amount in Cereal. One half cup skim milk contributes an additional 40 calories, 65 mg sodium, 6g total carbohydrate (6g sugars), and 4g protein.

**Percent Daily Values are based on a 2,000 calorie diet. Your daily values may be higher or lower depending on your calorie needs.

	Calories	2,000	2,500
Total Fat	Less than	65g	80g
Sat Fat	Less than	20g	25g
Cholesterol	Less than	300mg	300mg
Sodium	Less than	2,400mg	2,400mg
Total Carbohydrate		300g	375g
Dietary Fiber		25g	30g

Calories per gram:
Fat 9 • Carbohydrate 4 • Protein 4

Pretzels
Nutrition Facts

Serving Size: 7 Pretzels (30g)
Servings Per Container: 9.4

Amount Per Serving

Calories 120	
Calories from Fat 10	

	% Daily Value*
Total Fat 1g	**2%**
Saturated Fat 0g	**0%**
Cholesterol 0g	**0%**
Sodium 360mg	**15%**
Total Carbohydrate 24g	**8%**
Dietary Fiber 1g	**4%**
Sugars 1g	
Protein 3g	

Vitamin A 0%	Σ	Vitamin C	0%
Calcium 0%	Σ	Iron	2%

*Percent Daily Values are based on a 2,000 calorie diet. Your daily values may be higher or lower depending on your calorie needs:

	Calories	2,000	2,500
Total Fat	Less than	65g	80g
Sat Fat	Less than	20g	25g
Cholesterol	Less than	300mg	300mg
Sodium	Less than	2,400mg	2,400mg
Total Carbohydrate		300g	375g
Dietary Fiber		25g	30g

Calories per gram:
Fat 9 Σ Carbohydrate 4 Σ Protein 4

Ingredients: Unbleached Wheat Flour, Water, Corn Syrup, Partially Hydrogenated Vegetable Oil (Soybean), Yeast Salt, Bicarbonates and Carbonates of Sodium.

Case Studies

CASE STUDY 1

Dr. Elizabeth King has confirmed that patient Mary O'Keefe is pregnant with her third child.

CASE STUDY REVIEW QUESTIONS

1. Name two minerals that Mary must increase the intake of in her diet.

   _____

2. Name three reasons why a woman needs to increase her intake of nutrients and calories when she is pregnant.

   _____

   _____

   _____

   _____

3. What dietary supplements usually need to be added to a baby's diet?

   _____

CASE STUDY 2

Lourdes Austen, a breast cancer survivor, regularly attends a support group for breast cancer patients and survivors held once a month. Lourdes finds the group a great source of encouragement, information, and support—a safe place to discuss her feelings and concerns about breast cancer. The group is planning a session to talk about nutrition issues, and Lourdes asks clinical medical assistant Audrey Jones, RMA (AMT), if she would like to attend the meeting with her to contribute to the group's discussion. With permission from office manager Marilyn Johnson and Lourdes's provider Dr. Elizabeth King, Audrey attends the meeting. The group members are enthusiastic and ask Audrey many questions, including the following: "Why is good nutrition important for cancer patients?" "I don't have much appetite anymore and get nauseous all the time. What can I do?" "I keep hearing about those macrobiotic diets. Are they any good? Should I try them?"

CASE STUDY REVIEW QUESTIONS

1. What information can Audrey give in answer to the question regarding the importance of good nutrition for cancer patients?

_____

_____

_____

_____

_____

_____

_____

2. What suggestion can Audrey offer to patients who have no appetite and have nausea or vomiting?

_____

_____

_____

3. What can Audrey tell the group about macrobiotic diets?

_____

_____

_____

_____

_____

_____

4. What is the role of the medical assistant in attending the breast cancer support group meeting?

_____

_____

_____

Calorie Calculating Activity

1. An 8-fluid-ounce serving of 1% fat soy milk contains 110 calories with 2 grams of total fat, 20 grams of total carbohydrates, and 4 grams of total protein. Calculate the total number of calories from each energy nutrient; show your calculations in the space provided below.

   Number of calories from fat: __

   Number of calories from carbohydrates: __

   Number of calories from protein: __

   _____

   _____

   _____

2. Now calculate the percentage of total calories due to each energy nutrient.

   Percentage of calories from fat: __

   Percentage of calories from carbohydrates: __

   Percentage of calories from protein: ____

   _____

   _____

   _____

3. Compare the percentages of total calories due to fat, carbohydrates, and protein found in soy milk with the percentages you calculated for one serving of peanut butter in the textbook's Critical Thinking box on page 1025. How do the percentages relate to the ideal percentages for optimum energy balance in the body?

   _____

   _____

   _____

   _____

CHAPTER POST-TEST

Perform this test without looking at your book.

1. Pellagra is a disease that is caused by the deficiency of Vitamin _____.
   a. A
   b. B_3
   c. B_6
   d. B_{12}

2. Chloride is important in the _____ space.
   a. intracellular
   b. intravascular
   c. extracellular
   d. none of the above

3. The abbreviation Na stands for which of the following?
   a. niacin
   b. neoplasm
   c. sodium
   d. magnesium

4. Copper, chromium, molybdenum, and selenium are examples of:
   a. proteins
   b. amino acids
   c. electrolytes
   d. trace minerals

5. Food that has been cooked or packaged with parts removed is considered:
   a. organic
   b. preserved
   c. processed
   d. diuretics

6. Atherosclerosis includes the deposition of _____ on the inner walls of arteries.
   a. blood
   b. fat
   c. protein
   d. insulin

7. A patient with loss of appetite, malnutrition, and wasting, commonly associated with a diagnosis of cancer, is termed:
   a. candidiasis
   b. cachectic
   c. bulimic
   d. cheilosis

8. The disease beriberi is caused by a deficiency of _____.
   a. riboflavin
   b. biotin
   c. thiamin
   d. niacin

9. Another name for Vitamin B_{12} is:
   a. cobalamin
   b. riboflavin
   c. pyridoxine
   d. folic acid

10. The level of energy required for activities that occur when the body is at rest is known as:
    a. caloric requirement
    b. metabolism
    c. basal metabolic rate
    d. basal body temperature

SELF-ASSESSMENT

1. Keep track of your diet for a couple of days. Track everything you eat and drink and the amounts of each item.

   _____

   _____

   _____

2. Either use the Internet to research the nutritional value of each item or look in a good dietary resource for the information. Figure the number of calories you ate each day, the amount of fiber, the amount and types of fats, how much protein, how many carbohydrates and sugars, and which vitamins and minerals you consumed. Hint: There are specific Web sites that can help you with this project. One example is http://www .calorie-count.com. This Web site allows you to search through hundreds of different foods and drinks to find the "labels" for them. It is free! You can even create your own personal profile.

   A. Now figure in any vitamins and supplements you ingested.

   B. Is there any particular part of a nutritious diet that you are lacking?

   C. Are there any components that you ate too much of?

CHAPTER **35**

Basic Pharmacology

CHAPTER PRE-TEST

Perform this test without looking at your book.

1. The *Physician's Desk Reference* contains which of the following information?
   a. Brand and generic names of medications
   b. Classification or category
   c. Product information
   d. All of the above

2. An agent that produces numbness is called an:
   a. Analgesic
   b. Anesthetic
   c. Anticoagulant
   d. Antidote

3. Ibuprofen is considered which classification of medications?
   a. Sedative
   b. Nonsteroidal anti-inflammatory
   c. Vasopressor
   d. Decongestant

4. A liquid preparation of a drug is one that has been:
   a. Dissolved
   b. Suspended
   c. Crushed
   d. a and b

5. Misuse or overuse of medications is termed:
   a. Medication error
   b. Diversion
   c. Abuse
   d. All of the above

6. Hydromorphone, oxycodone, and morphine are Schedule _____ drugs.

   a. I

   b. II

   c. III

   d. IV

7. A drug's official name assigned by the U.S. Adopted Names Council is:

   a. The generic name

   b. The brand name

   c. The chemical name

   d. All of the above

8. Which of the following are the responsibilities of the medical assistant as they relate to controlled substances?

   a. Provide security for prescription pads

   b. Properly dispose of and document the disposal of expired drugs

   c. Maintain legal inventories of medications

   d. All of the above

9. What is true about over-the-counter drugs?

   a. They require a prescription.

   b. They are safe to use without the provider's supervision.

   c. They can be taken in unlimited quantities.

   d. None of the above.

10. Penicillin and Augmentin are considered which drug category:

    a. Antibiotic

    b. Anti-inflammatory

    c. Antiviral

    d. Antipyretic

VOCABULARY BUILDER

Misspelled Words I

Find the words in Column A that are misspelled; circle them, and then correctly spell them in the spaces provided. Then match each of the vocabulary terms below with the correct definition in Column B.

Column A	Correct Spelling	Column B
___ 1. Abuse	_____	A. Term used to describe when a licensed practitioner gives a written order to be taken to a pharmacist to be filled
___ 2. Administer	_____	B. An allergic hypersensitivity reaction of the body to a foreign protein or drug
___ 3. Anaphalaxis	_____	C. To give the medication to the patient to be used at another time
___ 4. Contradication	_____	D. The study of drugs; the science dealing with their history, origin, sources, physical and chemical properties, uses, and effects on living organisms

	Column A	Correct Spelling	Column B

____ 5. Dispense

_____

E. To give a medication to a patient by mouth, injection, or any other method of delivery

____ 6. Perscribe

_____

F. Any symptom or circumstance for which an otherwise approved form of treatment is inadvisable

____ 7. Pharmacology

_____

G. The misuse of legal and illegal drugs

Misspelled Words II

Find the words in the list below that are misspelled; circle them, and correctly spell them in the spaces provided. Then insert the proper terms into the spaces provided in the following text, which discusses medical uses of drugs, name of drugs, and sources of drugs.

animal	generic	replacement
chemicel	genetic engineering	sinthetic
curative	mineral	therepuetic
diagnostic	plant	trade name
jean splicing	prophalactic	

_____   _____   _____

_____   _____

A drug is a medicinal substance that may be used to vary or modify the functions of a living being. Of the five basic medical uses for drugs, antibiotics are an example of _____ drugs (agents used for the killing or removal of the causative agent of a disease). An immunizing agent is an example of a preventive or _____ drug, which is one used to stave off or abate the severity of a disease. Another medical use for drugs is in the treatment of a condition to provide symptomatic relief; this is known as _____. Insulin and hormones are examples of the medical use of drugs known as _____ drugs. A fifth basic medical use of drugs is in conjunction with radiology and allows providers to pinpoint the location of diseases' manifestations. This usage is known as _____.

The knowledge of the names of drugs is as essential to the medical assistant as the knowledge of basic uses for drugs. The majority of drugs have three types of names. The _____ name is the drug's official name assigned by the U.S. Adopted Names Council. *Aspirin* is an example of this type of name. The drug's _____ name describes its molecular structure and identification of its chemical structure. *Acetylsalicylic acid* is an example of this type of name. *Ecotrin* is an example of a _____ or brand name, which is registered by the U.S. Patent Office and approved for usage by the U.S. Food and Drug Administration.

Medical assistants must also have a comprehensive understanding of the five basic sources of drugs. The source of digitalis, the dried leaf of a foxglove plant, is an example of a _____ source. Insulin, a hormone derived from the pancreas of cows and hogs, is an example of a drug derived from an _____ source. Drugs that are artificially prepared in pharmaceutical laboratories are known as _____ drugs. Synthetically prepared sulfur, used in pharmaceutical products (such as certain bacteriostatic drugs), is an example of a drug derived from a _____ source. One of the latest sources for drugs has been provided by _____. Using a technique called _____, scientists are able to create hybrid forms of life that can treat certain diseases; interferon for cancer treatment is an example of this process.

LEARNING REVIEW

Short answer

1. Under federal law, providers who prescribe, administer, or dispense controlled substances must register with the DEA and renew their registration as required by state law. Describe the five schedules of classification for controlled substances and give an example for each.

_____

_____

_____

_____

_____

_____

2. For each of the following, identify whether the drug involved is an OTC medication (OTC) or a prescribed medication (PM). What patient guidelines for proper use are illustrated in each example?

_____   A. Nora Fowler insists that Dr. Winston Lewis cannot help her rheumatoid arthritis and that simple ibuprofen is all she needs. Nora buys bulk generic bottles of ibuprofen at the drugstore for her rheumatoid arthritis and takes as many as she needs to help ease the painful inflammation in her joints and tissues.

_____

_____

_____

_____   B. When Jim Marshall experiences extreme stress while finishing the architectural designs for a new office building in the community, his girlfriend offers him a tablet or two of lorazepam, a benzodiazepine drug used to treat anxiety and insomnia. "Here, Dr. King gave me these, and they work great," she says. "You can't drive when you take this stuff, though. Oh, and these pills are about 2 years old, but I'm sure they'll still work fine."

_____

_____

_____

_____   C. At the slightest sniffle or sneeze, Lenore McDonell takes the strongest multisymptom cold medication she can find. Her philosophy is: "I might as well knock it out of my system."

_____

_____

_____

_____   D. Abigail Johnson hates taking so many medications. So every now and then, when she feels especially good, Abigail just decides to stop taking the antihypertensive drug that is part of Dr. Elizabeth King's treatment plan to control Abigail's high blood pressure. On a bad day, she'll take an extra pill.

_____

_____

_____

_____   E. Patty McLean is susceptible to recurrent colds and ear infections. Patty's symptoms are hard to control because she will almost always stop taking the antibiotics when she starts to feel better and she does not finish the entire regimen recommended by Dr. Lewis.

_____

_____

_____

3. Proper disposal of drugs has become increasingly important. How should outdated medications be disposed of?

_____

_____

_____

4. The most frequently used routes of administering medication are oral and parenteral. List seven additional routes of administration.

_____

_____

_____

5. Name three recently developed systems of drug delivery. Describe each and note their specific advantages.

_____

_____

_____

_____

_____

_____

_____

_____

_____

6. List four examples of the ways in which drugs may be classified, or arranged, in groups.

_____

_____

_____

7. For each drug action, identify the correct drug classification. Then list one example of a drug contained in each class. The first row has been completed as an example for you.

Action	Classification	Drug Example
Controls or stops bleeding	_____	_____
Prevents or relieves nausea and vomiting	_____	_____
Neutralizes acid	_____	_____
Decreases blood pressure	_____	_____
Reduces fever	_____	_____
Loosens and promotes normal bowel elimination	_____	_____
Prevents conception	_____	_____

Kills or destroys malignant cells   _____   _____

                                                               _____

Prevents or relieves diarrhea   _____   _____

                                                               _____

Produces a calming effect without causing sleep   _____   _____

                                                               _____

CERTIFICATION REVIEW

These questions are designed to mimic the certification examination. Select the best response.

1. All drugs available for legal use are controlled by the:
   a. Federal Food, Drug, and Cosmetic Act
   b. Council on Pharmacy of the American Medical Association
   c. Controlled Substance Act of 1970
   d. Americans with Disabilities Act of 1990

2. Federal law requires that at the end of the workday, controlled substances that are used on the premises must be:
   a. locked in a provider's office by a provider
   b. counted, verified by two individuals, and recorded on an audit sheet
   c. discarded by flushing down the toilet or hopper
   d. returned to a pharmacy

3. An inventory record of Schedule II drugs must be submitted to the Drug Enforcement Administration (DEA) every:
   a. week
   b. month
   c. year
   d. 2 years

4. An example of a drug requiring a prescription is the:
   a. antibiotic penicillin
   b. antihistamine Benadryl®
   c. analgesic acetaminophen
   d. antacid cimetidine

5. An example of an OTC drug is the:
   a. analgesic ibuprofen
   b. vasodilator nitroglycerin
   c. antitussive codeine
   d. narcotic morphine

6. When a drug acts on the area to which it is administered, it has what is known as a:
   a. systemic action
   b. remote action
   c. local action
   d. none of the above

7. The four principal factors that affect drug action are absorption, distribution, biotransformation, and:

    a. elimination

    b. interaction

    c. contraindication

    d. excretion

8. By law, outdated and expired controlled substances must be:

    a. handed over to your local law enforcement agency

    b. thrown away

    c. returned to the pharmacy

    d. flushed down a toilet

9. Patients need to realize that OTC drugs can:

    a. interact with other drugs and cause undesirable or adverse reactions or complications

    b. mask symptoms and exacerbate an existing condition

    c. have little or no effect on disease processes

    d. a and b

10. The most frequently used routes of administering medication are:

    a. inhalation and sublingual

    b. parenteral and inhalation

    c. oral and parenteral

    d. transdermal and oral

LEARNING APPLICATION

Critical Thinking

1. What factor in determining the route selection for administering a medication is illustrated by each example below, and why?

    A. A patient diagnosed with insulin-dependent diabetes mellitus performs three self-injections of insulin daily, according to the provider's treatment plan.

    _____

    _____

    _____

    B. Chemotherapeutic drugs are used to attack cancer cells that may be traveling throughout a patient's body, and usually they are administered intravenously.

    _____

    _____

    _____

    C. A patient in a nursing home who is in the end stages of Parkinson's disease is bedridden, has trouble swallowing, and suffers from dementia. The patient, who is also suffering from angina as a result of poor blood circulation, is prescribed a nitroglycerin transdermal system instead of a sublingual dosage, to be held under the tongue, or time-released capsule to swallow.

    _____

    _____

    _____

Case Studies

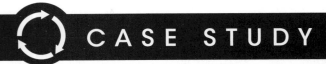

CASE STUDY

While Anna Preciado RMA, a clinical medical assistant newly hired at the clinic of Drs. Lewis and King, is performing her shift duties, she notices a fellow employee exhibiting strange behavior. Audrey Jones, CMA (AAMA), is usually the model of efficiency. Since Anna began working at the Northborough Family Medical Group, she has always known Audrey to be alert, friendly, and able to handle difficult clinical situations with grace under pressure. Lately, however, when Anna asks Audrey questions, Audrey seems irritable and easily confused. Anna also notices Audrey exhibiting a sloppy technique during routine clinical procedures. Anna is disturbed by Audrey's erratic behavior but does not mention anything to anyone. After all, Anna is new to the job. But while counting the contents of the controlled substance cabinet in preparation for the end of her shift, Anna notices that a bottle of phenobarbital is missing. Anna knows that office manager Marilyn Johnson will arrive shortly to verify and record the inventory count. Anna is now worried that perhaps Audrey is to blame for the missing drugs but is afraid of jumping to conclusions and of angering Audrey. Anna knows Audrey is in the staff lounge preparing to leave for a dinner break.

CASE STUDY REVIEW QUESTIONS

1. What is Anna's first action under the circumstances? Should she confront Audrey?

_____

_____

_____

_____

_____

2. What special responsibilities do health care professionals, including medical assistants, have regarding the misuse or abuse of legal or illegal drugs?

_____

_____

_____

_____

_____

_____

_____

Research Activities

The PDR is an invaluable resource and one of the most widely used publications in the medical industry. The annually updated publication is usually available in most clinics and medical offices. It provides medical professionals with practical information about thousands of medications and includes other useful data, such as lists of drugs new to the market and those that have been discontinued. It is essential that medical assistants become familiar with the publication and learn how to access the wealth of information stored within.

1. Use the PDR to locate the pertinent information for each of the following scenarios. Then identify the drug's source or method of production.

   A. Herb Fowler, Dr. Winston Lewis's patient, calls to report he is experiencing nausea, a symptom he believes may be a negative reaction to the Chronulac Syrup® Dr. Lewis recently prescribed for Herb's chronic constipation. Using the PDR, locate the following information:

Chronulac Syrup's generic name: _____

The sugar that Chronulac Syrup contains is _____

Identify the drug's source or method of production: _____

B. Another patient of Dr. Lewis's, Michael Zamboni, has recently been diagnosed with insulin-dependent type II diabetes. Dr. Lewis prescribes Humulin®. Using the PDR, find the following information: Humulin's® generic name: _____

The source from which Humulin® is derived: _____

Identify the drug's source or method of production: _____

C. Susan Marshall, a new patient of Dr. Elizabeth King, acquired a high-pressure job about 1 month ago. Recently, she has been reporting an upset stomach, which has been attributed to her stressful job and poor eating habits. Dr. King orders prescription-strength Pepcid® for Susan. Using the PDR, locate the following information:

Pepcid's® generic name: _____

Pepcid's® active ingredient: _____

Identify the drug's source or method of production: _____

2. Camille Saunders, another patient of Dr. King, has been taking Ortho Tri-Cyclen®, an oral contraceptive, for 6 months. It has just been discovered that Camille has epilepsy. Using the PDR, locate the following information:

A. Does Ortho Tri-Cyclen® have any known contraindications to any drugs used in the treatment of epilepsy, and if so, which drugs?

_____

_____

B. Identify the drug's source or method of production.

_____

_____

CHAPTER POST-TEST

Perform this test without looking at your book.

1. Hybrid forms of life have been created that benefit human beings by providing an alternative source of drugs; an example is:

   a. ibuprofen

   b. interferon

   c. digitalis

   d. epinephrine

2. If the symbol ® follows a drug name, no other manufacturer can make or sell the drug for:

   a. 7 years

   b. 10 years

   c. 20 years

   d. 17 years

3. One compound extracted from the adrenal gland of animals and used therapeutically is:

   a. cortisone

   b. acetaminophen

   c. insulin

   d. piroxician

4. Those drugs with a potential for abuse and dependency are monitored by the:

   a. FDA

   b. AAMA

   c. DEA

   d. CDC

5. An inventory record of Schedule II drugs must be submitted to appropriate authorities every:

   a. 2 years

   b. 1 year

   c. 5 years

   d. 7 years

6. The medication Isuprel is used to treat:

   a. seizures

   b. allergies

   c. heart block

   d. diabetic coma

7. The _____ name describes the drug's molecular structure and identifies its chemical structure.

   a. chemical

   b. trade

   c. generic

   d. brand

8. Schedule _____ drugs have low-to-moderate potential for physical dependence.

   a. I

   b. II

   c. III

   d. IV

9. An agent that prevents or relieves cough is classified as:

   a. expectorant

   b. antipsychotic

   c. antitussive

   d. laxative

10. Medications for respiratory diseases such as asthma may require direct delivery of medications using which method:

    a. transdermal

    b. inhalation

    c. rectal

    d. eye-curing lens

SELF-ASSESSMENT

Organize your medicine cabinet. Or, with permission, organize the medicine cabinet of a close family member.

1. First, determine which drugs are out of date and destroy them properly.

   _____

   _____

   _____

   _____

2. Next, determine which drugs are no longer being prescribed, but rather are basically "left over" from a previous illness.

   _____

   _____

   _____

   _____

3. Make a decision. Should those leftover drugs be disposed of, or was it the intention of the provider for those medications to be available to you (or your family member) in the future? If they are not to be used in the future, dispose of them properly.

   _____

   _____

   _____

   _____

4. Separate the OTC drugs from the prescription drugs. Organize the OTC medications into categories of actions (the analgesics together, cough and cold medicines together, etc.).

   _____

   _____

   _____

   _____

5. If you (or your family member) are on a long-term drug therapy, make up a medicine card to be carried with you (or your family member) at all times. On the card, list the drug, strength, and dosage. Place this card in your wallet or purse (or that of your family member), so the medicine list is available at all times. Keep the list updated as prescriptions change.

   _____

   _____

   _____

   _____

CHAPTER **36**

Calculation of Medication Dosage and Medication Administration

CHAPTER PRE-TEST

Perform this test without looking at your book.

1. When prescribing for an adult, the age range generally considered "adult" is:
   a. 15 to 40 years
   b. 20 to 60 years
   c. 25 to 80 years
   d. 20 to 45 years

2. The abbreviation for grains is:
   a. gr
   b. GR
   c. Gr
   d. any of the above

3. One microgram is equal to _____ milligram(s).
   a. 0.01
   b. 0.001
   c. 0.0001
   d. 1000

4. Insulin-dependent diabetes is termed:
   a. Type I
   b. Type II
   c. Gestational
   d. Diabetes insipidus

5. Which of the following insulins have the most rapid onset?
   a. Humalog
   b. Humulin R
   c. Lente L
   d. Humulin 70/30

6. One of the most accurate methods for calculating dosage for infants and children up to 12 years of age uses:
   a. Weight
   b. BMI
   c. Kilograms
   d. BSA

7. Guidelines for the administration of medications include:
   a. It is acceptable to administer a medication that has become cloudy.
   b. If you are busy, it is allowable for your co-worker to administer a medication that you have prepared.
   c. Always check the expiration date on a medication that is to be given.
   d. If a medication is dropped, it is still permissible to administer the medication.

8. Disadvantages to oral medication are:
   a. Irritation of the stomach
   b. Easy absorption by the digestive tract
   c. Discoloration of the teeth
   d. a and c

9. Injections should be avoided in which areas?
   a. Burns
   b. Inflamed areas
   c. Previous injection sites
   d. All of the above

10. Rapid response to a medication can be expected with which method of administration?
    a. Oral
    b. Intravenous
    c. Intramuscular
    d. b and c

VOCABULARY BUILDER

Misspelled Words

Find the words below that are misspelled, underline them, and correctly spell them in the spaces provided. Then fill in the blanks in the sentences below with the correct vocabulary term.

administer	hypoxemia	precipitate
apnea	meniskis	taut
body surface area	namogram	unit dose
dispense	parentral	

_____   _____   _____

1. The absence of breathing is termed _____.

2. _____ is a highly accurate method for calculating medication dosages for infants and children up to 12 years of age.

3. A lack of oxygen in the blood is _____.

4. The convex or concave upper surface of a column of liquid in a container is known as the _____.

5. A _____ is a graph that shows the relationship among numerical values; an estimate of body surface area (BSA) of a patient can be determined by using a nomogram.

6. The term _____ describes a route other than the alimentary canal for injection of a liquid substance into the body.

7. _____ is a substance in the form of fine particles that separates from a solution that is allowed to stand for a period of time.

8. Stretch the skin _____, pulling it tight, when giving an intramuscular injection.

9. A _____ is a premeasured amount of medication, individually packaged on a per dose basis.

LEARNING REVIEW

Short Answer

1. Identify the following measures as weight (W) or volume (V). Then name the measure each abbreviation stands for and what system of measurement it belongs to. The first row has been completed as an example for you.

Weight	Volume	Abbreviation	Measure	System
		g	Gram	Metric
		tbsp	_____	_____
		mL	_____	_____
		qt	_____	_____
		gtt	_____	_____
		µg	_____	_____

2. Perform the following conversions:
   a. 4 tsp = ____ mL
   b. 7 kg = ____ lb
   c. 3.5 in. = ____ cm
   d. 1,200 mg = ____ g
   e. 8 mL = ____ gtt

3. What are proportions? How are proportions useful in calculating dosages of medication?

_____

_____

_____

_____

_____

4. Identify the type of syringe typically used for each of the following; list the size and calibration as well.

Purpose	Type	Size	Calibration
Venipuncture	_____	_____	_____
Insulin administration	_____	_____	_____
Allergy testing	_____	_____	_____

5. For each syringe-needle combination below, identify the most likely parenteral route: subcutaneous injection (SC), intramuscular injection (IM), or intradermal injection (ID). Also identify the proper angle of injection.

	Route	Angle of Injection
3-mL syringe/22-G, 1½-inch needle	_____	_____
1-mL syringe/25-G, ¾-inch needle	_____	_____
U-100 (1 mL)/26-G, ½-inch needle	_____	_____
3-mL syringe/25-G, ¾-inch needle	_____	_____

CERTIFICATION REVIEW

These questions are designed to mimic the certification examination. Select the best response.

1. The hard copy of a prescription is filed and kept for a minimum of:
   a. 10 years
   b. 7 years
   c. 5 years
   d. indefinitely

2. The portion of the prescription that gives directions to the patient is called the:
   a. superscription
   b. inscription
   c. subscription
   d. signature

3. The metric prefix that refers to 1,000 units is:
   a. kilo-
   b. milli-
   c. micro-
   d. deca-

4. Dosage of insulin is always measured in:
   a. cubic centimeters
   b. milliliters
   c. units
   d. milliequivalents

5. The hollow core of a needle is called the:
   a. bevel
   b. gauge
   c. lumen
   d. hilt

6. The following is a part of a syringe:
   a. barrel
   b. hub
   c. plunger
   d. a and c

7. A potential hazard of medication administration by intramuscular injection is:
   a. injury to bone, nerve, or blood vessel
   b. breaking of the needle
   c. injecting into a blood vessel
   d. all of the above

8. The gentle pulling back on the plunger of the syringe to assure the needle tip is not in a blood vessel is called:
   a. injection
   b. aspiration
   c. instillation
   d. infusion

9. A disposable plastic tube that has small holes to be inserted in the nares is called:
   a. mask
   b. nasal cannula
   c. nasal catheter
   d. trach

10. Medications that are irritating to the tissues should be injected using what method?
    a. Intramuscular
    b. Slow
    c. Z-track
    d. Subcutaneous

LEARNING APPLICATION

Critical Thinking

1. Describe the process to follow to determine the state law regarding a medical assistant administering medications.

   _____

   _____

   _____

2. What is a medication order? Describe its purpose.

   _____

   _____

   _____

   _____

   _____

   _____

   _____

   _____

   _____

   _____

3. Name and describe factors that can affect medication dosage. Explain why and how the dosage is affected.

   _____

4. Name two methods used to calculate pediatric dosages of medication.

   _____

   _____

   _____

5. List and describe the "six rights".

   _____

6. A fellow student tells you that she accidentally gave a patient the incorrect dose of medication. Explain in detail what should be done.

   _____

   _____

   _____

   _____

   _____

   _____

7. You accidentally stick yourself with a contaminated needle. What are the correct steps to take?

   _____

   _____

   _____

Calculation Problems

1. Calculate the following dosages according to body surface area (BSA):

   a. If the adult dose of E.E.S. tabs is 400 mg every 6 hours, what is the dosage for a child who is 35 inches tall and weighs 28 lb (BSA 0.57)?

   _____

   _____

   _____

   _____

   _____

   _____

   b. If the adult dose of penicillin V potassium, USP, is 250 mg every 6 to 8 hours, what is the dosage for a child who is 24 inches tall and weighs 35 lb (BSA 0.56)?

   _____

   _____

   _____

   _____

   _____

   _____

2. Calculate the following dosages according to kilogram of body weight:

   a. The provider orders Augmentin 20 mg/kg/day for Sally Whitney, who weighs 72 pounds. The dose is to be divided and given every 8 hours. What is the total dose? What is the dose to be given every 8 hours?

      _____

      _____

      _____

      _____

      _____

      _____

   b. The provider orders Cefadyl 40 mg/kg for George Kipperley, who weighs 78 lb. The dosage is to be divided into four equal doses. What is the total dosage? What is the amount to be given in four equal doses?

      _____

      _____

      _____

      _____

      _____

      _____

      _____

      _____

3. The provider orders 125 mg Diamox. On hand you have 250 mg tablets. How many tablets will you give to your patient?

      _____

      _____

      _____

      _____

      _____

      _____

4. The provider orders 250 mg of Tagamet liquid. On hand you have 300 mg/5 mL. How many milliliters will you give?

      _____

      _____

      _____

      _____

      _____

      _____

      _____

Case Studies

CASE STUDY

Louise Kipperley comes to the urgent care center at Inner City Health Care when she experiences the third severe migraine headache in only 1 month. The headache has lasted 2 days, and Louise has experienced symptoms of nausea and vomiting. Dr. Rice gives written orders to administer Imitrex 25 mg IM stat, together with a prescription for the patient to fill and use at home. Liz Corbin, CMA (AAMA), makes a medicine card from the provider's order sheet of Louise's medical record and prepares the STAT dosage for Louise according to the correct procedure for administering oral medications. Liz is about to transport the medication to Louise in examination room 3 when she reads the provider's order for Louise, which calls for 25 mg IM STAT. The written prescription is for Imitrex every 4 hours as needed. Liz discards the dosage she has prepared for the patient and instead gives Louise Dr. Rice's prescription and tells her to have it filled immediately.

CASE STUDY REVIEW QUESTIONS

1. What medication error has Liz made? What effect will the error likely have on the patient?

_____

_____

_____

_____

2. What should Liz have done? What standard procedures should be followed when a medication error occurs?

_____

_____

_____

_____

_____

_____

_____

Reading Prescriptions

1. A prescription is a written legal document that gives directions for compounding, dispensing, and administering to a patient. Refer to the prescriptions shown below, and in the spaces provided, "decode" the prescriptions into layperson's terms and answer the questions that follow.

_____

_____

_____

_____

Dr. King prescribes an adult dosage for epilepsy.

Dr. Lewis prescribes a child's dosage for an ear infection.

```
┌─────────────────────────────────────┐
│  ◆L&K◆   LEWIS & KING, MD            │
│          2501 CENTER STREET          │
│          NORTHBOROUGH, OH 12345      │
│  ═══════════════════════════════     │
│  Name      Lourdes Austin            │
│  Address 821 Spring Lane, Apt. 12    │
│                        Date 3/1/XX   │
│  ℞                                    │
│  Dilantin      100 mg      tab       │
│  #90                                 │
│  Sig   100 mg   p.o.  tid            │
│                                      │
│  Generic Substitution Allowed        │
│          Susan King           M.D.   │
│  Dispense As Written _____ M.D.  │
│  REFILL 0 1 2 3 p.r.n.               │
│  [✓] LABEL                           │
└─────────────────────────────────────┘
```
© Cengage Learning 2014

```
┌─────────────────────────────────────┐
│  ◆L&K◆   LEWIS & KING, MD            │
│          2501 CENTER STREET          │
│          NORTHBOROUGH, OH 12345      │
│  ═══════════════════════════════     │
│  Name      Felicia Lawrence          │
│  Address 362 Owen's View Way         │
│                        Date 3/1/XX   │
│  ℞                                    │
│  Amoxicillin   250 mg/5 mL.          │
│  #150 mL                             │
│  Sig   500 mg   p.o.  tid            │
│                                      │
│  Generic Substitution Allowed        │
│          Winston Lewis        M.D.   │
│  Dispense As Written _____ M.D.  │
│  REFILL 0 1 2 3 p.r.n.               │
│  [✓] LABEL                           │
└─────────────────────────────────────┘
```
© Cengage Learning 2014

2. How many grams are in each dose of Dilantin? _____

3. How many days of Dilantin are dispensed? _____

4. How many teaspoons are in 5 mL? _____

5. How many doses of amoxicillin are included in the amount dispensed? _____

Web Activities

1. Search for a website to explore the various types of safety needles available for injection and venipuncture. What is the most recent ruling by OSHA in regard to safety needles?

2. Check the website http://www.cerner.com and search for the following:
   a. What is the most common medication error?
   b. Which group of medical professionals makes the most medication errors?
   c. How can medication errors be prevented?

3. Use the Google search engine and enter Top 10 Medication Errors and how to prevent them. List the errors and the keys to prevention.

4. Practice calculations of medications at the following sites:
   a. http://publichealth.lacounty.gov/phn/medication%20exam.htm
   b. http://www.dosagehelp.com/practice-questions

CHAPTER POST-TEST

Perform this test without looking at your book.

1. An intramuscular injection is given at what angle?
   a. 15 degrees
   b. 30 degrees
   c. 45 degrees
   d. 90 degrees

2. The abbreviation for intravenous is:
   a. IM
   b. IV
   c. INV
   d. IRQ

3. Pharmacokinetics is defined as:
   a. the average dosage of a drug
   b. the way the drug is handled by the body
   c. the indications for administration of a medication
   d. the half-life of a medication

4. Approximately _____ of the drugs approved by the FDA are indicated for pediatric use.
   a. ⅛
   b. ¼
   c. ½
   d. ¾

5. One kilogram is equal to _____ pound(s).
   a. 1
   b. 2.2
   c. 3.5
   d. 4.2

6. Precautions when administering insulin include which of the following?
   a. One insulin may be substituted for another.
   b. Check the label for the name and type of insulin.
   c. Store at room temperature.
   d. Always shake the insulin to mix.

7. The nine parts of a prescription include:
   a. drug name
   b. allergies of the patient
   c. dose
   d. a and c

8. The medical abbreviation pc indicates:

   a. before meals

   b. after meals

   c. at bedtime

   d. by mouth

9. A medication error might be which of the following?

   a. Drug given to the wrong patient

   b. Incorrect drug given

   c. Drug given at the incorrect time

   d. Any of the above

10. The point, the lumen, and the bevel are components of:

   a. a syringe

   b. a needle

   c. a sharps container

   d. none of the above

SELF-ASSESSMENT

1. Have you ever been given a shot? Do you remember how you felt just before the injection? Most people are more afraid of the pain of the injection than anything having to do with the medication. Do you think there are ways you can behave that will help your fearful patients feel less afraid? What could you do or say to alleviate their fears? Do you think only children are afraid of needles? Write down a couple of things you will do and say to help your patients. Discuss your ideas with a few classmates and listen to their ideas.

   _____

   _____

   _____

   _____

   _____

C H A P T E R **37**

Electrocardiography

CHAPTER PRE-TEST

Perform this test without looking at your book.

1. The abbreviation MI indicates:
   a. Mental illness
   b. Myocardial infarction
   c. Heart attack
   d. b or c

2. The _____ divides into the left and right bundle branch fibers.
   a. Purkinje fibers
   b. sinoatrial node
   c. bundle of His
   d. atrioventricular node

3. Blood that has been circulated through the body and returned to the right atrium is _____ blood.
   a. oxygenated
   b. deoxygenated
   c. arterial
   d. anticoagulated

4. Contraction of the ventricles is reflected in the _____ on an ECG.
   a. P wave
   b. R wave
   c. QRS Complex
   d. ST segment

5. The _____ detect the electrical impulses on the body surface.
   a. leads
   b. channels
   c. sensors
   d. galvanometer

6. Limb electrodes that record simultaneously are called _____ leads.
   a. augmented
   b. sensored
   c. bipolar
   d. precordial

7. Leads placed on the chest wall are known as _____ leads.
   a. augmented
   b. sensored
   c. bipolar
   d. precordial

8. _____ lead is placed at the fourth intercostal space at the right margin of the sternum.
   a. V_1
   b. V_2
   c. V_3
   d. V_4

9. Muscle tremor is a type of artifact that is also known as _____.
   a. involuntary
   b. voluntary
   c. somatic
   d. stable

10. An ECG that reflects a normal tracing in all parameters demonstrates a rhythm called:
    a. Atrial fibrillation
    b. Normal sinus rhythm
    c. PVC
    d. Asystole

VOCABULARY BUILDER

Misspelled Words

From the following terms, find the misspelled words, underline them, and spell them correctly in the spaces provided. Then, fill in the blanks in the sentences below.

amplytude   deoxygenated   electrocardiography
cardiac catheterization   diastole   Halter monitor
cardiac cycle   electrocardigraph   isoelectic
defibrilation

_____   _____   _____

_____   _____

1. _____ blood enters the right side of the heart.

2. The entire route of the electrical impulses through the heart is referred to as the _____.

3. _____ refers to the height of the ECG tracing.

4. Using an AED to restore a regular heart rhythm is called _____.

5. The _____ is a machine used to perform the ECG procedure.

6. The _____ line is another name for the baseline on an ECG tracing.

7. The word for the lowest amount of pressure on the vessel during a blood pressure reading is _____.

8. Ultrasonography and _____ are noninvasive diagnostic procedures commonly used in the clinical setting.

9. The study of the coronary arteries using a radiopaque medium is called a _____.

10. A _____ is utilized to record heart rate and rhythm for a 24-hour period.

LEARNING REVIEW

Short answer

1. List five reasons why electrocardiography is performed.

   _____

   _____

   _____

   _____

   _____

2. The first three leads recorded on a standard ECG are lead I, lead II, and lead III. These leads are called _____ leads because each of them uses two-limb electrodes that record simultaneously. For each lead, what electrical activity of the heart is recorded? Draw it on each figure.

Lead I   Lead II   Lead III

© Cengage Learning 2014

3. Fill in the blanks:
   a. Lead I records electrical activity between the _____ and the _____.
   b. Lead II records electrical activity between the _____ and the _____.
   c. Lead III records electrical activity between the _____ and the _____.

4. The next group of leads recorded on a standard ECG are augmented leads, designated aV$_R$, aV$_L$, and aV$_F$. These are called _____ leads. For each lead, what electrical activity of the heart is recorded? Draw it on each figure.

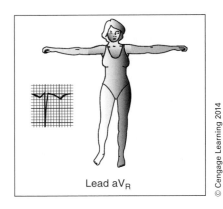

Lead aV$_R$

© Cengage Learning 2014

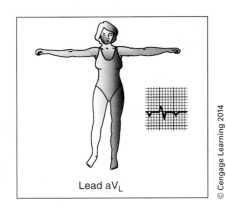

Lead aV$_L$

© Cengage Learning 2014

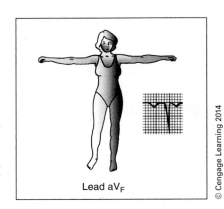

Lead aV$_F$

© Cengage Learning 2014

5. Fill in the blanks:

   a. Lead aV$_R$ records electrical activity from the _____ and the

   _____.

   b. Lead aV$_L$ records electrical activity from the _____ and the

   _____.

   c. Lead aV$_F$ records electrical activity from the _____ and the

   _____.

6. The remaining 6 leads of the standard 12-lead ECG are called the chest leads, or _____ leads. These leads are (*circle the correct one*) unipolar/bipolar. Where are the leads placed on the body?

   V$_1$: _____

   V$_2$: _____

   V$_3$: _____

   V$_4$: _____

   V$_5$: _____

   V$_6$: _____

Identifying Artifact Activity

Artifacts are unusual and unwanted activity in the ECG tracing not caused by the electrical activity of the heart. Match each circumstance below to the artifact ECG tracing it would produce and identify the type of artifact in the space provided.

A. A broken patient cable or lead wire has become detached from an electrode.

B. The patient sings to himself during the ECG procedure.

C. The patient uses body lotion.

D. The lead wires are crossed and do not follow the patient's body contour.

	Type of Artifact	**Circumstance**
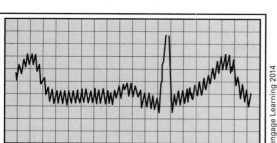		
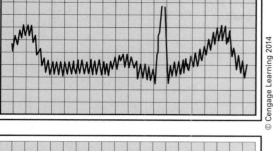		
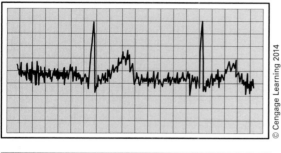		
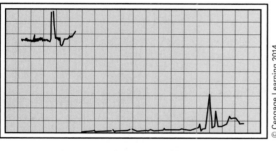		

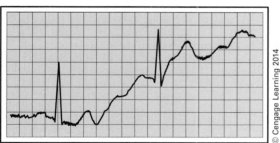

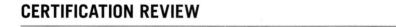

CERTIFICATION REVIEW

These questions are designed to mimic the certification examination. Select the best response.

1. Repolarization takes place while the heart muscle:

   a. contracts

   b. stops

   c. skips a beat

   d. relaxes

2. Chest leads are also called _____ leads.

   a. precordial

   b. limb

   c. augmented

   d. bipolar

3. Augmented leads are also called:

   a. unipolar

   b. bipolar

   c. precordial

   d. standard

4. One millivolt of cardiac electrical activity will deflect the stylus exactly:

   a. 5 mm high

   b. 10 mm high

   c. 25 mm high

   d. 40 mm high

5. A wandering baseline may be caused by:

   a. lotions, creams, or oils on the patient's skin

   b. electrical interference

   c. crossed lead wires

   d. improper grounding

6. Symptoms of syncope, fatigue, chest pain, and vertigo might indicate:

   a. influenza

   b. cardiac arrhythmia

   c. dehydration

   d. defibrillation

7. A surgical procedure that takes a portion of a vein and grafts it to a coronary artery is called:

   a. stenting

   b. angioplasty

   c. bypass

   d. merging

8. Interference with the ECG tracing from other electrical sources is called:

   a. wandering baseline

   b. AC interference

   c. arrhythmia

   d. somatic tremor

9. A life-threatening arrhythmia in which the ventricles contract wildly is:

   a. premature ventricular contractions

   b. ventricular fibrillation

   c. ventricular tachycardia

   d. all of the above

10. A continuous record of cardiac activity is provided by:

    a. ECG

    b. Holter monitor

    c. defibrillator

    d. cardioversion

LEARNING APPLICATION

Critical Thinking

1. The provider wants you to explain to Mrs. Johnson (see Case Study 2) what behaviors she can adopt to have a healthy heart. With a partner, role-play medical assistant and patient and explain to the patient what she can do to improve her heart's health.

   _____

   _____

   _____

   _____

2. Name four cardiac abnormalities that can be diagnosed using an ECG.

   _____

   _____

   _____

3. Identify the placement of the leads for a 12-lead ECG.

   _____

   _____

   _____

   _____

   _____

   _____

   _____

   _____

   _____

   _____

   _____

   _____

   _____

   _____

   _____

4. If a patient coughs or talks during an ECG. What effect with this have on the tracing?

   _____

   _____

   _____

Case Studies

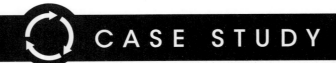

Jim Marshall, a prominent local architect in his late 30s, stays in good physical condition, works out regularly at the gym, and maintains a low-fat, low-cholesterol, low-sodium diet. Aggressive and ambitious, Jim enjoys pushing his mind and body to the limit. His favorite sports are skiing and sailing. At work, Jim is a perfectionist who puts in long hours and demands the same of his employees. Lately, though, Jim is more aware of the high-stress lifestyle he is leading and is worried about his family history of heart failure and diabetes. During periods of high physical exertion, Jim experiences mild chest pain and palpitations. Dr. Lewis prescribes an exercise tolerance test for Jim.

CASE STUDY REVIEW QUESTIONS

1. What is an exercise tolerance test? How is it performed?

_____

_____

_____

_____

_____

_____

2. Under what conditions would the test be discontinued?

_____

_____

_____

3. At the conclusion of the test, what patient care is given? What special instructions for home care should the patient observe?

_____

_____

_____

Web Activities

Search the Internet for a national organization that focuses on heart and blood vessel disorders such as the American Heart Association or the American College of Cardiology.

1. Print information about risk factors for cardiovascular heart disease.

2. What is the mortality rate for first-time myocardial infarctions for men versus women? Is there any difference in the mortality rate?

3. Are the symptoms identical in male and female patients when they are experiencing a myocardial infarction? Explain the similarities/differences between them.

4. Determine if there are newer types of 24-hour cardiac monitoring devices. How are they the same or different from the Holter monitor?

CHAPTER POST-TEST

Perform this test without looking at your book.

1. Oxygenated blood returns from the lungs and flows from the pulmonary veins into:
   a. the right atrium
   b. the left atrium
   c. the right ventricle
   d. the left ventricle

2. Tachycardia is defined as a heart rate greater than _____ bpm.
   a. 50
   b. 75
   c. 100
   d. 125

3. A 12-lead ECG is called such because:
   a. there are 12 lead wires
   b. there are 12 sensors
   c. it produces 12 views of the electroconduction of the heart
   d. none of the above

4. Voltage is changed into mechanical motion by the _____ in the ECG machine.
   a. stylus
   b. lead wire
   c. sensor
   d. galvanometer

5. Because the skin is a poor conductor of electricity, a(n) _____ substance is applied with each electrode.
   a. electrolyte
   b. adhesive
   c. amplified
   d. viscous

6. Augmented limb leads are:
   a. aVR
   b. aVL
   c. aVF
   d. all of the above

7. Health heart behaviors include:
   a. eating a low-fat diet
   b. using tobacco
   c. rest and sleep
   d. a and c

8. Treatment of life-threatening arrhythmias can be delivered using a(n) _____ to deliver countershocks.

   a. electrocardiograph

   b. defibrillator

   c. galvanometer

   d. ultrasound

9. A device that is surgically implanted to provide a regular, steady heartbeat is:

   a. venous filter

   b. AID

   c. pacemaker

   d. transducer

10. A _____ stress test is one in which the patient exercises on a treadmill after injection of a radioactive substance.

    a. thallium

    b. barium

    c. nitrous oxide

    d. bismuth

SELF-ASSESSMENT

Keep a strict diary of everything you eat and drink for the next 3 days (a week is better).

1. Count up the total fats you have eaten each day.

   _____

   _____

   _____

   _____

2. Separate the types of fats and total each type for each day.

   _____

   _____

   _____

   _____

3. Go online and use search words such as "saturated fats" or "trans fats" to learn more about the different fats.

   _____

   _____

   _____

   _____

4. Find out about omega-3 fatty acids. Are you eating enough? How could you take in more?

_____

_____

_____

_____

5. What else should you be doing to stay "heart healthy"?

_____

_____

_____

_____

C H A P T E R **38**

Regulatory Guidelines in the Medical Laboratory

CHAPTER PRE-TEST

Perform this test without looking at your book.

1. "Aegis" means:
   a. Sponsorship or protection
   b. The part of the laboratory sample that is discarded
   c. A reagent or chemical used in laboratory tests
   d. A region or area of concern

2. Quality control is a way of:
   a. Ensuring that the chemicals or reagents used are of good quality
   b. Ensuring the test is run correctly
   c. Ensuring that the patient sample is stored correctly
   d. All of the above

3. MSDS stands for:
   a. Material Safety Data Sheet
   b. Manual for Safety Documents/Sheets
   c. Mandated Standards for Documentation and Safety
   d. Manual of Supplies and Data for Safety

4. MSDS information must be:
   a. Read by all employees
   b. Indexed and alphabetized in a notebook or manual
   c. Made readily available to all employees
   d. All of the above

5. Which federal agency enforces regulations requiring the labeling of hazardous materials?
   a. CDC
   b. EPA
   c. NFPA
   d. OSHA

6. All of the following laboratory tests are PPMP levels of testing except:

    a. Urine sediment examinations

    b. Qualitative semen analysis

    c. Urine pregnancy test

    d. Wet mount preparations

7. CLIA certification for laboratories must be recertified:

    a. Every year

    b. Every 2 years

    c. Every 3 years

    d. Every 5 years

8. Records of test results reported within the laboratory are to be retained:

    a. 2 years

    b. 5 years

    c. 10 years

    d. Indefinitely

9. The blue color in the NFPA labeling system signifies what type of hazard?

    a. Reactivity hazard

    b. Health hazard

    c. Flammability hazard

    d. Hazard requiring use of PPE

10. The chemical warning label does not include:

    a. Manufacturer's name

    b. Chemical names

    c. Common name

    d. Product distributor

VOCABULARY BUILDER

Misspelled Words

Correct the spelling of the following terms and then define each term in the space provided.

1. Body flued _____ _____

    _____

    _____

2. Comunicible _____ _____

3. Excresion _____ _____

Matching

Match each of the vocabulary terms below with the correct definition in Column B.

Column A

____ 1. Spill kit

____ 2. Standards

____ 3. Proficiency testing

____ 4. Waived

____ 5. Fume hood

____ 6. *Federal Register*

____ 7. Calibration

____ 8. Requisition

____ 9. Mandate

____ 10. Quality control

Column B

A. Rules set up and established to measure quality, weight, extent, or value

B. The determination of the accuracy of an instrument by comparing the information provided with an accepted standard known to be accurate

C. Used to describe a category of clinical laboratory tests that are simple and unvarying and require a minimum of judgment and interpretation

D. Measures used to monitor the processing of laboratory specimens

E. Commercially packaged materials containing supplies and equipment needed to clean a biohazard spill

F. Formal order to obey certain rules and regulations

G. A written request for laboratory analysis to be performed on a specimen

H. A barrier used in the laboratory to capture chemical vapors

I. Federal agency from which written CLIA '88 documents may be obtained

J. Sample tests performed in a clinical laboratory to determine that a specific degree of accuracy is achieved

LEARNING REVIEW

Short answer

1. CLIA '88 requires that every facility that tests human specimens for diagnosis, treatment, and prevention of disease meet specific federal requirements. Name five specific duties a medical assistant may perform that will make an impact on the medical facility's compliance with CLIA '88 regulations.

_____

_____

_____

_____

_____

_____

2. To comply with OSHA regulations, chemicals must be labeled using the color and number symbols of the National Fire Protection Association (NFPA). Match the symbolic colors below to the type of hazard each signifies.

____ Blue   1. Fire

____ White   2. Reactivity

____ Yellow   3. Use of personal protective equipment (PPE)

____ Red   4. Health hazard

3. How does CLIA regulate quality control of automated hematology instruments?

_____

_____

_____

4. What are the three categories of testing? List three examples from the waived category.

_____

_____

_____

5. Describe the CMS 116 Form and explain its purpose.

_____

_____

_____

6. What are some personal safety precautions established by OSHA?

_____

_____

_____

7. Why are MSDS important?

_____

_____

_____

8. Name some unsafe working conditions and safety techniques that can be used to prevent accidents.

_____

_____

_____

CERTIFICATION REVIEW

These questions are designed to mimic the certification examination. Select the best response.

1. CLIA was passed in an effort to:
   a. teach staff how to read test results accurately
   b. establish standards to ensure the confidentiality of test results
   c. establish standards to ensure accurate test results
   d. all of the above

2. CLIA was passed in what year?
   a. 1902
   b. 1975
   c. 1988
   d. 1999

3. Which of the following procedures is a requirement of qualifying protocol for automated hematology instruments?
   a. Control samples
   b. Proficiency testing
   c. Calibration
   d. All of the above

4. Material Safety Data Sheets (MSDSs) do *not* contain:
   a. product/chemical information
   b. emergency response procedures
   c. manufacturer information
   d. training information for using the product/chemical

5. When skin comes into contact with chemicals, it is best to:

   a. wash the area with water immediately

   b. apply a neutralizing agent to the site

   c. consult the MSDS before treatment

   d. rinse area with vinegar

6. Which federal agency oversees the safety of health facilities including protection against occupational hazards such as BBPs?

   a. OSHA

   b. CLIA'88

   c. FDA

   d. CDC

7. Waived tests used in the medical facility are all of the following except?

   a. Urine glucose dipstick

   b. Pregnancy test

   c. QuickVue Strep test

   d. KOH preparations

8. Which profession obtains specific formal training in waived category testing procedures?

   a. Physicians

   b. Registered nurses

   c. Medical technicians

   d. Medical assistants

9. If any lab changes the tests performed, the lab must contact the CMS within what amount of time?

   a. 1 year

   b. 2 years

   c. 6 years

   d. 12 years

10. What regulating agency approves the proficiency programs that medical facilities are to be enrolled in?

    a. OSHA

    b. DHHS

    c. CMS

    d. FDA

LEARNING APPLICATION

Critical Thinking

1. Explain the purpose of CLIA '88 and why the law was amended.

   _____

   _____

   _____

2. Describe quality control and quality assurance. Why are they important?

_____

_____

_____

3. You have been asked to develop a manual for your provider–employer. The manual is to detail a chemical hygiene plan (CHP) for all employees in the office. How would you proceed? What should be included in the plan? In the CHP include three major goals that will ensure the provider–employer's compliance with the hazard standard.

_____

_____

_____

_____

_____

_____

_____

_____

_____

_____

_____

_____

_____

_____

_____

_____

4. You have been asked to compile a manual of the MSDSs. What must be included in the manual and from where does the information come?

_____

_____

_____

_____

_____

_____

_____

_____

_____

_____

Web Activities

1. Using the Internet, go to http://www.cms.hhs.gov and search for the list of CLIA waived tests. Is this list extensive/brand specific or general?

2. Go into the FDA's website at http://www.fda.gov and see if the list of CLIA waived tests on that site differs. What do you think is the reason for the lists being different or the same?

3. While you are searching those two websites, find out what language(s) is acceptable for labels on hazardous chemicals.

4. Go to the CDC website at http://www.cdc.gov/mmwr and find the report on Good Laboratory Practices. Find the seven important criteria to be considered before introducing a new waived test.

CHAPTER POST-TEST

1. "Aegis" means:
   a. sponsorship or protection
   b. the part of the laboratory sample that is discarded
   c. a reagent or chemical used in laboratory tests
   d. a region or area of concern

2. Quality control is a way of:
   a. ensuring that the chemicals or reagents used are of good quality
   b. ensuring the test is run correctly
   c. ensuring that the patient sample is stored correctly
   d. all of the above

3. MSDS stands for:
   a. Material Safety Data Sheet
   b. Manual for Safety Documents/Sheets
   c. Mandated Standards for Documentation and Safety
   d. Manual of Supplies and Data for Safety

4. MSDS information must be:
   a. read by all employees
   b. indexed and alphabetized in a notebook or manual
   c. made readily available to all employees
   d. all of the above

5. Which federal agency that enforces regulations requiring the labeling of hazardous materials?
   a. CDC
   b. EPA
   c. NFPA
   d. OSHA

6. All of the following laboratory tests are PPMP levels of testing except:
   a. urine sediment examinations
   b. qualitative semen analysis
   c. urine pregnancy test
   d. wet mount preparations

7. CLIA certification for laboratories must be recertified:
   a. every year
   b. every 2 years
   c. every 3 years
   d. every 5 years

8. Records of test results reported within the laboratory are to be retained:
   a. 2 years
   b. 5 years
   c. 10 years
   d. indefinitely

9. The blue color in the NFPA labeling system signifies what type of hazard?

   a. Reactivity hazard

   b. Health hazard

   c. Flammability hazard

   d. Hazard requiring use of PPE

10. The chemical warning label does not include:

    a. manufacturer's name

    b. chemical names

    c. common name

    d. product distributor

SELF-ASSESSMENT

1. Choose a chemical you have at home or in the basement, garage, or storage area.

   _____

   _____

   _____

2. Look at the label.

   a. Does it have any precautionary statements or warnings?

   _____

   _____

   _____

   b. Does it have any fire hazard information?

   _____

   _____

   _____

3. Complete the following:

   Name of chemical (brand name) _____

   What chemicals are included in the active ingredients? _____

   What precautions are listed? _____

   What instructions are listed for contamination of eyes or skin, ingestion, and so forth? _____

   What is the number in your area for Poison Control? _____

CHAPTER **39**

Introduction to the Medical Laboratory

CHAPTER PRE-TEST

1. A urine culture would be performed in which department of a regional laboratory?
   a. Bacteriology department
   b. Urinalysis department
   c. Culture department
   d. Cytology department

2. Which of the following is a description of a panel
   a. Many tests all billed together at one time
   b. All the tests for one patient during one calendar year
   c. All the tests a doctor orders consistently throughout her or his practice
   d. A related set of tests about an organ, system, or function

3. A low-powered objective lens on a microscope allows the specimen to magnified to what size for viewing?
   a. 10 times larger than life
   b. 100 times larger than life
   c. 1000 times larger than life
   d. 10,000 times larger than life

4. What is the meaning of the medical abbreviation NPO?
   a. Patient is not to ingest any food for 12 hours
   b. Patient is not to ingest food or drink fluids for 12 hours
   c. Patient is not to drink fluids for 12 hours
   d. None of the above

5. Many clinics require that pending lab reports contained within the EMR are to be reviewed and signed by a provider within what length of time?

   a. 6–12 hours

   b. 12–24 hours

   c. 24–36 hours

   d. 36–48 hours

6. POCT testing is also called:

   a. Patient office care testing

   b. Bedside testing

   c. At home testing

   d. Pharmacy testing

7. During a physical examination, healthy or normal test results are also known as?

   a. Metabolic level

   b. Calibration level

   c. Reference values

   d. Starting results

8. If a TDM specimen is drawn 30 minutes after the last dosage of medication was given to a patient, what would you be testing for?

   a. Trough level

   b. Random level

   c. Peak level

   d. Toxicity

VOCABULARY BUILDER

Misspelled Words

Find the words below that are misspelled; circle them, and correctly spell them in the spaces provided.

assey	diagnosis	qualitative tests
baseline	differential diagnosis	quantative tests
biopsy	electrolites	reagents
clinical diagnosis	glucose	requisition
control test	invasive	serum

_____   _____   _____

Fill in the Blanks

From the list above, insert the correct vocabulary terms into the sentences below. Each sentence describes a situation you might find in a POL or in a reference laboratory.

1. Dr. Mark Woo orders laboratory tests for a female patient experiencing severe abdominal cramps in order to make a _____ that will distinguish between a diagnosis of appendicitis and a diagnosis of an ovarian cyst.

2. Richard Butts receives a job offer from a construction company that requires all employees to be tested for general overall health before they can work on the site. Bruce Goldman, CMA (AAMA), performs Richard's blood test under the direction of Dr. Whitney; his test comes back 'within normal limits'. The results of Richard's test can be used in the future as a _____ measurement, a record of healthy normal results.

3. Dr. King needs a red blood cell (RBC) count, a white blood cell (WBC) count, and a platelet count for Melinda Cool. Joe Guerrero, CMA (AAMA), performs a venipuncture on Melinda and sends a tube of her blood to the laboratory, together with a written _____ containing specific information and instructions about what tests to perform on the specimens.

4. Dr. Lewis asks Audrey Jones, CMA (AAMA), to send a tube of Herb Fowler's blood to the laboratory for analysis. Dr. Lewis wants to determine the constituents and relative proportion of each of the enzymes in Herb's serum; this type of analysis is called an _____.

5. Hematology laboratories count the WBCs or RBCs in a sample of a patient's blood. In general, these types of counting tests with numerical results are known as _____.

6. As a method of quality control, a _____ sample is tested together with a patient's sample as a method of ensuring the accuracy of test results.

7. Joe Guerrero, CMA (AAMA), asks Abigail Johnson, whom he knows is diagnosed with diabetes mellitus, whether she regularly tests her blood at home to measure her _____ level.

8. The hematology laboratory performs tests that measure characteristics of blood such as size, shape, and maturity of cells. These types of tests are known in general as _____.

9. Histology is the study of tissue samples to determine disease. In most cases, a tissue sample or _____ is frozen, sliced, stained, and microscopically examined for anomalies.

10. Most of the patient samples that Audrey Jones, CMA (AAMA), prepares to send to the laboratory are samples of _____, the liquid portion of blood obtained after blood has been allowed to clot or has been separated.

11. If a control sample shows inaccurate results after testing, one possible explanation is that the _____ are faulty or have expired.

12. Fine-needle aspiration is an _____ procedure used in a preliminary diagnosis of breast cancer; the test involves inserting a needle into the suspicious breast lump and extracting cells for analysis under a microscope.

13. A _____ of Lyme disease can be confirmed by performing laboratory tests on patient blood specimens.

14. Dr. Rice makes a _____ of asthma for patient Yuping Chen, based on subjective and objective information gathered after obtaining an in-depth patient history and performing a complete physical examination.

15. _____ are substances that split into electrically charged particles, or ions, when dissolved or melted. These electricity conductors are important in maintaining fluid and acid-base homeostasis in the body.

LEARNING REVIEW

Matching

Match each laboratory facility or department to the statement below that best describes it.

A. Reference laboratories

B. Clinical chemistry

C. Cytology

D. Hematology

E. Histology

F. Immunology/immunohematology

G. Hospital-based laboratories

H. Parasitology

I. Microbiology

J. Mycology

K. Physician's office laboratories (POLs)

L. Procurement stations

M. Urinalysis

_____ 1. This laboratory department performs blood typing procedures, cross-matching, and the separation and storage of blood components for transfusion, as well as antibody-antigen reactions.

_____ 2. This subdivision of the microbiology department detects the presence of disease-producing human parasites or ova present in patient specimens such as feces and blood.

_____ 3. Independent laboratories often have smaller satellites or these offices located near isolated medical facilities or in areas convenient to patients.

_____ 4. This laboratory department performs qualitative and quantitative tests on blood and blood components.

_____ 5. This subdivision of the microbiology department is where fungi are grown and identified.

_____ 6. These laboratories are independent, regionally located, and used by hospitals and providers for complex, expensive, or specialized tests.

_____ 7. Some procedures performed by this department include assays of enzymes in the serum, serum glucose, or electrolyte levels.

_____ 8. This laboratory department analyzes patient specimens for the presence of disease-producing microorganisms.

_____ 9. These laboratories perform medical laboratory tests easily and inexpensively in the office by the medical assistant.

_____ 10. These laboratories perform most of the tests required in inpatient settings and hospitals.

_____ 11. This is the microscopic study of the form and structure of the various tissues making up living organisms. Tissue analysis and biopsy studies are performed in this area of the laboratory.

_____ 12. This laboratory department performs microscopic examinations of cells to detect irregularities in growth and development.

_____ 13. This involves the physical, chemical, and microscopic examination of urine as a diagnostic tool for physicians.

Short Answer

1. Identify each abbreviated test named below.

Hgb	_____
Diff	_____
ESR	_____
Hct	_____
O&P	_____
C&S	_____

2. What is the most important patient preparation question that should be asked prior to obtaining a blood specimen for chemistry testing?

   _____

   _____

3. Name five tests commonly performed in a physician's office laboratory (POL).

   _____

   _____

4. Name three criteria that would justify using point-of-care testing.

   _____

   _____

5. The accuracy of any laboratory test result depends on the performance of quality controls by all health care workers who handle a specimen. Medical assistants must have a thorough knowledge of quality controls and standards. List five factors that can compromise the accuracy of laboratory test results.

   _____

   _____

   _____

   _____

6. What is the reason for using a control test sample? Explain in detail.

   _____

   _____

   _____

   _____

   _____

7. Knowing how to perform tasks safely is critical when working in a medical laboratory. Medical assistants must understand the different types of hazards present in a medical laboratory and know how to protect themselves and other health care professionals from possible harm.

   A. It is important to avoid ingestion or exposure to chemicals and pathogens. Name four ways this can be avoided.

      _____

      _____

      _____

      _____

B. What is the first action to take when a surface becomes contaminated?

_____

_____

C. Explain why it is important to avoid wearing loose clothing or accessories in the laboratory.

_____

_____

D. In terms of safety issues, why is it important to properly maintain laboratory equipment?

_____

_____

8. Name the five parts of a microscope.

_____

_____

9. What type of microscope is the most commonly used in a medical laboratory?

_____

_____

10. Name three other types of microscopes and explain what each is designed for viewing.

_____

_____

_____

11. Name the two adjustments found on a microscope and explain the purpose of each.

_____

_____

12. Name six practices that should always be followed to properly care for a microscope.

_____

_____

_____

_____

_____

_____

CERTIFICATION REVIEW

These questions are designed to mimic the certification examination. Select the best response.

1. Choosing to perform the simplest and least invasive procedure to rule out a particular disease before requiring more extensive testing is known as obtaining a:
   a. clinical diagnosis
   b. cumulative diagnosis
   c. developmental diagnosis
   d. differential diagnosis

2. _____ involve actual number counts such as are done in WBC counts, RBC counts, and platelet levels.
   a. Qualitative tests
   b. Quantitative tests
   c. CLIA waived tests
   d. Functional tests

3. The area of the clinical laboratory where organisms such as bacteria and fungi are grown and identified is called the:
   a. cytology department
   b. chemistry department
   c. microbiology department
   d. histology department

4. A hepatic function panel will include a:
   a. creatinine level
   b. rheumatoid factor
   c. cholesterol level
   d. bilirubin level

5. Analysis of abnormal tissue cells is performed in which department of the laboratory?
   a. Hematology
   b. Serology
   c. Microbiology
   d. Cytology

6. Which of the following panel tests are ordered for diagnostic testing on the liver?
   a. Hepatic function panel
   b. Arthritis panel
   c. Renal function panel
   d. Cholesterol screening panel

LEARNING APPLICATION

Critical Thinking

1. A patient asks you to recommend a laboratory for the tests ordered by the provider. How will you respond to the request? What are some factors that will influence your response?

_____

_____

_____

_____

2. A patient performed a pregnancy test at home, but her provider has requested a pregnancy test in the office. How will you explain to the patient why the home test may not be as accurate as the test performed in the office?

_____

_____

_____

_____

Case Studies

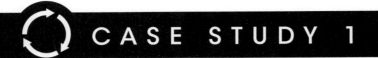

CASE STUDY 1

You come to work one morning to discover the electricity has gone off in the refrigerator in the laboratory. This refrigerator houses the reagents needed to perform the laboratory tests.

CASE STUDY REVIEW QUESTIONS

1. How will you proceed?

_____
_____
_____
_____
_____

2. Is there a way to determine whether or not the reagents are still acceptable?

_____
_____
_____

3. How could this have been prevented?

_____
_____
_____
_____
_____
_____

Hands-on Activity

At Abigail Johnson's annual physical examination on June 5, 20xx, at 2 PM, Dr. Elizabeth King orders several laboratory tests to monitor Abigail's diagnosed conditions of hypertension, diabetes mellitus, and moderate angina pectoris. Dr. Frank Jones, Abigail's cardiologist, will also receive a copy of the final laboratory report. Ellen Armstrong, CMA (AAMA), prepares the laboratory requisition form. Complete Ellen's laboratory requisition form for Abigail's laboratory work.

Patient:	Physicians:
Abigail Johnson	Dr. Elizabeth King
225 River Street	Northborough Family Medical Group
Northborough, OH 12336	2501 Center Street
Phone: 389-2631	Northborough, OH 12345
Date of Birth: March 1, 1940	Phone: 651-8000
Social Security Number: 011-11-1231	
Medicare #: 021-45-6712-D	Dr. Frank Jones
	815 Heart Health Blvd
	Northborough, OH 12339
	Phone: 655-7000

Physician's Order for Laboratory Testing: Blood panel to include BUN, chloride, cholesterol, creatinine, glucose, LDH, potassium, SGOT (AST), SGPT (ALT), sodium, and triglycerides.

NORTHBOROUGH REFERENCE LABORATORIES
128 Analysis Way
Northborough, OH 12468

❏ GROUP ACCOUNT ❏ PATIENT

LAST NAME	FIRST NAME	MI	SEX	DATE OF BIRTH

Ordering Physician Signature

PRIMARY CARE PHYSICIAN

_____

ADDRESS	CITY	STATE	ZIP

SPECIMEN INFORMATION

❏ **STAT**
Date of Collection _____

PHONE # Home	SOC. SEC #
Work	

Time of Collection _____

❏ Serum   ❏ Plasma
❏ Urine (Volume) _____
           Hours _____
❏ Other _____

COMPLETE SHADED BOX BELOW FOR PATIENT AND THIRD PARTY BILL ONLY

RESPONSIBLE PARTY	LAST NAME	FIRST NAME	MI	MEDICARE ❏ AMERICAID ❏
				#
ADDRESS	CITY	STATE	ZIP	PHONE #
INSURED NAME		INSURANCE CO. NAME/ADDRESS		
INSURED'S EMPLOYER		RELATIONSHIP TO PATIENT	CONTRACT #	GROUP #
		❏ Self ❏ Spouse ❏ Dependent		

CALL RESULTS TO:

Phone #:(   ) _____
Copy Results to:
_____
_____
_____

REASON FOR TEST (A DIAGNOSIS IS NECESSARY FOR ALL INSURANCE CLAIMS) *SEE REVERSE FOR CODES*

SPECIMEN CODES: G - GEL, L - LAVENDER, R - RED, B - BLUE, BK - BLACK, U - URINE

PROFILES

❏ BIOCHEM BASIC	1G	❏ BIOCHEM PROFILE III	2G, 1L	❏ LIPID	1G	❏ THYROID	1G
❏ BIOCHEM PROFILE I	1G, 1L	❏ ARTHRITIS	2G,1BK	12-16 HOUR FAST REQUIRED		❏ HYPERTHYROID	1G
❏ BIOCHEM PROFILE II	1G, 1L	❏ HEPATITIS	1G	❏ LIVER	1G	❏ HYPOTHYROID	1G
				❏ PRENATAL	1G, 1L, 1R	❏ TORCH PROFILE	1G

INDIVIDUAL TESTS

❏ ALBUMIN		❏ FSH	G
❏ ALK. PHOSPHATASE	G	❏ GC CULTURE, SOURCE _____	
❏ AMYLASE	G	❏ GLUCOSE	G
❏ ANA SCREEN	G	❏ GLYCATED HEMOGLOBIN	L
❏ BILIRUBIN, TOTAL	G	❏ hCG, BETA SUBUNIT QUANT.	G
❏ BILIRUBIN, TOTAL + DIRECT	G	❏ HDL	G
❏ BILIRUBIN, NEONATAL	G	❏ HEPATITIS B SURF. ANTIBODY	G
❏ BUN	G	❏ HEPATITIS B SURF. ANTIGEN	G
❏ CALCIUM, TOTAL	G	❏ HEPATITIS C ANTIBODY	G
❏ CBC W/AUTOMATED DIFF	L	❏ HIV ANTIBODY (SIGNED CONSENT REQUIRED)	G
❏ CBC W/MANUAL DIFF	L	❏ LACTIC DEHYDROGENASE	G
❏ CHLAMYDIA SCREEN, SOURCE _____		❏ LEAD, PEDIATRIC	L
❏ CHOLESTEROL	G	❏ LH	G
❏ CREATININE	G	❏ LIPASE	G
❏ CULTURE, SOURCE _____		❏ LITHIUM	G
❏ ELECTROLYTES	G	❏ OVA & PARASITE PREP.	
❏ ESTRADIOL	G	❏ PHOSPHORUS	G
❏ FERRITIN	G	❏ PREGNANCY TEST, BLOOD	G
❏ FOLIC ACID	G	❏ PROGESTERONE	G
❏ FREE T4	G	❏ PROLACTIN	G

❏ PROSTATE SPECIFIC ANTIGEN	G
❏ PT W/INR	B
❏ PTT	B
❏ RHEUMATOID FACTOR	G
❏ RPR	G
❏ RUBELLA IgG ANTIBODY	G
❏ SEDIMENTATION RATE	BK
❏ SGOT	G
❏ SGPT	G
❏ SPUTUM CULTURE	
❏ STOOL CULTURE	
❏ THROAT, GROUP A STREP CULTURE	
❏ TOTAL PROTEIN	G
❏ TSH	G
❏ URIC ACID	G
❏ URINALYSIS	U
❏ URINE CULTURE	U
❏ VITAMIN B12	G

ICD-9-CM DIAGNOSIS CODES

☐ 648.80	ABN GLUC TOL/PREG OR PP	☐ 250.00	DIABETES	☐ 487.1	INFLUENZA	☐ 486	PNEUMONIA
☐ 682.9	ABSCESS	☐ 558.9	DIARRHEA	☐ 774.6	JAUNDICE OF NEWBORN	☐ V22.2	PREGNANCY, NORMAL
☐ 042	AIDS	☐ 562.11	DIVERTICULITIS	☐ 782.4	JAUNDICE NOT NEWBORN	☐ 593.9	RENAL DISEASE
☐ 477.9	ALLERGIC RHINITIS	☐ 780.4	DIZZINESS	☐ V72.6	LAB EXAMINATION	☐ 461.9	SINUSITIS
☐ 626.0	AMENORRHEA	☐ 276.9	ELECTROLYTE IMBALANCE	☐ 709.8	LESION, SKIN	☐ 462	SORE THROAT
☐ 285.9	ANEMIA	☐ 259.9	ENDOCRINE DISORDERS	☐ 573.9	LIVER DISEASE	☐ V67.0	SURGICAL FOLLOW UP
☐ 413.9	ANGINA	☐ 530.10	ESOPHAGITIS	☐ 785.6	LYMPHADENOPATHY	☐ 780.2	SYNCOPE
☐ 716.90	ARTHRITIS	☐ 780.6	FEVER	☐ 780.7	MALAISE & FATIGUE	☐ 465.9	URI
☐ 414.00	ASHD	☐ 558.9	GASTROENTERITIS	☐ 382.9	OTITIS MEDIA	☐ 599.0	UTI
☐ 493.90	ASTHMA	☐ 784.0	HEADACHE	☐ 789.0	PAIN, ABDOMEN	☐ 616.10	VAGINITIS
☐ 600	BENIGN PROSTATIC HYPERTROPHY	☐ 599.7	HEMATURIA	☐ 724.5	PAIN, BACK	☐ 079.9	VIRAL SYNDROME
☐ 466.0	BRONCHITIS	☐ 573.3	HEPATITIS	☐ 723.1	PAIN, CERVICAL NECK	☐ 998.5	WOUND INFECTION
☐ 199.1	CA SPECIFY SITE:_____	☐ 070.9	HEPATITIS, VIRAL	☐ 786.50	PAIN, CHEST	☐	OTHER: _____
☐ 428.0	CHF	☐ 272.4	HYPERLIPIDEMIA	☐ 719.40	PAIN, JOINT	☐	_____
☐ 496	COPD	☐ 401.9	HYPERTENSION	☐ V76.2	PAP SMEAR	☐	_____
☐ 436	CVA	☐ 244.9	HYPOTHYROID	☐ 614.9	PID	☐	_____
☐ E934.9	COUMADIN THERAPY	☐ 626.9	INFERTILITY, FEMALE	☐ 462	PHARYNGITIS		

PROFILES / CPT CODES

BIOCHEM BASIC / 80019

Albumin
Alkaline Phosphatase
Anion Gap
Bicarbonate
Bilirubin, Total
BUN
Calcium
Chloride
Cholesterol
Creatinine
GGTP
Glucose
LDH
Phosphorus
Potassium
Protein, Total
SGOT (AST)
SGPT (ALT)
Sodium
Triglycerides
Uric Acid

BIOCHEM PROFILE I / 80019, 85025, 85029

Biochem Basic
CBC w/Automated Diff

BIOCHEM PROFILE II / 80019, 85025, 85029, 83718

Biochem Basic
CBC w/Automated Diff
Lipid Profile

BIOCHEM PROFILE III / 80019, 85025, 85029, 83718, 80091

Biochem Basic
CBC w/Automated Diff
Lipid Profile
Thyroid Profile

ARTHRITIS PROFILE / 80072

ANA
Rheumatoid Factor
Sed Rate
Uric Acid

HEPATITIS PROFILE / 80059

Hepatitis A Ab (HAAB)
Hepatitis B Core Ab (HBCAB)
Hepatitis B Surf Ab (HBSAB)
Hepatitis B Surf Ag (HBSAG)
Hepatitis C Ab (HCAB)

LIPID PROFILE / 80061
12-16 Hour Fast Required

Cholesterol
HDL
LDL
Triglycerides

LIVER PROFILE / 80058

Albumin
Alkaline Phosphatase
Bilirubin, Total
SGOT (AST)
SGPT (ALT)

PRENATAL PROFILE / 80055

ABO/Rh type
Antibody Screen
CBC w/Automated Diff
Hepatitis B Surf Antigen
Rubella IgG Antibody
RPR

THYROID PROFILE / 80091

Free Thyroxine Index
T_3 Uptake
T_4

HYPERTHYROID PROFILE / 80091, 84480

Thyroid Profile
T_3 Total

HYPOTHYROID PROFILE / 80092

Thyroid Profile
TSH

TORCH PROFILE / 80090

CMV IgG Ab
Herpes I and II Ab
Rubella IgG Antibody
Toxoplasma IgG Ab

Web Activities

1. For each group of credentialed laboratory personnel discussed in this chapter, search the Internet for a website that pertains to it. What kind of information does it offer?

2. Locate a local hospital's website. Does it outline all the specialty departments described in this chapter? What unique services do they offer?

3. Visit your insurance company's website. Does it specify which laboratories must be used by its subscribers?

CHAPTER POST-TEST

1. A urine culture would be performed in which department of a regional laboratory?
   a. Bacteriology department
   b. Urinalysis department
   c. Culture department
   d. Cytology department

2. Which of the following is a description of a panel?
   a. Many tests all billed together at one time
   b. All the tests for one patient during one calendar year
   c. All the tests a doctor orders consistently throughout her or his practice
   d. A related set of tests about an organ, system, or function

3. A low-powered objective lens on a microscope allows the specimen to be magnified to what size for viewing?
   a. 10 times larger than life
   b. 100 times larger than life
   c. 1000 times larger than life
   d. 10,000 times larger than life

4. What is the meaning of the medical abbreviation NPO?
   a. Patient not to ingest any food for 12 hours
   b. Patient not to ingest food or drink fluids for 12 hours
   c. Patient not to drink fluids for 12 hours
   d. Any of the above

5. Many clinics require that pending lab reports contained within the EMR are to be reviewed and signed by a provider within what length of time?
   a. 6–12 hours
   b. 12–24 hours
   c. 24–36 hours
   d. 36–48 hours

6. POCT testing is also called:
   a. patient office care testing
   b. bedside testing
   c. at home testing
   d. pharmacy testing

7. During a physical examination, healthy or normal test results are also known as:

    a. Metabolic level

    b. Calibration level

    c. Reference values

    d. Starting results

8. If a TDM specimen is drawn 30 minutes after the last dose of medication was given to a patient, you would be testing for:

    a. Trough level

    b. Random level

    c. Peak level

    d. Toxicity

SELF-ASSESSMENT

Working in a medical laboratory requires spending large amounts of time performing extremely detail-oriented procedures, such as observing specimens through a microscope for signs of disease. Laboratory analysis also involves maintaining high-quality controls and safety standards to ensure the accuracy and reliability of results. The way you deal with details in your everyday life can reveal much about your predisposition for detail-oriented analytic tasks. For each statement, circle the response that best describes you.

1. When walking along a city street, I:

    a. notice each person who passes me, remember details from storefronts, and even recognize the make and model of cars as they drive by

    b. like to listen to other people's conversations and enjoy interacting with friends who are accompanying me

    c. usually spend my time daydreaming

2. If I think about the way a pine tree looks, I:

    a. visualize the rough texture of its bark and see its long, thin leaves perfectly in my head

    b. think about the great Christmas trees my family always had when I was a kid

    c. see two blobs of color, green and brown

3. I prefer working in an atmosphere:

    a. that is structured and involves analytic thinking

    b. where the decision-making process is cut-and-dry and the options are well defined

    c. where I do not have to make decisions or interpret anything

4. When preparing a meal or recipe, I:

    a. am very careful to make sure I read the recipe over twice before I start and have each of the ingredients on hand

    b. read the recipe quickly just to make sure I understand the basics

    c. just wing it; I cook by intuition

5. When preparing for a trip or vacation, I:

    a. know exactly where my passport and other important papers are located, make a list of all essential items to bring and check off the list as each is packed, and leave detailed written instructions for the house sitter

    b. know pretty much what I need and where I can find it; but I wait until the day before to get it all together

    c. let someone else do all the packing and handle all the arrangements; too many details for me

6. After a conversation with someone I have just met, I:

   a. remember the exact color of his or her eyes

   b. would be able to make a pretty good guess about what color his or her eyes are

   c. have no idea what color his or her eyes are

7. When giving people driving directions to a destination, I:

   a. make sure to give detailed instructions, using at least two different routes, noting landmarks and the location of gas stations along the way

   b. say basically what area of town they need to head toward and the street address; I know they can figure out the rest on their own

   c. usually give people the wrong directions, so I tell them to ask someone else

8. In regard to friends' birthdays, I:

   a. have them all written down in my calendar, and I send cards out 4 days before the date

   b. know what month they fall in, and make sure to wish them a happy birthday somewhere around the middle of the month

   c. am usually embarrassed when I find out a friend's birthday has passed; I can never remember dates

Scoring

If most of your answers were A's, you are an extremely detail-oriented and observant person. You are well suited to the tasks performed in the medical laboratory. If your answers were mostly B's, you can be observant, but you do not always pay close attention to details. If your answers were mostly C's, you will need to work on your observation skills and pay special attention to details while working in the laboratory.

CHAPTER **40**

Phlebotomy: Venipuncture and Capillary Puncture

CHAPTER PRE-TEST

1. Red blood cells (RBCs) are produced in the:
   a. Liver
   b. Lymph nodes
   c. Spleen
   d. Bone marrow

2. What type of blood is most commonly used for laboratory tests?
   a. Arterial blood
   b. Venous blood
   c. Capillary blood
   d. Coronary blood

3. What is a buffy coat made of?
   a. White blood cells (WBCs)
   b. RBCs
   c. Platelets
   d. a and c

4. Which way should the bevel of the needle be held when performing venipuncture?
   a. Up
   b. Down
   c. Sideways
   d. Any of the above

5. Which of the following tubes contains no anticoagulants?

a. Green

b. Red

c. Gray

d. Lavender

6. What position should patients be in while they are having their blood drawn?

a. Standing

b. Lying down

c. Sitting

d. Either b or c

7. What is the maximum amount of time a tourniquet should be left on?

a. 30 seconds

b. 60 seconds

c. 90 seconds

d. 120 seconds

8. What is the most common method used to draw blood from an adult?

a. Syringe

b. Vacuum tube

c. Butterfly

d. Intravenous needle

VOCABULARY BUILDER

Misspelled Words and Definitions

Find the words listed below that are misspelled; circle them, and correctly spell them in the spaces provided. Then match the vocabulary terms with the correct definitions below.

additive	hemotoma	thirotrophic gel
aliquet	palpatate	thrombocytes
hemoconcentration	plasma	venipuncture
hemololysis	serum	

_____   _____   _____

_____   _____

1. _____ The fluid portion of blood from an anticoagulated tube

2. _____ The process of collecting blood

3. _____ A portion of the blood that has been taken off for use or storage

4. _____ Any material placed in a tube that maintains or facilitates the integrity and function of the specimen

5. _____ To feel, as in feeling for a vein

6. _____ An accumulation of blood around the venipuncture site during or after venipuncture, caused by the leakage of blood from where the needle punctured the vein

7. _____ The destruction of blood in a sample; the rupture of the red blood cells

8. _____ The fluid portion of the blood after clotting has taken place

9. _____ A gel material capable of forming an interface between the cells and fluid portion of the blood as a result of centrifugation

10. _____ Platelets

11. _____ Leaving a tourniquet on the arm longer than 1 minute, causing an increased concentration of constituents in the blood sample, resulting in inaccurate test results

LEARNING REVIEW

Short Answer

1. Identify and describe the first, second, and third choices of sites on the human body used to perform venipuncture.

   _____

   _____

   _____

   _____

2. Tourniquets play a critical role in venipuncture and must be applied and used properly to obtain a blood specimen for analysis.

   A. What is the purpose of a tourniquet?

   _____

   _____

   B. Where is the tourniquet placed?

   _____

   _____

   C. How long should the tourniquet remain on the arm during the procedure?

   _____

   _____

   D. At what point during the procedure should the tourniquet be removed? Why is the timing of removal so important?

   _____

   _____

3. Match the collection tubes containing anticoagulants with their corresponding color stoppers: green, gray, blue, and lavender.

   A. Coagulation "citrate" tube: _____

   B. EDTA tube: _____

   C. Oxalate/fluoride tube: _____

   D. Heparin tube: _____

4. Vein stimulation refers to techniques used when initial attempts to obtain a blood sample are not successful. What are five techniques used to stimulate veins?

_____

_____

5. Describe the characteristics of a vein versus an artery versus a tendon when palpating and drawing blood.

_____

_____

_____

6. Identify the recommended venipuncture method for each of the situations listed below.

   A. When drawing blood from a 75-year-old patient with thin veins   _____

   B. For collecting a blood specimen from children, who have small veins and a tendency to move during the venipuncture procedure   _____

   C. When multiple blood samples must be obtained from one venipuncture procedure   _____

7. What are two of the most common adverse reactions patients have during venipuncture?

_____

_____

8. In preparing a patient for venipuncture, why would it be helpful to know about the patient's past venipuncture experiences?

_____

_____

_____

9. Why does the appearance and attitude of the medical assistant matter when approaching a patient for a blood sample?

_____

_____

_____

10. If you sense that your patient does not understand that you are about to perform venipuncture, what would be some good actions to take?

_____

_____

Matching

Arteries and veins are crucial elements of the circulatory system. Indicate which of the following are functions or characteristics of arteries (A) and which are functions of veins (V).

_____ 1. Blood is brighter in color

_____ 2. No pulse

_____ 3. Carry blood to heart; carry deoxygenated blood (except pulmonary)

_____ 4. Thin wall and less elastic

_____ 5. Carry blood from heart; carry oxygenated blood (except pulmonary)

_____ 6. No valves

CERTIFICATION REVIEW

These questions are designed to mimic the certification examination. Select the best response.

1. To speed removal of serum from a tube of blood, an instrument called a(n) ___ is used.
   a. Autoclave
   b. Centrifuge
   c. Calibrator
   d. Incubator

2. Plasma differs from serum in that it contains:
   a. fibrinogen
   b. a buffy coat
   c. RBCs
   d. a clot

3. Needle insertion for venipuncture should be at an angle of:
   a. 90 degrees
   b. 30 degrees
   c. 45 degrees
   d. 15 degrees

4. The first step in a successful venipuncture is to:
   a. select the site
   b. put the patient at ease
   c. apply the tourniquet appropriately
   d. apply gloves

5. Syncope refers to:
   a. fasting
   b. relaxation
   c. fainting
   d. reclining

6. Certain levels of blood components are decreased in capillaries except:
   a. potassium
   b. total protein
   c. calcium
   d. glucose

7. All of the following additives bind with calcium when mixed with the blood specimen, except:
   a. sodium fluoride
   b. potassium oxalate
   c. sodium citrate
   d. EDTA

8. TDM specimens require that blood be collected in what types of tube?
   a. Light blue
   b. Green
   c. Red
   d. Lavender

9. Which circulating blood cell has no nucleus?

    a. Erythrocyte

    b. Leukocyte

    c. Thrombocyte

    d. Granulocyte

10. The most common size needle used for regular vacuum tube systems is:

    a. 16 G

    b. 18 G

    c. 21 G

    d. 22 G

LEARNING APPLICATION

Critical Thinking

1. Explain the difference between serum and plasma. Describe how serum and plasma samples are collected.

_____

_____

_____

_____

_____

_____

_____

_____

_____

2. How can vein collapse be avoided in a geriatric patient?

_____

_____

_____

_____

3. Discuss how clots are formed and what can be done to stop the clotting process.

_____

_____

_____

4. The patient cries out in pain when you insert the needle into the vein. What will you do to make the patient more comfortable? If you decide to try another site, how will you locate it?

_____

_____

_____

_____

_____

_____

Case Studies

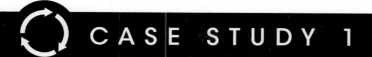

CASE STUDY 1

Wanda Slawson, CMA (AAMA), performs a successful venipuncture on Jaime Carrera using the vacuum tube system and a 21-G needle. Wanda is now preparing to label the tubes for laboratory analysis. She is careful to label all tubes at the patient's side before leaving the examination room.

CASE STUDY REVIEW QUESTIONS

1. What information must be included on the specimen labels for the specimen to be accepted for analysis?

_____

_____

_____

_____

2. What guidelines must Wanda follow during the venipuncture procedure to ensure that anticoagulated blood specimens are acceptable for analysis?

_____

_____

_____

3. Once Wanda has followed all procedures for correct labeling and processing of the blood specimens, what Standard Precautions must she perform?

_____

_____

_____

_____

CASE STUDY 2

After you have drawn two tubes of blood and the patient has left, you drop one of the tubes and it breaks, scattering glass and splashing blood all over the area. Fortunately this area is not in the main traffic flow of the office.

CASE STUDY REVIEW QUESTIONS

1. How do you proceed?

_____

_____

_____

_____

_____

_____

2. Could this have been prevented?

_____

_____

_____

Hands-on Activities

Make your own flashcards using the form on the last page of this chapter. Tear out the page of flashcards and copy them double-sided onto a cardstock or heavy-weight paper. Cut them apart. Color in the "O" with the same color as the vacuum tube tops (brick red, lavender, green, blue, etc.) and fill in the information. Use the cards to drill yourself and your classmates.

CHAPTER POST-TEST

Perform this test without looking at your book.

1. Red blood cells are produced in the:
   a. liver
   b. lymph nodes
   c. spleen
   d. bone marrow

2. The most common type of blood used for laboratory tests is:
   a. capillary blood
   b. venous blood
   c. arterial blood
   d. coronary blood

3. A buffy coat is a combination of:
   a. RBCs
   b. WBCs
   c. platelets
   d. b and c

4. The bevel of the needle should be held in which of the following positions when performing venipuncture?
   a. Up
   b. Down
   c. Sideways
   d. Any of the above

5. Which tube color contains no anticoagulants?
   a. Red top
   b. Gray top
   c. Green top
   d. Lavender top

6. Which of the following position(s) should patients be in while they are having their blood drawn?

    a. Lying down

    b. Standing

    c. Sitting

    d. Either a or c

7. What is the maximum amount of time a tourniquet should be left on?

    a. 30 seconds

    b. 60 seconds

    c. 90 seconds

    d. 120 seconds

8. The most common method used to draw blood from an adult is:

    a. syringe

    b. butterfly

    c. vacuum tube

    d. intravenous needle

SELF-ASSESSMENT

During your career as a medical assistant, you will probably run into a patient who refuses to have his or her blood drawn.

a. How will you calm the patient?

b. What measures will you take that might be different from typical blood draws?

c. What would make you decide not to continue with a blood draw?

d. How would you chart each situation? In the first situation, you are able to convince the patient and end up with a successful blood draw. In the other situation, you decide to stop the procedures without obtaining a blood draw.

On the lines below, chart both situations.

_____

_____

_____

_____

_____

_____

_____

_____

_____

_____

_____

(Date/time) Venipuncture attempted, but not performed because of uncooperative patient. Attempts were made to relieve patient apprehension but eventually the procedure was aborted. (Supervisor's name) was notified and ordering provider was sent a note of explanation. (signature/initials of supervisor)

O	Color: Additive: Specimen type: Tests:
O	Color: Additive: Specimen type: Tests:
O	Color: Additive: Specimen type: Tests:
O	Color: Additive: Specimen type: Tests:
O	Color: Additive: Specimen type: Tests:
O	Color: Additive: Specimen type: Tests:
O	Color: Additive: Specimen type: Tests:
O	Color: Additive: Specimen type: Tests:

C H A P T E R **41**

Hematology

CHAPTER PRE-TEST

Perform this test without looking at your book.

1. Which blood cell has the ability to travel through the vessel walls into the tissues?
   a. Thrombocytes
   b. Leukocytes
   c. Erythrocytes
   d. All of the above

2. When performing the Westergren method for ESR testing, the specimen is mixed with what anticoagulant?
   a. Sodium citrate
   b. Sodium heparin
   c. EDTA
   d. Sodium fluoride

3. Normal blood will clot within what amount of time?
   a. 11–13 seconds
   b. 20–30 seconds
   c. 45 seconds
   d. 60 seconds

4. Automated blood cell counts are considered by CLIA to be what level of complexity in testing?
   a. Waived
   b. Moderate-complexity
   c. High-complexity
   d. All of the above

5. Which blood cell is the most numerous and the heaviest?
   a. Erythrocytes
   b. Leukocytes
   c. Thrombocytes
   d. Platelets

6. What is the normal number of platelets found in a microliter of blood?
   a. 140–4000
   b. 1400–40,000
   c. 140,000–400,000
   d. 1,400,000–4,000,000

7. Which of the following WBCs is not a granulocyte?
   a. Eosinophil
   b. Neutrophils
   c. Basophils
   d. Lymphocytes

8. Two chemicals are contained within the blood system to prevent clotting of the blood while circulating through our bodies. One chemical is heparin and the second chemical is:
   a. Antithrombin
   b. C-reactive protein
   c. Thromboplastin
   d. Erythropoietin

9. Synthesis of the heme portion of a hemoglobin molecule requires the addition of what element or chemical?
   a. Calcium
   b. Sodium
   c. Iron
   d. Heparin

10. Which leukocytes are also known as "big eaters"?
    a. Leukocytes
    b. Monocytes
    c. Neutrophils
    d. Eosinophils

VOCABULARY BUILDER

Misspelled Words

Find the words in Column A that are misspelled; circle them, and correctly spell them in the spaces provided. Then match each of the vocabulary terms below with the correct definition in Column B.

	Column A	Correct Spelling	Column B
_____	1. Complete blood count	_____	A. A hormone triggered by the kidneys that helps produce RBCs
_____	2. Erythrocysts	_____	B. Having less color than normal
_____	3. Esinophil	_____	C. A larger than normal cell
_____	4. Microcytic	_____	D. A WBC without cytoplasmic granules that has a large, convoluted, nonsegmented nucleus
_____	5. Luekocytes	_____	E. A smaller than normal cell
_____	6. Hematacrit	_____	F. WBCs, one of the formed elements of blood

Column A	Correct Spelling	Column B
_____ 7. Hemaglobin	_____	G. WBC with a dense, nonsegmented nucleus that lacks granules in the cytoplasm
_____ 8. Basophil	_____	H. Platelets
_____ 9. Thrombocytes	_____	I. Granulocytic WBC with dark purple cytoplasmic granules
_____ 10. Lymphocytes	_____	J. Molecule of the RBC that transports oxygen
_____ 11. Monocytes	_____	K. Test to measure the percentage of RBCs within a specimen of anticoagulated whole blood
_____ 12. Macrocytic	_____	L. A granulocytic WBC with red-stained granules in the cytoplasm that is increased with allergies
_____ 13. Hypochromic	_____	M. RBCs, one of the formed elements of blood
_____ 14. Erythropotin	_____	N. Hematologic test consisting of Hct, Hgb, RBC and WBC counts, differential WBC count, and the erythrocyte indices

LEARNING REVIEW

Short Answer

1. When Dr. Winston Lewis orders CBCs on his patients, what are the general tests the provider will study to help him make a diagnosis?

   _____

   _____

   _____

2. While Dr. Elizabeth King is reviewing blood tests drawn on one of her patients, she notes the hematocrit is normal, yet the hemoglobin is low. This is an indication of which disease?

   _____

   _____

3. What two WBC features on a stained differential slide are studied to assist in the identification of the cell?

   _____

   _____

4. Identify and explain the following erythrocyte indices:

   _____   _____

   _____

   _____   _____

   _____

   _____   _____

5. Sedimentation-rate results vary with different states of health. Name two factors that influence the sedimentation rate. Why is the ESR a more accurate tool in diagnosing the onset of a disease than in checking on the progress of treatment?

   _____

   _____

_____

_____

_____

6. At Inner City Health Care, Mary Kilmer-Tice, CMA (AAMA), uses automated hematology instruments. Automated hematology procedures have many advantages over the manual methods. List five of these advantages.

_____

_____

_____

7. Name three procedures required by CLIA '88 regulations for automated hematology instruments.

_____

_____

_____

_____

8. Define hematopoiesis and describe where hematopoiesis occurs from the embryo through adulthood.

_____

_____

_____

Matching

Match the appropriate adult parameters with the following blood tests.

_____ 1. 36–55%

_____ 2. 80–100 fL

_____ 3. 4,500–11,000/mm^3

_____ 4. 32–36 g/dL

_____ 5. 4.0–6.0 million/mm^3

_____ 6. 12–18 g/dL

_____ 7. 27–33 pg

A. Hemoglobin

B. WBC count

C. Mean corpuscular volume

D. Hematocrit

E. Mean corpuscular hemoglobin concentration

F. RBC count

G. Mean corpuscular hemoglobin

CERTIFICATION REVIEW

These questions are designed to mimic the certification examination. Select the best response.

1. The central ion of each heme group is:

   a. magnesium

   b. calcium

   c. potassium

   d. iron

2. A buffy coat contains WBCs and:

   a. RBCs

   b. plasma

   c. platelets

   d. serum

3. When a patient has iron-deficiency anemia, the erythrocytes will appear:
   a. hyperchromic
   b. hypochromic
   c. polychromic
   d. bichromic

4. Increased eosinophils may indicate:
   a. hay fever or other allergic conditions
   b. leukemia
   c. appendicitis
   d. tuberculosis

5. When reading the packed cell volume of the hematocrit tube, what cells are you reading?
   a. Erythrocytes
   b. Leukocytes
   c. Thrombocytes
   d. All of the above

6. Which leukocyte is the most numerous within the body?
   a. Eosinophils
   b. Neutrophils
   c. Lymphocytes
   d. Monocytes

7. Erythrocytes of normal size are called:
   a. erythrocytic
   b. normocytic
   c. macrocytic
   d. microcytic

8. Erythropoietin is produced where in the body?
   a. Spleen
   b. Kidneys
   c. Bone marrow
   d. Pancreas

9. Which CLIA-certified laboratory is allowed to report normal and abnormal results of a manually performed CBC?
   a. Waived
   b. Moderate-complexity
   c. High-complexity
   d. PPMP

10. The most common type of anemia found in a clinical setting is:
    a. iron-deficiency anemia
    b. hemorrhagic anemia
    c. aplastic anemia
    d. nutritional anemia

LEARNING APPLICATION

Critical Thinking

1. What hematologic factors do the erythrocyte indices provide information about? List one example for each index in which a disease causes an elevation or decrease.

   _____

   _____

   _____

   _____

   _____

   _____

   _____

2. You are serving your practicum in a local clinic. A provider has made a tentative diagnosis of appendicitis for a patient. In addition to the urinalysis, what single hematologic test is most likely to confirm the diagnosis?

   _____

   _____

   _____

3. List the guidelines that must be followed to ensure accurate sed rate results.

   _____

   _____

   _____

4. How does aspirin interfere with clotting?

   _____

   _____

5. What test would have elevated results if a patient had lupus? Why?

   _____

   _____

   _____

Case Studies

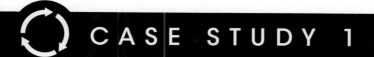

CASE STUDY 1

Jackson Tyndall is a regular patient at Inner City Health Care. Two days ago, he began to feel fatigued, experiencing development of a cough, fever, and chills. Dr. Rice has examined Mr. Tyndall and, based on the presented symptoms, makes a clinical diagnosis of influenza.

CASE STUDY REVIEW QUESTIONS

1. What type of blood test might Dr. Rice order to confirm his diagnosis?

   _____

   _____

2. What type of results are to be expected based on a diagnosis confirming clinical data?

   _____

   _____

   _____

CASE STUDY 2

Mary Manning is describing a constant rundown feeling. After examining her, Dr. Elizabeth King has ordered a hemoglobin determination and a thyroid panel. Also, because of a past history of a blood transfusion, she has ordered an HIV test to be done at an outside reference laboratory. Dr. King asks Ellen Armstrong, CMA (AAMA), to perform the venipuncture procedure on Mary to obtain the blood specimens for analysis.

CASE STUDY REVIEW QUESTIONS

1. What tube will Ellen use to collect the blood sample to be used for the hemoglobin determination test?

   _____

   _____

2. What is Dr. King hoping to learn from the hemoglobin test results?

   _____

   _____

   _____

3. With the fact that HIV infection cannot yet be ruled out, what Standard Precautions should Ellen follow in performing the venipuncture and the automated hemoglobin determination test?

   _____

   _____

   _____

   _____

CASE STUDY 3

During an ESR test, the rack that is holding the filled tubes is bumped and the entire rack, tubes and all, is knocked over. Fortunately, the tubes are securely capped so no blood has spilled.

CASE STUDY REVIEW QUESTIONS

1. Can you proceed with the test or must it be redone?

_____

_____

_____

_____

_____

2. Could this have been prevented?

_____

_____

_____

Web Activities

1. Review the CDC's Web site to review Standard Precautions required during blood collection.

2. Does the American Heart Association's Web site offer parameters for different blood counts and hematology values? Are guidelines and tips on specimen collection outlined?

CHAPTER POST-TEST

Perform this test without looking at your book.

1. Which blood cell has the ability to travel through the vessel walls into the tissues?
   a. Thrombocytes
   b. Leukocytes
   c. Erythrocytes
   d. All of the above

2. When performing the Westergren method for ESR testing, the specimen is mixed with what anticoagulant?
   a. Sodium citrate
   b. Sodium heparin
   c. EDTA
   d. Sodium fluoride

3. Normal blood will clot within what amount of time?
   a. 11–13 seconds
   b. 20–30 seconds
   c. 45 seconds
   d. 60 seconds

4. Automated blood cell counts are considered by CLIA to be what level of complexity in testing?
   a. Waived
   b. Moderate-complexity
   c. High-complexity
   d. All of the above

5. Which blood cell is the most numerous and the heaviest?
   a. Erythrocytes
   b. Leukocytes
   c. Thrombocytes
   d. Platelets

6. The normal number of platelets found in a microliter of blood is:
   a. 140–4000
   b. 1400–40,000
   c. 140,000–400,000
   d. 1,400,000–4,000,000

7. Which of the following WBCs is not a granulocyte?
   a. Eosinophil
   b. Neutrophils
   c. Basophils
   d. Lymphocytes

8. Two chemicals are contained within the blood system to prevent clotting of the blood while circulating through our bodies. One chemical is heparin and the second chemical is:
   a. antithrombin
   b. C-reactive protein
   c. thromboplastine
   d. erythropoietin

9. Synthesis of the heme portion of a hemoglobin molecule requires the addition of what element or chemical?
   a. Calcium
   b. Sodium
   c. Iron
   d. Heparin

10. Which leukocytes are also known as "big eaters"?
    a. Leukocytes
    b. Monocytes
    c. Neutrophils
    d. Eosinophils

SELF-ASSESSMENT

What are your personal feelings about performing venipuncture and testing the blood of individuals who may be infected with HIV?

1. Do you think you will be more cautious than with a non–HIV infected patient?

_____

_____

_____

_____

_____

_____

_____

2. Do you think you should be notified if the blood you are drawing or testing is known to be HIV positive?

_____

_____

_____

3. Do you have the same concerns with hepatitis-infected specimens?

_____

_____

_____

C H A P T E R **42**

Urinalysis

CHAPTER PRE-TEST

Perform this test without looking at your book.

1. Which part of the urinalysis is to be performed by the provider?
   a. The chemical examination
   b. The physical examination
   c. The specific gravity
   d. The microscopic examination

2. Ketones in urine indicate:
   a. Diabetes
   b. Glomerulonephritis
   c. Lipolysis
   d. Both a and c

3. If the patient brings a urine sample in a household container from home for a complete urinalysis, you would:
   a. Accept it this time, but after this, you will give them a proper container
   b. Provide the patient with an appropriate container and ask for a fresh sample
   c. Carefully and politely explain to the patient why you require a freshly voided specimen in a sterile container.
   d. Both b and c

4. The most common urine specimen type in the provider's office laboratory (POL) is the:
   a. Sterile specimen
   b. Timed specimen
   c. Random specimen
   d. Catheterized specimen

5. The written patient instructions for a midstream, clean catch urine specimen should be:
   a. Posted in the restroom behind the toilet
   b. Posted in the restroom beside the toilet
   c. Posted in the restroom behind the door
   d. Both a (for male patients) and b (for female patients)

6. Pyridium, a bladder analgesic, can:

   a. Increase urine flow

   b. Turn the urine a bright orange to red and may stain clothes

   c. Calm bladder irritation

   d. Both b and c

7. What is the recommended procedure for collecting a 24-hour urine sample?

   a. Collect all of the urine voided in any 24-hour period.

   b. Collect the first morning specimen and all other specimens, except the next morning specimen.

   c. Start the timing; collect the first morning specimen and all other specimens including the next morning specimen.

   d. Void the first morning specimen, start the timing, and collect all other specimens including the next morning's specimen.

8. Neutral pH is measured at 7. If a specimen has a pH of 5.3, what concentration is it?

   a. Alkaline

   b. Acidic

   c. Base

   d. None of the above

9. Transparency of urine is usually recorded as all of the following except:

   a. Clear

   b. Cloudy

   c. Hazy

   d. Musty

VOCABULARY BUILDER

Misspelled Words

Find the words in Column A that are misspelled; circle them, and then correctly spell them in the spaces provided. Then match each of the vocabulary terms below with the correct definition in Column B.

	Column A	Correct Spelling	Column B
_____	1. Ketones	_____	A. Urine testing that includes physical, chemical, and microscopic testing of a urine sample
_____	2. pH	_____	B. Crystalline material found in urine sediment; shapeless; possessing no definite form
_____	3. Sedament	_____	C. Compounds produced during increased fat metabolism; can be tested on a reagent strip
_____	4. Amorphus	_____	D. Transparent, clear casts that are often hard to see in urine; these casts should be examined under subdued lighting
_____	5. Casts	_____	E. The liquid (top) portion of centrifuged urine that is disposed of
_____	6. Urinelysis	_____	F. An infection of the urinary system

Column A	Correct Spelling	Column B
_____ 7. Specific gravity	_____	G. Scale that indicates the relative alkalinity or acidity of a solution; measurement of hydrogen ion concentration
_____ 8. Hyline	_____	H. Narrow strip of plastic used in urinalysis to detect a variety of substances and values
_____ 9. Crystals	_____	I. Insoluble matter that settles to the bottom of a liquid; material examined in the urinalysis microscopic examination
_____ 10. Midstream collection	_____	J. Opaque; lack of clarity
_____ 11. Supernatant	_____	K. Condition that occurs when the net rate at which the body produces acids or bases is equal to the net rate at which acids or bases are excreted
_____ 12. Regent test strips	_____	L. Tiny structures usually formed by deposits of protein (or other substances) within the walls of renal tubules
_____ 13. Urea	_____	M. Urine sample collected in the middle of the flow of urine
_____ 14. Turbid	_____	N. Principal end product of protein metabolism
_____ 15. Acid-base balance	_____	O. Found in normal urine sediment, these structures generally have no particular significance; the presence of a few should be noted because they may indicate disease states
_____ 16. UTI	_____	P. Ratio of weight of a given volume of a substance to the weight of the same volume of distilled water at the same temperature; test often performed during the urinalysis physical examination (can also appear on the reagent strip)

Terms

Fill in the proper terms relating to urinalysis.

_____ 1. Orange-yellow pigment that forms from the breakdown of hemoglobin in red blood cells. It usually travels in the bloodstream to the liver, where it is converted to a water-soluble form and excreted into the bile.

_____ 2. Abnormal presence of blood in urine, symptomatic of many disorders of the genitourinary system and renal diseases

_____ 3. Test on a reagent strip that indicates the presence of white blood cells in the urinary tract

_____ 4. Colorless compound produced in the intestine after the breakdown by bacteria of bilirubin

_____ 5. Accumulation of ketones in the body, occurring primarily as a complication of diabetes mellitus; if left untreated, it could cause coma

_____ 6. Pattern based on 24-hour cycle that emphasizes the repetition of certain physiologic phenomena such as eating and sleeping

_____ 7. Waste product formed in muscle that is excreted by the kidneys; increased in blood and urine when kidney function is abnormal

_____ 8. Instrument that measures the refractive index of a substance or solution; used in the urinalysis chemical examination to measure the urine specimen's specific gravity

_____ 9. Urine that appears to be above the sediment when centrifuged; poured off before sediment is examined in the urinalysis microscopic examination

LEARNING REVIEW

Short Answer

1. After passing through a healthy kidney, urine composition is approximately __ percent water and __ percent dissolved substances, which generally come from dietary intake or metabolic waste products.

2. Identify each substance below as a normal (N) or an abnormal (AB) substance found in urine.

   Urobilinogen ____

   Potassium ____

   Uric acid ____

   White blood cells ____

   Fat ____

   Protein ____

   Blood ____

   Creatinine ____

   Chloride ____

3. When handling urine specimens, Standard Precautions must be followed to ensure that proper infection control standards are observed. In the spaces provided below, list three precautions used when handling urine specimens.

   _____

   _____

   _____

4. List seven regulations of the Clinical Laboratory Improvement Act (CLIA) that apply to the clinical medical assistant performing urine testing.

   _____

   _____

   _____

5. What are the four steps in a physical examination of a urine specimen?

   _____

   _____

   _____

   _____

6. What does the specific gravity of urine indicate?

   _____

   _____

   _____

   _____

7. How should reagent test strips be handled and stored?

   _____

   _____

   _____

8. Crystals are the most insignificant part of urinary sediment and are not usually an important element of microscopic analysis, though many laboratories do report them. However, a few crystals may indicate disease states; name three crystals that need to be reported.

_____

_____

9. Casts are formed when protein accumulates and precipitates in the kidney tubules and are then washed into the urine. Identify each cast below and draw an example in the square provided.

Description	**Cast Name**	**Drawing**
These casts contain remnants of disintegrated cells that have a fine or coarse appearance.	_____	
These casts contain leukocytes, erythrocytes, or skin cells.	_____	
These casts are difficult to see under the microscope without some light adjustment because of their near transparency.	_____	

10. In the squares below, draw an example of the sediment as seen under a microscope.

Drawing	**Sediment**
	Spermatozoa, cotton fibers, and starch granules
	Yeast
	Squamous epithelial cells
	Bacteria

Matching

Microscopic examination of urine sediment is also a valuable diagnostic tool for providers. Match each type of sediment listed to the statement that best describes it.

A. White blood cells

B. Yeast

C. Squamous epithelial cells

D. Renal epithelial cells

E. Bacteria

F. Artifacts

G. Red blood cells

H. Parasite

I. Sperm

_____ Hair, fiber, air bubbles, and oil are common examples.

_____ These skin cells are not medically significant and are sloughed off continuously in urine.

_____ *Trichomonas vaginalis* is the most common example.

_____ Cocci, bacilli, and spirilla.

_____ These non-nucleated cells appear as pale, light-refractive disks; they are counted in a microscopic field and reported as cells per high-power field (HPF).

_____ These cells are larger than erythrocytes, have a visible nucleus, and may appear granular; they are reported as cells per HPF.

_____ These are reported when seen in urine, although they do not necessarily indicate a disorder.

_____ *Candida albicans* is the most common example.

_____ These cells can indicate kidney disease if present in large numbers and are easily confused with other surface cells. If suspected, the slide should be reviewed by the provider. They are reported as cells per HPF.

CERTIFICATION REVIEW

These questions are designed to mimic the certification examination. Select the best response.

1. The filtering unit of the kidney is called the:
   a. meatus
   b. glomerulus
   c. ureter
   d. urethra

2. A common medication that is used to treat bladder infections and that turns the urine bright orange is:
   a. Pyridium®
   b. Zestoretic®
   c. propranolol
   d. Neurontin

3. The urine of a diabetic patient with ketoacidosis may smell:
   a. musty
   b. sour
   c. putrid
   d. sweet

4. The curvature that appears in a liquid's upper surface when placed in a container is the:
   a. specific gravity
   b. urobilinogen
   c. meniscus
   d. buffy coat

5. The most common type of cast seen in urine sediment is:
   a. hyaline
   b. granular
   c. waxy
   d. cellular

LEARNING APPLICATION

Critical Thinking

1. What is the importance of proper urine collection?

   _____

   _____

2. When is a urine preservative necessary?

3. Why is the first morning specimen preferred for routine urinalysis?

4. What would give a urine sample a cloudy appearance?

Case Studies

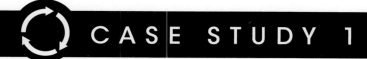

CASE STUDY 1

At Inner City Health Care, Wanda Slawson, CMA (AAMA), gives patient Wendy Janus written directions for a 24-hour urine collection to be performed at home, but Wendy misplaces them. Wanda must give directions to Wendy over the telephone.

CASE STUDY REVIEW QUESTIONS

1. What directions should be given to the patient to correctly perform the urine collection?

2. What communication techniques should Wendy use to make sure the patient understands the collection procedures? What other potential alternatives for communicating the information, besides the telephone, are available?

CASE STUDY 2

Wanda Slawson, CMA (AAMA), is asked to give a male adolescent patient the proper procedure for a clean-catch specimen. The 15-year-old boy is visibly embarrassed and will not hold eye contact with Wanda as she relates the instructions for collection to him.

CASE STUDY REVIEW QUESTIONS

1. What instructions are relevant for a clean-catch specimen for this patient?

_____

_____

_____

_____

_____

_____

_____

2. What communication techniques should Wanda use when working with this patient?

_____

_____

_____

_____

CASE STUDY 3

Your patient comes in with complaints of severe lower abdominal pain, burning, frequency, and blood in her urine. When you ask her for a urine sample for testing, she is able to give only about 6 mL because of the frequency of her urination.

1. Will you be able to perform any testing on the 6 mL specimen?

_____

_____

_____

_____

Hands-On Activities

1. One of the most important steps in the collection of urine specimens is to correctly identify the specimen through proper labeling. Make up your own identification number, using Dr. Mark Woo as your provider, and write out complete labeling information for a specimen of your own urine below.

2. What is the proper procedure for testing an unlabeled or incorrectly labeled specimen?

CHAPTER POST-TEST

Perform this test without looking at your book.

1. Which part of the urinalysis is to be performed by the provider?
   a. The chemical examination
   b. The physical examination
   c. The specific gravity
   d. The microscopic examination

2. Ketones in urine indicate:
   a. diabetes
   b. lipolysis
   c. cystitis
   d. both a & b

3. If the patient brings a urine sample in a household container from home for a complete urinalysis, you would:
   a. accept it this time, but after this, you will give them a proper container
   b. provide the patient with an appropriate container and ask for a fresh sample
   c. carefully and politely explain to the patient why you require a freshly voided specimen in a sterile container
   d. both b and c

4. The most common urine specimen type in the provider's office laboratory (POL) is the:
   a. sterile specimen
   b. timed specimen
   c. random specimen
   d. catheterized specimen

5. The written patient instructions for a midstream, clean catch urine specimen should be:
   a. posted in the restroom behind the toilet
   b. posted in the restroom beside the toilet
   c. posted in the restroom behind the door
   d. both a (for male patients) and b (for female patients)

6. Pyridium, a bladder analgesic, can:
   a. increase urine flow
   b. turn the urine a bright orange to red and may stain clothes
   c. calm bladder irritation
   d. both b and c

7. What is the recommended procedure for collecting a 24-hour urine sample?
   a. Collect all of the urine voided in any 24-hour period.
   b. Collect the first morning specimen and all other specimens, except the next morning specimen.
   c. Start the timing; collect the first morning specimen and all other specimens including the next morning specimen.
   d. Void the first morning specimen, start the timing, and collect all other specimens including the next morning's specimen.

8. Neutral pH is measured at 7. If a specimen has a pH of 5.3, what concentration is it?
   a. Alkaline
   b. Acidic
   c. Base
   d. None of the above

9. Transparency of urine is usually recorded as all of the following except:
   a. clear
   b. cloudy
   c. hazy
   d. musty

SELF-ASSESSMENT

1. Have you ever had a urinalysis performed?

   _____

   _____

   _____

   _____

2. Were you ever given proper instructions for a urinalysis? If not, why do you think you were not instructed properly? If you were, did you understand clearly what you were to do?

   _____

   _____

   _____

   _____

3. Were instructions clearly written and posted in the restroom at a location that was readable during the collection?

_____

_____

_____

_____

4. Do you think that good patient preparation and instructions influence the result of the test performed? In what way?

_____

_____

_____

_____

5. Now that you know the importance of proper patient teaching, how will your experience and training influence your work as a medical assistant in other areas of patient education?

_____

_____

_____

_____

C H A P T E R **43**

Basic Microbiology

CHAPTER PRE-TEST

Perform this test without looking at your book.

1. The field of microbiology does not include the study of:
   a. Plants
   b. Bacteria
   c. Fungi
   d. Parasites

2. Media is:
   a. The microscopic slide that is smeared with a specimen
   b. The laboratory chemical that is used in testing
   c. A nutritional mixture specific to a particular type of bacteria
   d. A sample of body secretions that contains harmful pathogens

3. Appropriate handling of specimens includes:
   a. Wearing personal protective equipment (PPE)
   b. Washing hands often
   c. Wearing gloves
   d. All of the above

4. Which of the following is *not* an important quality control measure?
   a. Monitoring the refrigerator temperatures daily
   b. Checking culture media for accuracy with positive and negative controls
   c. Updating Occupational Safety and Health Administration (OSHA) manuals periodically
   d. Respecting the expiration date of testing materials

5. What fluid is not collected in a sterile specimen container?
   a. Sputum
   b. Urine
   c. Cerebral spinal fluid
   d. Stool specimen

6. CSF cultures must be tested as:

   a. A timed specimen

   b. ASAP specimen

   c. STAT specimen

   d. Random specimen

7. All bacteria remain purple in the staining process if they are:

   a. Gram-positive

   b. Gram-negative

   c. Acid-fast

   d. None of the above

8. Dermophytes can cause what types of infections?

   a. Parasitic

   b. Fungal

   c. Viral

   d. Bacterial

9. Most fecal specimens being tested for ova or parasitic infestations are stored at what temperature?

   a. Room temperature

   b. Body temperature

   c. Refrigerated

   d. Frozen

10. Which organism is responsible for most yeast infections?

    a. *Candida albicans*

    b. *Trichomonas vaginalis*

    c. *Enterobius vermicularis*

    d. *Neisseria gonorrhoeae*

VOCABULARY BUILDER

Misspelled Words

Find the words in Column A that are misspelled; circle them, and then correctly spell them in the spaces provided. Then match each of the vocabulary terms below with the correct definition in Column B.

	Column A	Correct Spelling	Column B
_____	1. Erobic	_____	A. The science and study of fungi
_____	2. Culture	_____	B. The act of coughing up material from the air passages
_____	3. Genus	_____	C. Infection acquired in a hospital
_____	4. Anerobic	_____	D. A microorganism or substance capable of producing disease
_____	5. Mycology	_____	E. The study of parasites
_____	6. Dermataphyte	_____	F. Living only in the presence of oxygen
_____	7. Mordent	_____	G. A class that includes the true roundworm or threadworm

Column A	Correct Spelling	Column B
_____ 8. Inoculate	_____	H. Living only in the absence of oxygen
_____ 9. Nosacomal	_____	I. A fungal parasite that grows in the skin
_____ 10. Expectorate	_____	J. To place colonies of microorganisms onto nutrient media
_____ 11. Microbiology	_____	K. A substance that fixes a stain or dye
_____ 12. Morphology	_____	L. The scientific study of microorganisms
_____ 13. Nematode	_____	M. The science of structure and form without regard to function
_____ 14. Parasitology	_____	N. The classification between family and species
_____ 15. Pathogen	_____	O. The propagation of microorganisms in a special media conducive to growth

LEARNING REVIEW

Fill in the Blanks

1. Infections from parasites have increased as more people travel and public awareness of the symptoms grow. The most common parasite infections seen in the laboratory are _____, a nematode that causes pinworm infections, and _____, a flagellate that causes a sexually transmitted disease in both men and women.

2. Parasite tests are usually performed on body fluids/excretions such as _____, _____, and _____.

3. Labeling specimens sent for testing with _____, _____, and _____ collected is important, as well as noting if the patient has been _____ to a specific place and what the provider suspects.

4. To diagnose the presence of a parasite, either the _____ or _____ must be located in the specimen.

5. _____ should be worn when working with specimens. Assuming that all specimens are _____ is an important element of following Standard Precautions for infection control.

6. The practice of proper aseptic _____ several times a day, including after glove removal, is essential and should become a _____.

Short Answer

1. Specimen containers will arrive at the laboratory inside biohazard plastic transport bags to avoid danger to laboratory personnel. What precautions are taken before opening the bags?

_____

_____

_____

2. A laboratory's success in finding and identifying the pathogenic organism depends on multiple factors. Name nine.

_____

_____

_____

_____

_____

3. The medical assistant in a provider's office will most likely frequently assist in the care and treatment of patients with sore throats.

   A. Why is it necessary to rapidly identify the cause?

   _____

   _____

   _____

   B. What test would be used?

   _____

   _____

   _____

   C. What five rules should be followed?

   _____

   _____

   _____

4. Label the parts of the cell and check off "Sometimes" for the parts that are sometimes present and "Always" for the parts that are always present.

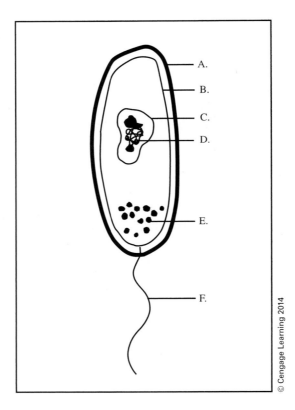

© Cengage Learning 2014

Label	Sometimes	Always
A. _____	_____	_____
B. _____	_____	_____
C. _____	_____	_____
D. _____	_____	_____
E. _____	_____	_____
F. _____	_____	_____

5. List two examples of stains used on microscope slides and explain why they are used.

_____

_____

_____

6. Describe the process of sensitivity testing and explain why it is an important tool.

_____

_____

_____

CERTIFICATION REVIEW

These questions are designed to mimic the certification examination. Select the best response.

1. Common nosocomial infections are caused by:
   a. *Salmonella*
   b. *Staphylococcus*
   c. *Shigella*
   d. Protista

2. Some bacteria produce _____, which are so resistant that they can live 150,000 years.
   a. flagella
   b. cell walls
   c. nuclei
   d. spores

3. Septicemia is a:
   a. blood infection
   b. throat infection
   c. urinary tract infection
   d. respiratory infection

4. Bacilli are:
   a. rod-shaped
   b. round
   c. spiral-shaped
   d. found in clusters

5. Gram-negative bacteria stain:
   a. purple
   b. pink
   c. red
   d. green

LEARNING APPLICATION

Critical Thinking

1. What is liquid suspension and what special situations make this a better aid than staining?

   _____

   _____

   _____

2. Define an aerosol and explain how protection is provided when working with an aerosol.

   _____

   _____

   _____

3. Identify one potential pathogen and list the specimen source, media for culture, microscopic appearance, and the disease it causes.

   _____

   _____

   _____

   _____

   _____

   _____

4. Explain why pinworm specimens are collected at a certain time of the day.

   _____

   _____

   _____

Case Studies

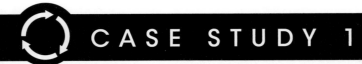

CASE STUDY 1

Winston Lewis, M.D., has ordered a series of three sputum cultures for Herb Fowler, who has been suffering with a productive cough for several months and extreme fatigue. Audrey Jones, CMA (AAMA), is assigned to obtain the cultures. When each culture is obtained from Mr. Fowler, Audrey brings it to the POL for culturing.

CASE STUDY REVIEW QUESTIONS

1. What is the procedure for obtaining a sputum specimen? Why are detailed patient instructions critical?

   _____

   _____

   _____

2. Mr. Fowler wishes to give all three specimens in one day to save on the transportation to and from the provider's office. Audrey explains that the specimens must be obtained one each day, on awakening, for three days. What is the reason for this?

_____

_____

_____

3. What microorganisms might the provider suspect, and how should the specimen be treated in the POL? Under what circumstances should the specimen be sent to an outside reference laboratory for further testing?

_____

_____

_____

⟳ CASE STUDY 2

A patient calls and shares with you that he thinks he has a toenail fungus. He has no insurance and needs to know what tests will be performed to diagnose the fungus. He also wants to know how long it will take to diagnose the problem. He has a friend who got a toenail fungus and had to have his toenail removed, so he is concerned that this will happen to him, too.

1. What will you be able to tell him?

_____

_____

_____

_____

_____

Research Activity

Make a list of all the things that are done to keep your food and environment free of pathogens. This would include water purification, food processing, homogenization, use of antibacterial soap and cleansers, immunizations, and any other process you can think of.

1. After each item on the list, place a check mark by those that are available only to certain populations but not to underdeveloped countries and areas.

_____

_____

_____

_____

2. Discuss with fellow students which of the things on your lists could be implemented fairly simply and inexpensively.

_____

_____

_____

_____

3. Reorganize the lists starting with the easiest to implement and going toward the most expensive/difficult.

_____

_____

_____

_____

_____

4. List other items or processes that would need to be done to implement each item on your list.

_____

_____

_____

_____

Web Activities

Visit the Centers for Disease Control and Prevention web site and other web sites to review guidelines on reportable diseases for your state.

CHAPTER POST-TEST

1. The field of microbiology does not include the study of:
   a. plants
   b. bacteria
   c. fungi
   d. parasites

2. Media is:
   a. the microscopic slide that is smeared with a specimen
   b. the laboratory chemical that is used in testing
   c. a nutritional mixture specific to a particular type of bacteria
   d. a sample of body secretions that contains harmful pathogens

3. Appropriate handling of specimens includes:
   a. wearing personal protective equipment (PPE)
   b. washing hands often
   c. wearing gloves
   d. all of the above

4. Which of the following is *not* an important quality control measure?
   a. Monitoring the refrigerator temperatures daily
   b. Checking culture media for accuracy with positive and negative controls
   c. Updating Occupational Safety and Health Administration (OSHA) manuals periodically
   d. Respecting the expiration date of testing materials

5. What fluid is not collected in a sterile specimen container?
   a. Sputum
   b. Urine
   c. Cerebral spinal fluid
   d. Stool specimen

6. CSF cultures must be tested as:
   a. a timed specimen
   b. ASAP specimen
   c. STAT specimen
   d. random specimen

7. All bacteria remain purple in the staining process if they are:
   a. gram-positive
   b. gram-negative
   c. acid-fast
   d. none of the above

8. Dermophytes can cause what types of infections?
   a. Parasitic
   b. Fungal
   c. Viral
   d. Bacterial

9. Most fecal specimens being tested for ova or parasitic infestations are stored at what temperature?
   a. Room temperature
   b. Body temperature
   c. Refrigerated
   d. Frozen

10. Which organism is responsible for most yeast infections?
    a. *Candida albicans*
    b. *Trichomonas vaginalis*
    c. *Enterobius vermicularis*
    d. *Neisseria gonorrhoeae*

SELF-ASSESSMENT

Describe how you feel about working with patients who have infections that are possibly communicable. What, if anything, concerns you? What resources do you have in addressing your concerns?

_____

_____

_____

_____

_____

_____

_____

_____

_____

C H A P T E R **44**

Specialty Laboratory Tests

CHAPTER PRE-TEST

Perform this test without looking at your book.

1. How many different blood types are there?
   a. 3
   b. 5
   c. 4
   d. 8

2. During pregnancy, hCG levels peak at about _____ weeks.
   a. 4
   b. 8
   c. 16
   d. 24

3. What percentage of North Americans are Rh-positive?
   a. 20%
   b. 45%
   c. 60%
   d. 85%

4. When performing a CTT on a patient, the fasting blood glucose must be lower than _____ to continue testing.
   a. 70 mg/dL
   b. 100 mg/dL
   c. 140 mg/dL
   d. 200 mg/dL

5. Of the following fats, which one is not polyunsaturated?
   a. Olive oil
   b. Corn oil
   c. Sunflower oil
   d. Safflower oil

6. Antigens that circulate within the blood system and are attached to RBCs are made of what?

   a. Carbohydrates

   b. Protein

   c. Serum

   d. None of the above

7. Patients who have a very high sugar level in their blood are diagnosed with the medical condition of:

   a. Hypoglycemia

   b. Hyperglycemia

   c. Diabetes insipidus

   d. Pancreatitis

8. If urine cannot be used immediately for pregnancy testing, it can be stored in the refrigerator for how long before the specimen is no longer viable?

   a. 4 hours

   b. 8 hours

   c. 16 hours

   d. 24 hours

9. All of the following are symptoms for IM except:

   a. Swollen extremities

   b. Swollen glands

   c. Swollen spleen

   d. Swollen lymph nodes

10. Prothrombin time testing is also called all of the following except:

    a. Coumadin levels

    b. INR

    c. Protime

    d. PT

VOCABULARY BUILDER

Misspelled Words

Find the words listed below that are misspelled; circle them, and correctly spell them in the spaces provided. Then insert the following correct vocabulary terms into the sentences that follow.

ABO blood group	homeopathy	Mantous test
billirubin	high-density lipoprotein	phenylketonuria (PKU)
blood urea nitrogin	human chorionic gonadotropin (hCG)	purified protein derivative (PPD)
cholestrol	low-density lipoprotein	Rh factor
Guthrie screening test		tryglicerides

_____   _____   _____

_____   _____

1. Although PPD is used to test for tuberculosis it is called the _____ test after the physician who developed it.

2. To evaluate a newborn for PKU, Audrey Jones, CMA (AAMA), uses the _____ to evaluate the baby's blood.

3. When Mary O'Keefe's enzyme immunoassay test is positive, Ellen Armstrong, CMA (AAMA), assumes that this positive reaction indicates a normal pregnancy. However, detection of hCG, _____, can also indicate abnormal conditions such as an ectopic pregnancy.

4. High levels of _____, the "bad" cholesterol, are associated with an increased risk for coronary artery disease. Cholesterol bound to _____, the "good" cholesterol, is transported to the liver, where it is excreted in the form of bile.

5. Serum _____ concentration will increase moderately after ingesting a meal containing fat, peaking 4 to 5 hours later.

6. Nora Fowler was born with _____, an inherited condition in which the amino acid phenylalanine is not metabolized.

7. When renal disease is suspected, a physician will order, as one of several tests, a _____ test, which measures the concentration of urea in the blood.

8. Patients exhibiting a positive or questionable _____ reaction should have a chest x-ray study to examine for tubercules, and a sputum sample should be stained to search for acid-fast rods. The presence of tubercules and acid-fast rods confirms active tuberculosis.

9. Two categories of blood typing are for the _____ and the _____.

LEARNING REVIEW

Short Answer

1. Name three reasons for performing a semen analysis on a male patient.

   _____

   _____

   _____

2. When a semen analysis is performed as part of a fertility workup, seminal fluid is analyzed to determine what four factors?

   _____

   _____

   _____

3. Name the four blood group categories.

   _____

   _____

   _____

4. Fill in the missing information in the chart below.

Blood Group/Type	Antigen on RBC	Serum Antibodies
AB	_____	_____
_____	B	_____
_____	_____	anti-B

5. How can most cases of hemolytic disease of the newborn (HDN) be prevented?

_____

_____

_____

6. Explain the difference between saturated, monounsaturated, and polyunsaturated fats and give an example of each.

_____

_____

_____

7. What are some ways that quality control can be maintained when performing waived category tests in the POL?

_____

_____

_____

8. List three specialty tests from the CLIA waived category that might be performed in the POL and what type of specimen is needed for each.

_____

_____

_____

Fill in the Blanks

Fill in the blanks with the correct term.

1. The Rh type of most North Americans is _____.

2. Glucose is the principal carbohydrate found circulating in the _____.

3. Excess glucose is converted into _____ for short-term storage in the liver and muscle cells.

4. The blood glucose level of _____ patients usually peaks 30 to 60 minutes after consumption of the glucose test solution, leading to a level of 160 to 180 mg/dL, and then returns to the fasting level after 2 to 3 hours.

5. A patient should be instructed to eat a diet high in _____ for 3 days before the glucose tolerance test.

6. To determine whether diabetic patients are consistently adhering to their diets, providers can administer the _____.

CERTIFICATION REVIEW

These questions are designed to mimic the certification examination. Select the best response.

1. Antigens present or absent on the surface of the red blood cell (RBC) are used to determine blood types. These are _____ molecules.
   a. carbohydrate
   b. protein
   c. fat
   d. electrolyte

2. A potentially life-threatening situation during incompatible blood transfusion is called:

   a. Epstein-Barr

   b. intravascular hemolysis

   c. hydatidiform mole

   d. phenylketonuria

3. Men with oligospermia should be evaluated for which type of disorder?

   a. Pancreatic

   b. Liver

   c. Thyroid

   d. Kidney

4. A negative reaction to a Mantoux test would include an induration of:

   a. 10 mm or more

   b. 5–9 mm

   c. 12–15 mm

   d. less than 5 mm

5. Postprandial refers to:

   a. after eating

   b. after medication

   c. after sleeping

   d. after urinating

6. Insulin is secreted by which organ?

   a. Liver

   b. Spleen

   c. Kidney

   d. Pancreas

7. When performing the Mantoux test, what size needle would you choose?

   a. 25 gauge, ½ inch

   b. 26 gauge, ⅜ inch

   c. 27–28 gauge, ½ inch

   d. 29–30 gauge, ⅜ inch

8. Which of the following factors can alter the results of semen analysis?

   a. Eating foods containing garlic

   b. Smoking cigarettes

   c. Riding a bicycle on the day of the analysis

   d. Drinking milk

9. The induration (raised hardened area) on a patient's arm in response to a Mantoux test is positive if it is:

   a. almost invisible

   b. 15 mm or more of induration

   c. 10 mm or more of induration

   d. exactly 2 mm of induration

LEARNING APPLICATION

1. What factors may alter the results of a blood glucose measurement?

_____

_____

_____

2. How can you distinguish between the diabetic and nondiabetic patient based on the results of the 2-hour postprandial glucose evaluation?

_____

_____

_____

3. What is the function of triglycerides in the body?

_____

_____

_____

4. What instructions should the patient be given in preparation for a triglyceride evaluation?

_____

_____

_____

5. What is the source of urea in the blood?

_____

_____

_____

Case Studies

 C A S E   S T U D Y   1

Mary Alexander is an established patient of Dr. Lewis's at Inner City Health Care. Mary, 32 years old, is about 10 pounds overweight for her height. Mary has been diagnosed with type 1 insulin-dependent diabetes mellitus since childhood. Dr. Lewis's treatment plan includes administration of 30 units of U-100 NPH insulin by injection every day. Dr. Lewis knows that Mary has trouble complying with the dietary restrictions included in her treatment plan and in observing regular mealtimes. Every now and then, the lifetime rigor of the diet wears Mary down and she begins to eat whatever she likes, whenever she feels like it. To guard against this, Mary must report her average glucose levels to Bruce Goldman, CMA (AAMA), twice monthly as a safeguard. At her next regular follow-up examination with Dr. Lewis, the physician orders a glycosated hemoglobin determination and discovers that Mary has been cheating on her diet again and has been reporting inaccurate glucose levels to the physician's office, hoping she would not get caught.

CASE STUDY REVIEW QUESTIONS

1. How is Dr. Lewis able to tell from the glycosylated hemoglobin determination that Mary is not adhering to her diet and health guidelines?

_____

_____

_____

2. What is glycosated hemoglobin?

_____

_____

_____

CASE STUDY 2

Your patient, a Vietnamese immigrant, is entering a medical assisting program and needs to be tested for TB. She is concerned because she received the BCG vaccination in Vietnam and was told by her friends that she will always react to the PPD test even if she doesn't have TB because of the BCG vaccination. She has many questions.

CASE STUDY REVIEW QUESTIONS

1. Why does she need to have the Mantoux test if she will always react because of the BCG?

_____

_____

_____

2. Will she always react to the PPD?

_____

_____

_____

3. Will she still need to have a chest x-ray study?

_____

_____

_____

4. Does she have TB?

_____

_____

_____

5. Is she protected from getting TB by the BCG vaccination?

_____

_____

_____

6. Does she need treatment?

_____

_____

_____

Research Activities

1. Do an Internet investigation to see if your state requires PKU testing on newborns.

   a. If not, why do you think it is not required? Is the test recommended? How much does it cost? What can you do to change the law?

   b. If your state does require it, are parents allowed to refuse? Why would a parent refuse?

   c. Role-play with another student: How would you react if a parent refused?

2. Look at Table 44-4 (Values for Cholesterol, HDL, LDL, and Triglycerides) in your textbook. What are the normal ranges of each for your gender?

_____

_____

CHAPTER POST-TEST

1. How many different blood types are there?

   a. 3

   b. 5

   c. 4

   d. 8

2. During pregnancy, hCG levels peak at about _____ weeks.

   a. 4

   b. 8

   c. 16

   d. 24

3. What percentage of North Americans are Rh-positive?

   a. 20%

   b. 45%

   c. 60%

   d. 85%

4. When performing a CTT on a patient, the fasting blood glucose must be lower than _____ to continue testing.

    a. 70 mg/dL

    b. 100 mg/dL

    c. 140 mg/dL

    d. 200 mg/dL

5. Of the following fats, which one is not polyunsaturated?

    a. Olive oil

    b. Corn oil

    c. Sunflower oil

    d. Safflower oil

6. Antigens that circulate within the blood system and are attached to RBCs are made of what?

    a. Carbohydrates

    b. Protein

    c. Serum

    d. None of the above

7. Patients who have a very high sugar level in their blood are diagnosed with the medical condition of _____?

    a. hypoglycemia

    b. hyperglycemia

    c. diabetes insipidus

    d. pancreatitis

8. If urine cannot be used immediately for pregnancy testing, it can be stored in the refrigerator for how long before the specimen is no longer viable?

    a. 4 hours

    b. 8 hours

    c. 16 hours

    d. 24 hours

9. All of the following are symptoms for IM except:

    a. swollen extremities

    b. swollen glands

    c. swollen spleen

    d. swollen lymph nodes

10. Prothrombin time testing is also called all of the following except:

    a. Coumadin levels

    b. INR

    c. protime

    d. PT

SELF-ASSESSMENT

1. Do you think all states should require PKU testing on all newborns? List three advantages and three disadvantages of each.

   _____

   _____

   _____

   _____

C H A P T E R   **45**

The Medical Assistant as Clinic Manager

CHAPTER PRE-TEST

Perform this test without looking at your book.

1. Which of the following is not a duty of a medical clinic manager?
   a. Supervising the purchase, repair, and maintenance of clinic equipment
   b. Arranging and maintaining practice insurance and developing risk management strategies
   c. Preparing patient education materials
   d. None of the above
   e. a and c only

2. Which of the following is a characteristic of an authoritarian rather than a leader?
   a. Not afraid of change
   b. Bottom line is all-important
   c. Inspires by example
   d. Does the right thing

3. One step in team development is to establish a _____ for achieving results and identifying the standards that must be maintained.
   a. timetable
   b. matrix
   c. schedule
   d. agenda

4. Solving problems between any two parties is known as:
   a. Brainstorming
   b. Benchmarking
   c. Conflict resolution
   d. Self-actualization

5. The student _____ provides an opportunity for the student to apply theory learned in the classroom to a health care setting through practical, hands-on experience.
   a. internship
   b. externship
   c. practicum
   d. All of the above

6. One of the key points to keep in mind when dismissal is necessary is:
   a. Take no longer than 20 minutes for the dismissal.
   b. Escort the employee out of the facility once they have finished their work for the day.
   c. Do not engage in an in-depth conversation of performance.
   d. Agree and empathize with all of the employee's opinions and rationalizations.

7. The process by which the provider of services makes the consumer aware of the scope and quality of services is known as:
   a. Marketing
   b. Advertising
   c. Strategizing
   d. Conference

VOCABULARY BUILDER

Misspelled Words

Find the words listed below that are misspelled; circle them, and correctly spell them in the spaces provided. Then insert the correct vocabulary terms beside the sentences that follow.

agenda	"going bare"	practicum
ancilliary services	itinerary	procedures manual
benchmarking	liability	professional liability insurance
benifits	marketting	risk managment
bond	minutes	teamwork
embezzel	negligance	work statement

_____   _____   _____

_____   _____   _____

1. _____ Professional occupational companies hired to complete a specific job such as janitorial services, laundry, or disposal of hazardous materials

2. _____ The situation of a provider who does not carry insurance to protect the provider's assets in the event of a liability claim

3. _____ Making a comparison between different organizations relative to how they accomplish tasks, remunerate employees, and so on

4. _____ Designed to protect assets in the event a liability claim is filed and awarded

5. _____ A written record of topics discussed and actions taken during meeting sessions

6. _____ This provides a concise description of the work you plan to accomplish

7. _____ A binding agreement with an employee ensuring recovery of financial loss should funds be stolen or embezzled

8. _____ A printed list of topics to be discussed during a meeting

9. _____ The process by which the provider of services makes the consumer aware of the scope and quality of those services. Examples might include public relations, brochures, patient education seminars, and newsletters.

10. _____ Involves persons synergistically working together

11. _____ A transitional stage providing an opportunity to apply theory learned in the classroom to a health care setting through practical, hands-on experience

12. _____ Remuneration that is in addition to a salary

13. _____ To appropriate fraudulently for one's own use

14. _____ Involves the identification, analysis, and treatment of risks within the medical clinic

15. _____ Performing an act that a reasonable and prudent provider would not perform or failure to perform an act that a reasonable and prudent provider would perform

16. _____ Provides detailed information relative to the performance of tasks within the facility in which one is employed

17. _____ A detailed plan for a proposed trip

LEARNING REVIEW

Short Answer

1. The manager of a medical clinic or ambulatory care facility can have many varied responsibilities based on individual facility needs. What are five duties that are the responsibility of the clinic manager in a health care setting?

   _____

   _____

   _____

   _____

   _____

   _____

   _____

2. What are five attributes needed to perform as a quality manager in any clinic setting?

   _____

   _____

3. List four suggestions that are proven means of managing your time whether in management or as a salaried employee.

   _____

4. What is the difference between authoritarian and participatory management styles?

_____

_____

_____

_____

5. What does "management by walking around" mean, and why would it be useful in a medical clinic setting?

_____

_____

6. The table below discusses some of the common risks for medical clinics, as well as risk control measures for each one. Fill in any missing information.

Risk	Risk Control Measures
_____	Train various employees to assume other duties and perform them when an employee is ill, on vacation, etc.
Failure of a supplier or contractor	_____
_____	Have protocols in place for handling this situation and make patients aware of the protocols; notify patients immediately if confidential information is disclosed and work with them toward resolution.
Computer failure	_____
_____	Continually review safety procedures; conduct safety surveys; always carry liability insurance; complete an Incident Report to signal the risk manager to implement existing protocols to minimize risk

7. Define harassment in the workplace.

_____

_____

8. List the steps that a manager should take if he or she is made aware of harassment in the medical clinic.

_____

_____

_____

_____

9. Why do some employers put new employees on probation? What is the usual length of an employee's probationary period?

_____

_____

_____

Ordering Activity

All administrative and clinical supplies and equipment in the facility must be inventoried. The following tasks are performed when new supplies and/or equipment are received. Put the tasks in the correct order, from 1 to 5.

_____ A. Unpack each item, checking against the packing slip.

_____ B. Write the date the shipment was received and who verified it.

_____ C. Stock each item appropriately.

_____ D. Verify that no items have been substituted or back-ordered.

_____ E. Find the packing slip listing the items ordered.

Matching

Most marketing tools used in a medical environment provide educational and clinic services information to patients, potential patients, and the local community. Match the following marketing tools with their potential use in the ambulatory care facility setting.

A. Seminars

B. Brochures

C. Newsletters

D. Press releases

E. Special events

_____ 1. These are used for announcing new equipment, new staff, expanded or remodeled clinic space, and so on.

_____ 2. These typically come in two types—patient education and clinic services—and present a professional image of the ambulatory care setting.

_____ 3. These provide an effective way to join with other community organizations to promote wellness.

_____ 4. These can educate patients and provide goodwill in the community. All facility staff can work as a team to organize these.

_____ 5. These can include a wide range of information from health-related topics to staff introductions to insurance updates. They may form the nucleus of a marketing program.

CERTIFICATION REVIEW

These questions are designed to mimic the certification examination. Select the best response.

1. There is a direct correlation between a person's management style and his or her:
    a. technical expertise
    b. educational level
    c. personality
    d. salary

2. Most conflicts occur between employees and supervisors or providers because of:
   a. attitude
   b. poor communication
   c. a misunderstanding
   d. b and c

3. The person who applies the team-oriented management style is often comfortable with:
   a. teaching and coaching
   b. building, constructing, and modeling
   c. ideas, information, and data
   d. all of the above

4. A comprehensive safety program is essential to:
   a. marketing functions
   b. team building
   c. risk management
   d. equipment and supply maintenance

5. Leadership for the twenty-first century includes components of flexibility, mentoring, and:
   a. networking
   b. domination
   c. hierarchy
   d. rigidity

6. A rule that defines almost all of the ethical qualities of a manager is:
   a. Murphy's law
   b. the Rule of Nines
   c. the Golden Rule
   d. none of the above

7. The _____ management style is based on the premise that the worker is capable and wants to do a good job.
   a. walking around
   b. participatory
   c. risk
   d. authoritarian

8. The most significant task(s) of the team leader or clinic manager is (are):
   a. getting the team members to understand and support the specifics of the problem they are asked to solve
   b. enabling the team to develop their own work statement where they will assume ownership of the goals and objectives
   c. establishing a timetable for achieving results and identifying the standards that must be maintained
   d. all of the above

9. The documentation of policies and procedures that make up the clinic HIPAA manual should be:
   a. filed in a locked cabinet
   b. kept for six years, even though wording has been changed or has been eliminated
   c. made available for all employees
   d. b and c

10. If malpractice litigation should occur, the best protocol to follow is to:

    a. be honest with the patients and insurance carriers

    b. let the HR person handle the situation

    c. notify the provider

    d. not get involved

LEARNING APPLICATION

Critical Thinking

1. How would you, as the clinic manager, handle someone who is spreading an awful rumor about another employee in the clinic?

2. How can the clinic manager promote open and honest communication?

3. The student practicum can be a stressful time for the extern. As the clinic manager, how can you help the extern feel more at ease the first day of "work"?

4. Describe how a procedure manual for a single-provider practice would differ from a procedure manual for a multiprovider practice.

5. Describe how a procedure manual could become outdated and need revisions.

Case Studies

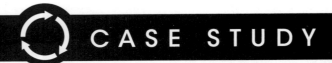

CASE STUDY

Clinic manager Shirley Brooks is responsible for the preparation and distribution of payroll checks at the clinics of Drs. Lewis and King. Because the group practice is in the process of upgrading the computer system to accommodate a recent influx of new patients, Shirley is temporarily preparing the payroll using the manual write-it-once bookkeeping system. She is careful to consult payroll records for each employee, which include the employee's name, address, telephone number, and Social Security number; number of exemptions claimed on the W-4 form; gross salary; deductions withheld for all taxes, including Social Security, federal, state, and local; deductions withheld for health insurance and disability insurance; and date of employment.

CASE STUDY REVIEW QUESTIONS

1. As Shirley writes out the payroll check for Audrey Jones, CMA (AAMA), what information should be included on the paycheck stub?

   _____

   _____

   _____

   _____

2. What must the provider's clinic have to process payroll?

   _____

   _____

3. What responsibility does the clinic manager have with regard to the confidentiality of payroll records? How might employees' rights to privacy be maintained?

   _____

   _____

   _____

   _____

   _____

Web Activities

Use the websites given in the text or alternative sites you know about to plan a trip between two cities within the United States. Compare the fares for Sunday departure and Friday return dates with the fares for low-volume days as obtained from the Priceline.com site. Also compare fares on flights purchased within one week of departure with fares on flights purchased one month before departure. Follow the instructor's instructions on completing and turning in your results.

CHAPTER POST-TEST

Perform this test without looking at your book.

1. Examples of marketing tools include which of the following?
   a. Newsletters
   b. Press releases
   c. Seminars
   d. All of the above

2. What is the action that should be taken by the clinic manager when handling personnel data?
   a. Review if patient demographics and HIPAA requirements are current
   b. Progress reviews, salary reviews, W-4 forms, corrective actions, licenses, and malpractice insurance contracts
   c. Hire or terminate employees, and obtain additional clinic space
   d. Payroll authorization and corrective action for missed work

3. Magazine subscriptions and health-related literature are the responsibility of:
   a. the clinic manager
   b. the provider
   c. the medical assistant
   d. the custodial staff

4. Performing an act that a reasonable and prudent provider would not perform or failure to perform an act that a reasonable and prudent provider would perform is known as:
   a. liability
   b. malpractice
   c. negligence
   d. going bare

5. The _____ provides detailed information relative to the performance of tasks within the facility in which one is employed.
   a. policy manual
   b. procedures manual
   c. facility handbook
   d. job description

SELF-ASSESSMENT

Put yourself in the place of the clinic manager.

1. What type of management style do you think you are the most comfortable with?

   _____
   _____
   _____

2. Carefully read about each type of style and explain why you think you are or are not that type.

   _____
   _____

3. What skills will come naturally to you?

   _____
   _____

4. What skills will you have to work on the most?

   _____
   _____

C H A P T E R **46**

The Medical Assistant as Human Resources Manager

CHAPTER PRE-TEST

Perform this test without looking at your book.

1. Which of the following is *not* a function of the human resources (HR) manager?
   a. Creating and updating a policy manual
   b. Recruiting and hiring clinic personnel
   c. Orienting new personnel
   d. Training new personnel

2. A job description must include:
   a. Necessary work experience
   b. Any special certification or licensure
   c. Basic qualifications for the position
   d. All of the above

3. A suggested item for the interview worksheet would include which of the following?
   a. Ability to problem solve when given a scenario
   b. Description of a work-related decision
   c. Identifying what is most important in a job
   d. Strengths and weaknesses

4. All personal reference information is to be kept:
   a. Concealed
   b. Confidential
   c. Private
   d. Protected

5. _____ usually occurs when an employee's performance is poor or there has been a serious violation of the clinic policies or job description.
   a. Involuntary dismissal
   b. Voluntary dismissal
   c. Probation
   d. Written advisement

6. The _____ prohibits discrimination by all private employers with 15 or more employees.
   a. Immigration Reform Act
   b. Anti-Kickback Statute
   c. Americans with Disabilities Act
   d. Health Insurance Portability and Accountability Act

7. The Equal Pay Act of 1963 prevents _____ for jobs that require equal skill, effort, and responsibility.
   a. age discrimination
   b. wage discrimination
   c. sexual discrimination
   d. reference verification

8. Which of the following is not a question to ask when checking references?
   a. Would you rehire?
   b. Describe the job performed.
   c. Can you comment on attendance and dependability?
   d. What were the wages of the employee?

VOCABULARY BUILDER

Misspelled Words

Find the words listed below that are misspelled; circle them, and correctly spell them in the spaces provided. Then, insert the correct vocabulary terms into the following sentences.

exit interveiw	letter of refeaence	overtime
involuntary dismisal	letter of resignation	probation
job desciption	menter	résumés

_____   _____   _____

_____   _____

1. Because of an unexpected staffing shortfall, Audrey Jones, CMA (AAMA), has volunteered to work _____ this week. She will receive 1½ times the regular rate of pay for hours above her regular 40-hour week.

2. An _____ has been scheduled for administrative/clinical medical assistant Liz Corbin, CMA (AAMA), before she leaves the clinic to continue her education. This session will give Liz an opportunity to provide her positive and negative opinions of the position and the facility.

3. Clinic manager Marilyn Johnson CMAS (AMT) has received a _____ from the former instructor of a current job applicant describing the applicant's performance, attitude, and qualifications.

4. The violation of clinic policies at Inner City Health Care led to the _____ of one of the part-time employees.

5. Liz Corbin, CMA (AAMA) submitted a _____ to her current employer when she decided to leave her present position to return to school to pursue an advanced degree.

6. Clinic manager Marilyn Johnson CMAS (AMT) will inform all of the job applicants that they will be on _____ for their first 30–60 days in the position. During this period, the employee and supervisory personnel can determine if the environment and the position are satisfactory for the employee.

7. Clinic manager Jane O'Hara, CMA (AAMA), updating the employee manual, includes a _____ for every position in the clinic, which details tasks, duties, and responsibilities.

8. Administrative medical assistant Ellen Armstrong RMA (AMT) considers clinic manager Marilyn Johnson CMAS (AMT) as her _____, since Marilyn has been instrumental in Ellen's training, coaching, and guidance in her newly acquired position.

LEARNING REVIEW

Short Answer

1. The manual that identifies clear guidelines and directions required of all employees is known as the policy manual. What are four topics identified in this chapter that would be included in a policy manual, regardless of the size of the practice?

_____

_____

2. Clinic manager Marilyn Johnson CMAS (AMT) has the responsibility of dismissing an employee for a serious violation of clinic policies. From the list below, select key points to keep in mind when dismissal is necessary by circling the letters of the statements that apply.

   a. Have employee pack his or her belongings from desk.

   b. The dismissal should be made in private.

   c. Take no longer than 20 minutes for the dismissal.

   d. Be direct, firm, and to the point in identifying reasons.

   e. Explain terms of dismissal (keys, clearing out area, final paperwork).

   f. Do not listen to the employee's opinion and emotions.

   g. If he or she insists, allow the employee to finish the work of the day.

   h. Do not engage in an in-depth discussion of performance.

3. Compare and contrast voluntary and involuntary separation.

_____

_____

_____

_____

_____

4. The job description must have enough information to provide both the supervisor and the employee with a clear outline of what the job entails. Name four items that must be included in a job description.

_____

5. The interview worksheet is an excellent tool to make certain that the interviews with each candidate are fair and equitable. Provide six items that should be included on any interview worksheet.

_____

_____

_____

_____

CERTIFICATION REVIEW

These questions are designed to mimic the certification examination. Select the best response.

1. A salary review is:
   a. usually conducted at the beginning of the new year
   b. virtually the same as the performance review
   c. conducted on the anniversary date of hire
   d. normally done every three years

2. Questions regarding substance abuse, arrest records, and medical history during an interview are:
   a. appropriate
   b. inappropriate
   c. illegal
   d. none of the above

3. Title VII of the Civil Rights Act addresses:
   a. overtime pay
   b. discrimination based on race, age, and sex
   c. hiring and firing practices
   d. sexual harassment

4. When a candidate accepts a position, the HR manager should write a letter outlining the specifics of the position. This letter is called a:
   a. confirmation letter
   b. congratulatory letter
   c. recommendation letter
   d. reference letter

5. A person with AIDS who satisfies the necessary skills for a position and has the experience and education required will be protected from discrimination by:
   a. OSHA
   b. CLIA
   c. AAMA
   d. ADA

6. A job description should be reviewed and updated:
   a. every 2 years
   b. every 90 days
   c. every year
   d. every 5 years

7. Voluntary separation usually occurs when:
   a. advancing to another position
   b. there is a violation of clinic policies
   c. the employee is relocating
   d. a and c

8. Verifying that all potential new employees are authorized to work is done by
   a. asking for verbal clarification
   b. having the candidate complete an I-9 form
   c. having the candidate provide a notarized statement
   d. having the candidate fill out an attestation form

9. What documents should be included in the personnel file? *(circle all that apply)*
   a. Application
   b. Formal review
   c. Awards
   d. Employee handbook

10. What act was established to prevent injuries and illnesses resulting from unsafe and unhealthy working conditions?
    a. Americans with Disabilities Act
    b. Civil Rights Act
    c. OSHA
    d. Equal Pay Act

LEARNING APPLICATION

Critical Thinking

1. You have just accepted a position to work in a larger, more specialized clinic where you will be able to use skills you are not currently able to exercise. Identify two or three main points for the letter of resignation you will prepare.

   _____

   _____

   _____

   _____

2. An employee approaches you, the HR manager, identifying that he or she has just become responsible for the care of an aging parent and may require occasional time away from work. You have no policy about how this absence should be treated. What kind of policy might be helpful? Where would you look for suggestions?

   _____

   _____

   _____

   _____

   _____

3. An exit interview form has been introduced in this chapter. Another simple form for an exit interview is to use the ABCs. A stands for "awesome." What do we do that is awesome? B stands for "better." What could we do better in our organization? C stands for "change." What would you recommend we change? Discuss the merits of both forms for an exit interview.

_____

_____

_____

_____

4. What might employers and HR managers do to make certain they keep valued employees? Is salary really the most important issue?

_____

_____

_____

_____

_____

_____

_____

_____

Case Studies

CASE STUDY

Since the clinics of Drs. Lewis and King have expanded to cover a rapidly growing patient load, including the hiring of a co-clinic manager and a new clinical medical assistant, the work pace has been hectic, but challenging. At the suggestion of Dr. Lewis, the clinic managers decide to hold a staff meeting to talk about ways to keep the lines of communication open and to process the many changes occurring at the growing medical practice. Marilyn Johnson CMAS (AMT) and Shirley Brooks RMA (AMT) encourage staff to be vocal with their feedback, suggestions, and concerns.

CASE STUDY REVIEW QUESTIONS

1. What other techniques can the clinic managers use to prevent or solve conflicts in the workplace during the period of growth and transition?

_____

_____

_____

_____

_____

_____

2. Why is effective communication one of the most important goals of the HR manager?

_____

_____

Web Activities

1. Research the Centers for Medicare and Medicaid Services Web site (http://www.cms.hhs.gov) for information related to the prohibition of discrimination on the basis of sexual orientation. What do you find? Are there other sources on this subject that are helpful? Can the manager choose not to hire a person who is otherwise qualified on the basis of sexual orientation? Why or why not?

2. Research the ADA Web site to determine if there are any examples of accommodations made in the medical setting. If yes, describe them. Are all provider-employers covered by the ADA? If not, how might discrimination be prevented?

CHAPTER POST-TEST

Perform this test without looking at your book.

1. Which of the following are functions of the HR manager? *(Circle all that apply)*
   a. Creating and updating a policy manual
   b. Training new personnel
   c. Recruiting and hiring clinic personnel
   d. Orienting new personnel

2. A job description must include:
   a. any special certification or licensure
   b. necessary work experience
   c. basic qualifications for the position
   d. all of the above

3. A suggested item for the interview worksheet would include which of the following?
   a. Identifying what is most important in a job
   b. Ability to problem solve when given a scenario
   c. Description of a work-related decision
   d. Strengths and weaknesses

4. All personal reference information is to be kept:
   a. protected
   b. concealed
   c. confidential
   d. private

5. _____ usually occurs when an employee's performance is poor or there has been a serious violation of the clinic policies or job description.
   a. Probation
   b. Involuntary dismissal
   c. Voluntary dismissal
   d. Written advisement

6. The _____ prohibits discrimination by all private employers with 15 or more employees.
   a. Americans with Disabilities Act
   b. Immigration Reform Act
   c. Anti-Kickback Statute
   d. Health Insurance Portability and Accountability Act

7. The Equal Pay Act of 1963 prevents _____ for jobs that require equal skill, effort, and responsibility.
   a. sexual discrimination
   b. age discrimination
   c. wage discrimination
   d. reference verification

8. Which of the following is not a question to ask when checking references?
   a. Would you rehire?
   b. What were the wages of the employee?
   c. Describe the job performed.
   d. Can you comment on attendance and dependability?

SELF-ASSESSMENT

1. If you were put into the position of hiring a new employee, what attributes would you be looking for?
   a. Make a list of the technical skills your new employee would need.

   _____

   _____

   b. Make a list of the affective (behavior) skills your new employee would need, including a positive attitude, a good work ethic, and so forth.

   _____

   _____

   _____

   c. Determine how you could measure the technical skills you listed.

   _____

   _____

   d. Determine how you could quantify the affective (behavior) skills you listed in item b. above. How could you determine those qualities?

   _____

   _____

   e. Which is more difficult to measure: technical or behavioral qualities? Which is more difficult to teach?

   _____

2. When you interview for a job, what technical and behavioral skills on your lists will you need to improve on?

   _____

C H A P T E R **47**

Preparing for Medical Assisting Credentials

CHAPTER PRE-TEST

Perform this test without looking at your book.

1. The _____ is an organization whose objectives are to promote skills and professionalism, protect the medical assistant's right to practice, and encourage consistent health care delivery through professional certification.
   a. ABHES
   b. CAAHEP
   c. AAMA
   d. AMT

2. _____ can be achieved either by reexamination or by the continuing education method.
   a. Continuing education units
   b. Accreditation
   c. Licensure
   d. Recertification

3. On the RMA examination, areas of general medical assisting knowledge include:
   a. Financial bookkeeping
   b. Therapeutic modalities
   c. Insurance
   d. Patient education

4. The NHA stands for:
   a. National Health Association
   b. National Healthcareer Association
   c. National Hospital Association
   d. National Hospital Accreditation

5. The major test areas of the AAMA examination include:

   a. Clinical

   b. Administrative

   c. Technical

   d. All of the above

   e. a and b only

6. Only graduates of CAAHEP- and _____-accredited medical assistant programs may sit for the CMA examination.

   a. ABHES

   b. AAMA

   c. NHA

   d. AMT

7. The American Medical Technologists (AMT) offers examinations to certify the:

   a. CMA

   b. RMA

   c. AAMA

   d. CEU

8. On successfully passing the certification examination and earning the CMA (AAMA) credential, one should begin to document all _____ earned.

   a. CMASs

   b. citations

   c. CEUs

   d. points

VOCABULARY BUILDER

Matching

Match each correct vocabulary term to the aspect of the certification process that best describes it.

___ 1. Certification examination

___ 2. Certified medical assistant (CMA [AAMA])

___ 3. Continuing education units (CEUs)

___ 4. Certified clinical medical assistant (CCMA)

___ 5. Recertification

___ 6. Registered medical assistant (RMA)

___ 7. Task Force for Test Construction

A. Method for earning points toward recertification

B. A standardized means of evaluating medical assistant competency

C. Maintaining current CMA (AAMA) status

D. Credential awarded for successfully passing the AAMA certification examination

E. Committee of professionals whose responsibility is to update the CMA (AAMA) examination annually to reflect changes in medical assistants' responsibilities and to include new developments in medical knowledge and technology

F. Credential awarded for successfully passing the AMT examination

G. One of the credentials awarded for passing the National Healthcare Association exam

LEARNING REVIEW

Short Answer

1. Name the three major areas tested in the AAMA certification examination and describe what each includes.

   _____
   _____
   _____
   _____
   _____
   _____
   _____

2. What are the addresses, telephone numbers, and Web sites for obtaining applications for the certification examinations of the AAMA, AMT, and NHA?

   AAMA _____
   _____
   _____

   AMT _____
   _____
   _____

   NHA _____
   _____
   _____

3. To keep their CMA (AAMA) credentials current, how often are individuals required to recertify? How many continuing education units (CEUs) are necessary to recertify?

   _____
   _____

4. What are the criteria that have been established for applicants to be able to sit for the RMA examination?

   _____
   _____
   _____
   _____
   _____
   _____
   _____

5. In addition to the RMA credential, what is the credential that the AMT offers for those who primarily want to be employed in the front offices of provider offices, clinics, or hospitals?

   _____

6. List the criteria an applicant must possess for taking the NHA certification exam.

   _____
   _____
   _____
   _____

CERTIFICATION REVIEW

These questions are designed to mimic the certification examination. Select the best response.

1. General medical assisting knowledge on the AMT certification examination includes anatomy and physiology, medical terminology, and:
   a. insurance and billing
   b. medical ethics
   c. bookkeeping and filing
   d. first aid

2. The AMT registration exam consists of:
   a. 300 multiple choice questions
   b. 250 multiple choice questions
   c. 200–210 four-option multiple choice questions
   d. 500 multiple choice questions

3. A total of how many questions are on the CMA (AAMA) certification examination?
   a. 100
   b. 200
   c. 1,000
   d. It varies year to year.

4. How often does an RMA need to recertify?
   a. Every year
   b. Every 6 years
   c. Every 5 years
   d. Every 3 years

5. A total of how many CEUs are required to recertify the CMA (AAMA) credential?
   a. 45
   b. 60
   c. 100
   d. 120

6. When recertifying through the AAMA, a minimum of _____ points is required in each of the three categories. The remaining _____ points may be accumulated in any of the three content areas or from any combination of the three categories.
   a. 15, 60
   b. 20, 40
   c. 10, 30
   d. 30, 60

7. The purpose of certification is that it:
   a. acknowledges that you are a professional with standard entry-level knowledge and skills
   b. builds your personal self-esteem and confidence in knowing that you can do the job asked of you
   c. helps in your career advancement and compensation
   d. all of the above

LEARNING APPLICATION

Critical Thinking

1. You are a recent high school graduate and have decided to pursue medical assisting as a career. What will you do to find a school offering an accredited program? Is accreditation important? How might your school selection impact your future as a professional medical assistant?

_____

_____

_____

_____

_____

2. After graduation you plan to sit for the certification examination. How will you prepare for the examination to ensure a positive outcome and earn your CMA/RMA credential?

_____

_____

_____

_____

_____

_____

_____

_____

_____

3. After graduating from an accredited program, you immediately went to work as a medical assistant. Now that you have been working several years you decide to become credentialed. How will you achieve this?

_____

_____

_____

_____

_____

_____

_____

Case Studies

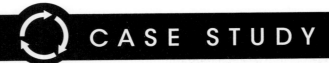

CASE STUDY

Michele Lucas is performing her practicum at Inner City Health Care under the direction of office manager Jane O'Hara. Michele has purchased a certification review study guide and has taken the sample 120-question certification examination available from the AAMA. From her studies, she has determined that she needs more work in the areas of collections and insurance processing. Part-time administrative medical assistant Karen Ritter is responsible for these duties at Inner City Health Care, under Jane's supervision.

CASE STUDY REVIEW QUESTIONS

1. How can Michele use her practicum experience to help her concentrate on improving her skills in the area of collections and insurance processing?

   _____

   _____

   _____

   _____

   _____

2. What are your own personal strengths and weaknesses in preparing for a certification examination through AAMA, AMT, or NHA? What can you do to improve your areas of weakness?

   _____

   _____

   _____

Web Activities

Using the Internet, search your local and state AAMA or AMT Web sites. Print and turn in to your instructor the location, meeting schedules, and any upcoming events planned for your state. Review the certification process that applies to your program.

CHAPTER POST-TEST

Perform this test without looking at your book.

1. 35 percent of the examination given by the AMT consists of:
    a. physical examinations
    b. general medical assisting knowledge
    c. administrative medical assisting
    d. clinical medical assisting

2. _____ through the AAMA can be achieved either by reexamination or by the continuing education method.

   a. Credentialing

   b. Recertification

   c. Certification

   d. Registration

3. Only graduates of CAAHEP- and _____-accredited medical assisting programs may sit for the Certified Medical Assistant exam.

   a. NHA

   b. AAMA

   c. ABHES

   d. CMAS

4. The AAMA certification examination questions are formulated by the:

   a. TFTC

   b. NHA

   c. CAAHEP

   d. ABHES

5. A total of _____ points are necessary to recertify the CMA (AAMA) credential.

   a. 50

   b. 70

   c. 65

   d. 60

SELF-ASSESSMENT

1. Think of two different places where you could get continuing education credits.

   a. Investigate each one.

   b. Write a paragraph on the benefits and disadvantages of each method for you and your lifestyle.

2. Find out when and where your local chapter meetings are held.

   a. Attend a meeting with a classmate.

   b. Discuss what you learned from the meeting.

3. What can you do to prepare for the national certification examination?

   a. Write a plan in which you determine how much time you have to prepare and what you will accomplish each week/month in preparation.

   b. Make a calendar showing the steps toward your examination date.

   c. Try to stick with the plan as you progress closer to the examination date.

CHAPTER **48**

Employment Strategies

CHAPTER PRE-TEST

Perform this test without looking at your book.

1. Medical insurance, a 401K program, and stock options are all examples of:
   a. Bullet points
   b. Benefits
   c. Transferable skills
   d. Accomplishment statements

2. A(n) _____ is a summary data sheet or a brief account of qualifications and progress in a career you have chosen.
   a. résumé
   b. contact tracker
   c. cover letter
   d. accomplishment statement

3. Which of the following is not an advantage of a functional resume?
   a. You want to emphasize a management growth pattern
   b. You are changing careers
   c. You have extensive specialized experience
   d. You are reentering the job market after an absence

4. The _____ is best for focusing on a clear, specific job target.
   a. functional resume
   b. chronological resume
   c. targeted resume
   d. basic resume

5. Which of the following are top errors found in resumes?

   a. Lack of power verbs and keywords

   b. Typographical errors

   c. Stating objectives that do not focus on the needs of the employer

   d. All of the above

VOCABULARY BUILDER

Misspelled Words

Find the words listed below that are misspelled; circle them, and correctly spell them in the spaces provided. Then match each correct vocabulary term to the aspect of the job-seeking process that best describes it.

accomplishment statement	cover letter	refrences
application form	cronological résumé	résumé
bullat point	functional résumé	targeted résumé
career objective	intervue	
contact tracker	power verbs	

_____   _____

_____   _____

_____   1. Expresses your career goal and the position for which you are applying

_____   2. Résumé format used to highlight specialty areas of accomplishments and strengths

_____   3. A form devised by a prospective employer to collect information relative to qualifications, education, and experience in employment

_____   4. Individuals who have known or worked with you long enough to make an honest assessment and recommendation regarding your background history

_____   5. Résumé format used when focusing on a clear, specific job

_____   6. A statement that begins with a power verb and gives a brief description of what you did and the demonstrable results that were produced

_____   7. Asterisk or dot followed by a descriptive phrase

_____   8. A written summary data sheet or brief account of your qualifications and progress in your chosen career

_____   9. Action words used to describe your attributes and strengths

_____   10. A letter used to introduce yourself and your résumé to a prospective employer with the goal of obtaining an interview

_____   11. Résumé format used when you have employment experience

_____   12. A meeting in which you discuss employment opportunities and strengths that you can bring to the organization

_____   13. Form used to keep track of employment contact information, such as name of employer, name of contact person, address and telephone number, date of first contact, résumé sent, interview date, and follow-up information and dates

LEARNING REVIEW

Short Answer

1. List three types of professionals that would make excellent reference choices.

   _____

   _____

2. Identify an individual that you know personally, or have contact with, who fits each professional reference type listed above, and explain why you think they would be an excellent reference for you.

   _____

   _____

3. Identify the situations in which using a targeted résumé is advantageous by circling the number next to the statements that apply.

   (1) You are just starting your career and have little experience, but you know what you want and you are clear about your capabilities.

   (2) You want to use one résumé for several different applications.

   (3) You are not clear about your abilities and accomplishments.

   (4) You can go in several directions, and you want a different résumé for each.

   (5) You are able to keep your résumé on a computer or flash drive.

4. Identify the situations in which using a chronological résumé is advantageous by circling the number next to the statements that apply.

   (1) The position is in a highly traditional field.

   (2) Your job history shows real growth and development.

   (3) You are changing career goals.

   (4) You are looking for your first job.

   (5) You are staying in the same field as prior jobs.

5. Identify the situations in which using a functional résumé is advantageous by circling the number next to the statements that apply.

   (1) You have extensive specialized experience.

   (2) Your most recent employers have been highly prestigious.

   (3) You have had a variety of different, apparently unconnected, work experiences.

   (4) You want to emphasize a management growth pattern.

   (5) Much of your work has been volunteer, freelance, or temporary.

6. List four items that are important when completing a job application.

   _____

   _____

   _____

   _____

7. Bob Thompson has an interview at Inner City Health Care for a new clinical medical assisting position. He is confident that he has prepared well for the interview. On the way to the interview, Bob reminds himself of three principles he has learned about interviewing:

   (1) _____ before answering questions, and try to provide the information requested in a professional manner.

   (2) _____ carefully so that you understand what information the interviewer is requesting.

   (3) _____ if you are uncertain.

8. How would you "dress for success" when preparing for your interview?

   _____

   _____

   _____

   _____

   _____

   _____

CERTIFICATION REVIEW

These questions are designed to mimic the certification examination. Select the best response.

1. Telling your friends, family, personal provider, dentist, and ophthalmologist that you are looking for a position in health care is called:

   a. networking

   b. references

   c. professionalism

   d. critiquing

2. Summarizing employment is acceptable on a résumé if it is prior to how many years ago?

   a. 1 year

   b. 5 years

   c. 10 years

   d. 15 years

3. The type of résumé that should be developed by someone who is just starting a career and has little experience is a(n):

   a. targeted résumé

   b. chronological résumé

   c. functional résumé

   d. objective résumé

4. Poise includes such things as:

   a. skill level

   b. confidence and appearance

   c. a and b

   d. none of the above

5. Providing a second opportunity to express your interest in an organization and a position may be done with a:

   a. cover letter

   b. recommendation letter

   c. follow-up letter

   d. strategic letter

6. Your attitude is reflected in how you react to:

   a. taking direction

   b. seeking excellence or doing just enough to get by

   c. assuming responsibility for your actions and considering your problems not to be someone else's fault

   d. all of the above

7. Some examples of transferable skills are *(circle all that apply):*

   a. leadership

   b. communication

   c. keyboarding

   d. drawing blood

8. When using someone as a reference, you should:

   a. always ask permission first before the name is printed on the reference list

   b. use your relatives

   c. verify correct spelling, title, place of employment and position, and telephone number

   d. a and c

9. Circle the top errors found with résumés.

   a. Typographical and grammatical errors

   b. Not mentioning jobs having transferable skills

   c. Using the same résumé for all job applications

   d. Listing your credentials

10. During the interview, it is *not* appropriate to ask:

    a. if this is a newly created position

    b. if there are opportunities for advancement

    c. about salary, sick leave, benefits, or vacation

    d. what the interviewer considers to be the most difficult task on the job

LEARNING APPLICATION

Critical Thinking

1. Discuss the various resume styles with a classmate and how to determine which style best presents your knowledge and skills to a prospective employer.

   _____

   _____

   _____

   _____

   _____

   _____

_____
_____
_____
_____
_____

2. After reading the section discussing methods of researching a prospective employer, how will you proceed with your research?

_____
_____
_____
_____
_____

3. How will you prepare a budget for living expenses to determine job salary requirements?

_____
_____
_____

Case Studies

◯ CASE STUDY

CASE STUDY REVIEW QUESTION

1. You are the subject of this case study. Complete the Self-Evaluation Worksheet that follows. Use your answers to help you determine the working environment you are most interested in and that best suits you. The worksheet can become a useful tool when researching prospective employers to target for your exciting first job in the medical assisting profession.

SELF-EVALUATION WORKSHEET

Respond to the following questions honestly and sincerely. They are meant to assist you in self-assessment.

1. List your strongest attributes as related to people, data, or things. For example,

   Interpersonal skills related to people

   Accuracy related to data

   Mechanical ability related to things

   _____ related to _____

   _____ related to _____

   _____ related to _____

2. List your three weakest attributes related to people, data, or things.

   _____ related to _____

   _____ related to _____

   _____ related to _____

3. How do you express yourself? Excellent, good, fair, or poor?

    Orally _____ In writing _____

4. Do you work well as a leader of a group or team? Yes _____ No _____

5. Do you prefer to work alone and on your own? Yes _____ No _____

6. Can you work under stress/pressure? Yes _____ No _____

7. Do you enjoy new ideas and situations? Yes _____ No _____

8. Are you comfortable with routines/schedules? Yes _____ No _____

9. Which work setting do you prefer?

    Single-provider setting _____ Multiprovider setting _____

    Small clinic setting _____ Large clinic setting _____

    Single-specialty setting _____ Multispecialty setting _____

10. Are you willing to relocate? _____ Willing to travel? _____

Application Activities

1. In the Case Study, you completed a self-assessment form to help you find the type of working environment that you are most interested in and that best suits you. Create a contact tracker file for yourself, based on the one shown in Figure 48-2 in your textbook. Compile a list from the Yellow Pages, the Internet, want ads in your local paper, your program director, and other sources (hint: other sources are listed in the textbook).

2. Refer to Figure 48-11 in your textbook, which lists typical questions asked during an interview. Write what you would say to a potential employer in response to all of these questions. Then role play with another student, acting as interviewer and interviewee, with these questions and answers to gain confidence for an interview.

3. Recall that the interview process is a "two-way street." You, as the interviewee, should interview the employer. The text lists several example questions you might ask the interviewer during an interview. Develop a list of at least two additional questions that are important to you during the interview process.

Web Activities

1. Being prepared to answer and discuss interview questions is critical in the selection for the position opening. Using Google or your favorite search engine, search job interview questions. Many sites provide sample questions and appropriate answers. Study them and prepare a list of questions with personal responses you feel are appropriate.

2. There are some illegal interview questions based on Federal Discrimination Laws enforced by the Equal Employment Opportunity Commission. They are questions that specifically discriminate against you on the basis of:
   • Age
   • Color
   • Disability
   • Sex
   • National origin
   • Race, religion, or creed

   Using your favorite search engine, research these inappropriate questions and ways in which you might handle them appropriately. Compile a list of questions and your personal appropriate response to each. Discuss these with a classmate and role-play responding to the questions.

CHAPTER POST-TEST

Perform this test without looking at your book.

1. Which of the following is a question that should not be asked during a job interview?
   a. What is your personal mission statement?
   b. Are you married?
   c. What are your greatest strengths?
   d. How would you establish credibility quickly with our team?

2. A means of introducing yourself and submitting your resume to a potential employer with the goal of obtaining an interview:
   a. cover letter
   b. introduction
   c. bullet point
   d. functional resume

3. Keywords may include:
   a. job-specific skills
   b. types of degrees
   c. names of colleges
   d. all of the above

4. Your skills, capabilities, and any supporting accomplishments should relate to your _____:
   a. targeted résumé
   b. career objective
   c. mission statement
   d. cover letter

5. _____ should be listed on a separate sheet of paper that matches your resume.
   a. Qualifications
   b. Credentials
   c. References
   d. College degrees

SELF-ASSESSMENT

Imagine you are interviewing a recent graduate for a medical assisting position.

1. What questions might you ask during the interviewing process?

   _____

   _____

   _____

2. Do you think you could determine the best person for the job by meeting him or her just once? What else might you do to get to know the person better or get to know his or her work style better?

_____

_____

_____

3. Did the applicant use power verbs effectively? Did they pique your interest?

_____

_____

_____

_____

Comprehensive Examination

1. Which term describes false and malicious writing about another that constitutes defamation of character?
    a. Slander
    b. Assault
    c. Libel
    d. Invasion of privacy
    e. Battery

2. When reviewing a résumé, the human resources manager does NOT consider the applicant's:
    a. supplemental education
    b. unexplained gaps in employment
    c. training related to the position
    d. age, sex, and race
    e. previous experience

3. The standard of professional conduct for a certified medical assistant should be:
    a. in keeping with the AAMA Code of Ethics
    b. outlined by the provider or employer
    c. based on the Hippocratic oath
    d. in keeping with the AMA Principles of Medical Ethics
    e. determined by the state's medical practice act

4. After an interview, the applicant should:
    a. telephone to say thank you
    b. have his or her references call the interviewer
    c. telephone after 3 days to check the status of his or her application
    d. promptly send a follow-up letter
    e. send a lavish thank-you gift

5. A medical assistant must NEVER:
    a. perform a venipuncture
    b. perform a laboratory test
    c. imply that he or she is a nurse
    d. dispense a medication after a direct order from the provider
    e. give a medication after a direct order from the provider

6. Which legal principle is violated when a medical assistant practices outside his or her training?
    a. Public duty
    b. Consent
    c. Privacy rights
    d. Confidentiality
    e. Standard of care

7. Which manner of dress is appropriate for an interview?
    a. A medical assistant's uniform
    b. Evening makeup
    c. Spectacular nail polish
    d. Casual clothing
    e. Neat business attire

8. Which statement accurately describes ethics?
   a. Ethics are a personal moral philosophy of right and wrong.
   b. Ethics are a code of minimal acceptable behavior.
   c. Ethics are the state's legal standards established for a profession.
   d. Ethics are the federal legal standards established for a profession.
   e. Ethics are standards for personal behavior as established by organized religions.

9. When stressed, we may exhibit all of the following EXCEPT:
   a. anxiety
   b. objective thinking
   c. depression
   d. anger
   e. irrational behavior

10. All of the following statements about Good Samaritan laws are true EXCEPT:
    a. these laws do not provide legal protection to on-duty emergency care providers
    b. providers must act in a reasonable and prudent manner
    c. the conditions of these laws vary in each state
    d. no matter what their level of training, providers must do everything for the patient
    e. health care providers are ethically, not legally, obligated to assist in emergency situations

11. What is the purpose of the certification credential for medical assistants?
    a. The certification credential is required for graduation.
    b. The certification credential guarantees a job.
    c. The certification credential meets state registration requirements.
    d. The certification credential indicates a medical assistant's professional and technical competence.
    e. The certification credential meets state licensure requirements.

12. Consent for treatment may usually be given by:
    a. the patient's closest relative
    b. a patient in a mental institution
    c. any minor over 16
    d. the person accompanying the patient
    e. a legally competent patient

13. Who is the most important member of the health care team?
    a. The patient
    b. The provider
    c. The medical assistant
    d. The nurse
    e. The receptionist

14. All of the following cultural influences may affect communication EXCEPT:
    a. education
    b. sexual orientation
    c. ethnic heritage
    d. geographic location
    e. age

15. When the medical office wins in small claims court, the money is collected from the patient by:
    a. the bailiff
    b. the patient's insurance company
    c. the probate court
    d. the medical office
    e. the court-appointed collection agency

16. Which statement is accurate regarding the Americans with Disabilities Act (ADA)?
    a. The ADA applies only to medical practices and health care facilities.
    b. The ADA applies to all businesses.
    c. The ADA applies only to businesses with 15 or more employees.
    d. The ADA applies only to businesses with 50 or more employees.
    e. The ADA applies only to state and federal government agencies.

17. Which governmental agency requires employers to ensure employee safety concerning occupational exposure to potentially harmful substances?
    a. CDC
    b. HCFA
    c. OSHA
    d. USPS
    e. Department of Health and Human Services

18. The certifying board of which organization awards the CMA credential?
    a. AAMA
    b. AMT
    c. ABHES
    d. CAAHEP
    e. RMA

19. The certifying board of which organization awards the RMA credential?
    a. AAMA
    b. ABHES
    c. CAAHEP
    d. CMA
    e. AMT

20. How often must the CMA (AAMA) credential be renewed?
    a. Annually
    b. Every five years
    c. Biannually
    d. Every three years
    e. With every job change

21. What is the highest level in Maslow's hierarchy of needs?
    a. Safety needs
    b. Love needs
    c. Self-actualization
    d. Belongingness needs
    e. Esteem needs

22. Which of the following information is considered to be public domain?

    a. A person's sexual preference

    b. A person's police record

    c. A person's past drug addiction

    d. A person's HIV-positive status

    e. A person's alcoholism

23. The goal of the National Health Information Network is to create a:

    a. unified EMR for all health care facilities

    b. standard for computer hardware in health care facilities

    c. support network for health care facilities transitioning to EMR

    d. method of communicating EMR software program options

    e. system for exchange of health care information

24. Dr. Bennett's office will be switching to an EMR system. The office manager communicates to staff that they will be using a "remote hosted" system. This means that:

    a. the software will be run from a server in the office, which requires the purchase of only one software license

    b. the software will be installed on each individual computer, and each individual computer will require its own license

    c. the software is owned and maintained by another company, but the office will pay for the right to log in and use the system

    d. a software company will log in to the office computers in order to install and maintain the software

    e. the system will require the use of very complex hardware and additional training for staff

25. An individual who has done something that results in damage to another person or his or her property would be prosecuted under what type of law?

    a. Statute

    b. Case

    c. Breach of contract

    d. Tort

    e. Regulatory

26. Which of the following would NOT be considered an intentional tort?

    a. Defamation of character

    b. Invasion of privacy

    c. Assault

    d. Negligence

    e. Fraud

27. A patient who is undergoing a surgical procedure signs a consent for treatment. The consent would be referred to as a(n):

    a. expressed contract

    b. implied contract

    c. breach of contract

    d. tort contract

    e. consideration contract

28. Licensing for health care professionals, health department regulations, and regulations for mandatory reporting are all examples of:

    a. civil law

    b. administrative law

    c. criminal law

    d. negligent law

    e. contract law

29. A durable power of attorney document indicates:

    a. what type of medical treatment a patient wishes to have during end-of-life care

    b. who the patient would like to make decisions for him if he cannot make decisions himself

    c. what (if any) organs a patient would like to donate

    d. Do Not Resuscitate orders

    e. consent for surgical treatment

30. A medical professional who is convicted of nonfeasance would have:

    a. performed a treatment improperly

    b. performed an illegal act

    c. failed to perform necessary treatment

    d. violated confidentiality

    e. performed a duty outside her scope of practice

31. Statutes of limitation apply to everything but:

    a. negligence

    b. fraud

    c. malfeasance

    d. dereliction of duty

    e. murder

32. Health care workers are mandatory reporters in all BUT which of the following situations?

    a. Child abuse

    b. Elder abuse

    c. Alcoholism

    d. Communicable diseases

    e. Death

33. Which of the following is true of HIPAA?

    a. Hospitals are prevented from releasing homicide or other crime-related information to law enforcement agencies.

    b. Students performing internships may not have access to computer systems in health care facilities.

    c. The HIPAA prevents health care facilities from sharing information with health care providers who are not their employees even when the information is essential for patient treatment.

    d. Health care facilities should appoint a privacy officer and adopt procedures for handling requests.

    e. HIPAA regulations do not apply to patients seeking care under government assistance programs.

34. The stage of grief in which patients attempt to make promises in order to change their situation would be considered:

    a. denial

    b. bargaining

    c. anger

    d. depression

    e. acceptance

35. End-of-life palliative care is most often provided by:

    a. hospice

    b. acute care hospitals

    c. rehabilitation hospitals

    d. skilled nursing facilities

    e. assisted living facilities

36. The AAMA code of ethics for medical assistants includes statements about each of the following EXCEPT:

    a. honor

    b. confidentiality

    c. continuing education

    d. improving community

    e. supervising provider

37. A medical office that transmits information over a wireless network must ensure that:

    a. the network allows staff to transmit information from home

    b. the network allows the provider to transmit information while doing patient visits at the hospital

    c. each staff member understands the encryption of the network

    d. the network meets HIPAA guidelines

    e. the network can be accessed by the appropriate insurance companies

38. Advanced Beneficiary Notices must be used for patients with what type of insurance?

    a. Medicaid

    b. Workers Compensation

    c. Medicare

    d. Blue Cross/Blue Shield

    e. TRICARE

39. Which of the following helps a medical assistant to manage time well?

    a. Reading email while answering patient calls

    b. Asking patients to jot down their complaints in their charts

    c. Asking patients to email rather than call with questions

    d. Asking front office staff to obtain patients' complaint

    e. Identifying priorities

40. Which of the following is NOT an important quality for a medical assistant?

    a. Ability to manage time efficiently

    b. Ability to delegate

    c. Initiative

    d. Flexibility

    e. Ability to work as a team member

41. Which of the following is an important aspect of verbal communication?
    a. Facial expressions
    b. Appearance
    c. Tone of voice
    d. Body language
    e. Gestures

42. The most important component of the message you communicate is:
    a. perception of the person receiving the message
    b. tone of voice
    c. the vocabulary used
    d. facial expression
    e. body language

43. Nancy, the medical assistant you work with, always changes the subject when you bring up topics that she does not want to discuss. This behavior would be considered:
    a. assertive
    b. passive
    c. aggressive
    d. professional
    e. passive-aggressive

44. Which of the following is NOT considered a part of negligence?
    a. Duty
    b. Dereliction
    c. Denial
    d. Direct cause
    e. Damages

45. The "base" of a medical word is called the:
    a. prefix
    b. suffix
    c. combining form
    d. root
    e. anatomical

46. The provider you are working with asks you to place a bandage just proximal to the knee. You would place the bandage:
    a. just below the knee
    b. on the front of the knee
    c. on the back of the knee
    d. just above the knee
    e. covering the entire knee area from top to bottom

47. You read a medical report that indicates that a provider made an incision from the superior to the inferior portion of the heart during a surgery. This means that the incision was made in the:
    a. frontal plane
    b. coronal plane
    c. transverse plane
    d. superior plane
    e. horizontal plane

48. The sac that covers the heart is referred to as the:
    a. pericardium
    b. epicardium
    c. endocardium
    d. myocardium
    e. mediastinum

49. The structure that is responsible for the formation of urine is the:
    a. medulla
    b. cortex
    c. nephron
    d. major calyx
    e. minor calyx

50. The congenital disorder that involves one or more vertebrae that do not close is called:
    a. cerebral palsy
    b. muscular dystrophy
    c. Tay-Sachs disease
    d. spina bifida
    e. hydrocele

51. Which of the following is a characteristic of a malignant tumor?
    a. Smooth borders
    b. Irregular shape
    c. Slow growth
    d. Well-differentiated cells
    e. Encapsulation

52. Muscular movements that are out of conscious control (e.g., the heart beating) are called:
    a. voluntary
    b. involuntary
    c. agonist
    d. antagonist
    e. synergistic

53. The type of joint that allows for the greatest range of motion is the:
    a. hinge
    b. suture
    c. pivot
    d. cartilaginous
    e. ball and socket

54. The portion of the brain that is responsible for higher thought processes such as logical thinking is the:
    a. parietal lobe
    b. frontal lobe
    c. occipital lobe
    d. temporal lobe
    e. cerebellum

55. An individual with a blood type of O positive is considered:

    a. a universal recipient

    b. ineligible to donate

    c. able to donate only to people with O positive blood

    d. able to donate only to people with only O negative blood

    e. a universal donor

56. The type of immunity that is developed from being vaccinated is:

    a. naturally acquired active immunity

    b. artificially acquired passive immunity

    c. artificially acquired active immunity

    d. naturally acquired passive immunity

    e. naturally acquired active passive immunity

57. An X-ray study that is shot from the back of the person toward the front would be considered:

    a. AP

    b. lateral

    c. oblique

    d. PA

    e. transverse

58. Which of the following is NOT a portion of the large intestine?

    a. Duodenum

    b. Cecum

    c. Transverse colon

    d. Rectum

    e. Ascending colon

59. When performing screening, the medical assistant must:

    a. diagnose patients' symptoms

    b. prioritize patients' needs

    c. allow patients to determine their own needs

    d. schedule patients in the order in which they arrive

    e. evaluate patients' ability to pay

60. A person with a hypersensitivity to a bee sting may go into:

    a. cardiac arrest

    b. neurogenic shock

    c. anaphylactic shock

    d. seizures

    e. respiratory shock

61. All of the following statements about shock are accurate EXCEPT:

    a. there is inadequate circulation to body parts

    b. the patient's body is kept warm to prevent chilling

    c. the patient's pulse becomes rapid and weak

    d. the medical assistant can administer medication as ordered by the provider

    e. the patient's blood pressure increases

62. Which of the following is a major disadvantage of NOT seeking care for an illness until it becomes very advanced?

    a. The patient does not have time to deal with death.

    b. Pain management and treatment may not work as well as they could have.

    c. The family can prepare without frightening the patient.

    d. Denial postpones the inevitable.

    e. The patient does not have time to create advance directives.

63. Redirecting a socially unacceptable impulse into one that is socially acceptable is called:

    a. regression

    b. repression

    c. projection

    d. sublimation

    e. denial

64. You are a medical assistant in an ambulatory care facility, and an emergency situation arises. What should you do first?

    a. Notify the provider.

    b. Give first aid.

    c. Assess the patient.

    d. Call 911.

    e. Evaluate the causes.

65. The act of evaluating the urgency of a medical situation and prioritizing treatment is known as:

    a. screening

    b. empathy

    c. trauma

    d. diagnosing

    e. triage

66. Which condition is detected with the Mantoux test?

    a. HIV

    b. Syphilis

    c. PKU

    d. TB

    e. Infectious mononucleosis

67. Which of the following is used as a contrast medium for a radiographic lower GI examination?

    a. Air

    b. Iodine salts

    c. Water

    d. A barium swallow

    e. A barium enema

68. Which type of pathogen causes mumps, measles, and chickenpox?

    a. Bacteria

    b. Viruses

    c. Spirochetes

    d. Parasites

    e. Rickettsiae

69. Which body system does the acronym PERRLA refer to?

    a. Cardiovascular system

    b. Gastrointestinal system

    c. Nervous system

    d. Respiratory system

    e. Urogenital system

70. Which term means difficulty breathing?

    a. Apnea

    b. Bradypnea

    c. Tachypnea

    d. Eupnea

    e. Dyspnea

71. Which of the following statements is accurate regarding vitamins?

    a. Vitamins A, B, D, and E are fat soluble.

    b. Vitamins are needed in large quantities.

    c. Water-soluble vitamins are stored in fatty tissues.

    d. Vitamins are simple molecules.

    e. Vitamins B and C are water soluble.

72. Which statement is accurate regarding ventricular tachycardia?

    a. Ventricular tachycardia causes severe chest pain.

    b. Ventricular tachycardia is life threatening.

    c. Ventricular tachycardia is often seen in patients using depressants.

    d. Ventricular tachycardia has a cardiac cycle that occurs early.

    e. Ventricular tachycardia occurs in healthy people.

73. Which genetic disorder is characterized by mental retardation?

    a. Sickle cell anemia

    b. Huntington's disease

    c. Down syndrome

    d. Cystic fibrosis

    e. Pernicious anemia

74. Which type of nutrient contains the most calories per gram?

    a. Carbohydrate

    b. Protein

    c. Mineral

    d. Fat

    e. Vitamin

75. Which term describes a reason why a medication should NOT be administered?

    a. Side effect

    b. Contraindication

    c. Potentiation

    d. Idiosyncratic

    e. Cross-tolerance

76. Robby is coming down with chickenpox but does not have any symptoms yet. He is now at the:
    a. acute stage
    b. convalescent stage
    c. declining stage
    d. incubation stage
    e. prodromal stage

77. Which of the following statements about medical asepsis hand washing is accurate?
    a. Medical assistants should turn the faucet on with a clean, dry paper towel.
    b. Medical assistants should hold their hands upward.
    c. Medical assistants should scrub up to their elbows.
    d. Medical assistants should touch only the inside of the sink with their hands.
    e. Medical assistants should turn off the faucet with a used paper towel.

78. Which of these positions is used for the treatment and examination of the back and buttocks?
    a. Trendelenburg
    b. Dorsal recumbent
    c. Lithotomy
    d. Supine
    e. Prone

79. Which term describes a woman who has never been pregnant?
    a. Multigravida
    b. Nullipara
    c. Nulligravida
    d. Multipara
    e. Primipara

80. Which infection control guidelines are used by all health care professionals for all patients?
    a. Body substance isolation guidelines
    b. Standard Precautions
    c. OSHA guidelines
    d. Transmission-based precautions
    e. Universal Precautions

81. All of the following are acceptable wrappings for autoclaving EXCEPT:
    a. plastic pouches
    b. muslin
    c. paper bags
    d. aluminum foil
    e. paper wrapping

82. The most common disorder of the urinary system is:
    a. renal calculi
    b. urinary tract infection
    c. glomerulonephritis
    d. cystitis
    e. pyelonephritis

83. Which of the following diseases is sexually transmitted?
    a. Pelvic inflammatory disease
    b. Cervical cancer
    c. Endometriosis
    d. Prostatitis
    e. Ovarian cancer

84. Which term describes an infection of the middle ear?
    a. Otitis externa
    b. Otalgia
    c. Otitis media
    d. Otorrhagia
    e. Otosclerosis

85. Which condition is commonly known as fainting?
    a. Tinnitus
    b. Singultus
    c. Bruit
    d. Syncope
    e. Vertigo

86. Which of the following is a progressive degenerative disease of the liver?
    a. Hepatitis A
    b. Cholecystitis
    c. Hepatomegaly
    d. Hepatitis B
    e. Cirrhosis

87. Which type of injection is made into the fatty layer just below the skin?
    a. Intramuscular
    b. Subcutaneous
    c. Intradermal
    d. Intravenous
    e. Intermuscular

88. An elevation of which blood cell count indicates the presence of inflammation in the body?
    a. Platelet count
    b. Erythrocyte sedimentation rate
    c. Hematocrit
    d. Total hemoglobin
    e. White blood cell differentiation

89. What condition is characterized by an abnormal thickening and hardening of the skin?
    a. Acne
    b. Melanoma
    c. Dermatophytosis
    d. Scleroderma
    e. Psoriasis

90. Who discovered penicillin?

    a. Sir Alexander Fleming

    b. Robert Koch

    c. Louis Pasteur

    d. Joseph Lister

    e. Edward Jenner

91. Homeostasis refers to what?

    a. A sterile environment

    b. A complete procedure

    c. Everyone getting along

    d. Internal equilibrium

    e. Rapid heart rate

92. The classification of drugs with the lowest potential of abuse is:

    a. Schedule IV

    b. Schedule I

    c. Schedule V

    d. Schedule II

    e. Schedule III

93. The provider you are working with asks you to provide a patient with samples of a new medication. By doing so, you are:

    a. prescribing medication

    b. administering medication

    c. compounding medication

    d. mixing medication

    e. dispensing medication

94. Which of the following is information about a medication that is NOT found in the PDR?

    a. Indications for use

    b. The shape of each pill

    c. Dosage and administration route

    d. Precautions

    e. Generic name

95. A drug that increases the effect of another has which type of effect?

    a. Local

    b. Remote

    c. Synergistic

    d. Systemic

    e. Topical

96. A medication that is ordered to be delivered in a sublingual route would be:

    a. placed in the cheek

    b. swallowed

    c. inserted into the rectum

    d. placed under the tongue

    e. placed on top of the tongue

97. A medication that is classified as an expectorant would have what effect?

    a. Dilate bronchi

    b. Prevent coughing

    c. Relax blood vessels

    d. Decrease nausea

    e. Increase the amount of mucus being expelled

98. A medication that increases the amount of urine excreted by the body would be classified as a(n):

    a. diuretic

    b. antiarrhythmic

    c. antiemetic

    d. vasopressor

    e. muscle relaxant

99. All of the following are part of a medication order EXCEPT:

    a. name of drug

    b. who dispenses the medication

    c. form of drug

    d. route of administration

    e. prescribing provider's signature

100. A prescription that indicates a medication should be administered "OD" would go where?

    a. Left eye

    b. Right ear

    c. Left ear

    d. Right eye

    e. In the nose

101. The metric prefix which refers to one-millionth of a unit is:

    a. milli

    b. kilo

    c. meter

    d. gram

    e. micro

102. Pediatric medication dosages are figured based on the child's:

    a. height

    b. age

    c. weight

    d. gender

    e. chest circumference

103. A patient weighs 130 pounds. The provider asked you to convert that weight into kilograms. You know that there are 2.2 pounds in 1 kilogram. How many kilograms does this patient weigh?

    a. 4.55 kg

    b. 59.09 kg

    c. 286 kg

    d. .07 kg

    e. 260 kg

104. Which of the following is NOT 1 of the 6 rights of medication administration?

    a. Dose

    b. Provider

    c. Route

    d. Patient

    e. Drug

105. Parenteral medication is administered via:

    a. the mouth

    b. the rectum

    c. the skin

    d. inhalation

    e. an injection

106. The type of injection that is administered at a 90-degree angle is:

    a. subcutaneous

    b. intradermal

    c. intravenous

    d. inhaled

    e. intramuscular

107. Hypodermic needles are most appropriate for what?

    a. Venipuncture

    b. Aspirations

    c. Allergy injections

    d. Intramuscular and subcutaneous injections

    e. Insulin administration

108. Which of the following is NOT an appropriate injection site for an intramuscular injection?

    a. Dorsogluteal

    b. Biceps

    c. Ventrogluteal

    d. Deltoid

    e. Vastus lateralis

109. The yellow portion of the safety warning label indicates which of the following?

    a. Chemical instability

    b. Health hazard

    c. Fire hazard

    d. PPE requirements

    e. Biohazard level

110. A chemical that is extremely flammable would be given a safety rating of:

    a. 3

    b. 2

    c. 1

    d. 4

    e. 0

111. The component of blood that is responsible for clotting is:
    a. erythrocyte
    b. leukocyte
    c. plasma
    d. serum
    e. thrombocyte

112. Which of the following substances is NOT a normal component of urine?
    a. Ammonia
    b. Blood
    c. Creatinine
    d. Urea
    e. Water

113. The type of urine sample that requires a patient to avoid eating and drinking prior to voiding is:
    a. 24-hour
    b. first-morning
    c. fasting
    d. random
    e. catheter collection

114. Which of the following is NOT a component of the physical examination of urine?
    a. Volume
    b. Color
    c. Unusual
    d. Specific gravity
    e. pH

115. Casts found in urine are formed from:
    a. carbohydrates
    b. lipids
    c. calcium
    d. proteins
    e. potassium

116. Exposing bacterial growth to an antibiotic in order to determine effective treatment of an infection is called:
    a. culturing
    b. taxonomy
    c. sensitivity testing
    d. inoculation
    e. Gram stain

117. The disease of the eye that is characterized by an elevated intraocular pressure is:
    a. cataract
    b. glaucoma
    c. macular degeneration
    d. amblyopia
    e. strabismus

118. The mineral that is important for the formation of bone tissue is:
    a. calcium
    b. potassium
    c. zinc
    d. iron
    e. magnesium

119. Which of the following is a type of bacteria?
    a. Streptococci
    b. Helminth
    c. Protozoa
    d. Tinea
    e. Scabies

120. Diseases caused by which type of pathogen are treated by antibiotics?
    a. Protozoa
    b. Fungi
    c. Bacteria
    d. Virus
    e. Parasite

121. Personal protective equipment should always be used in each of the following situations EXCEPT:
    a. handling or processing a urine specimen
    b. taking vital signs
    c. performing venipuncture
    d. assisting with surgical procedures
    e. disinfecting instruments

122. A worker who is exposed to bodily fluids through an accidental needlestick from a contaminated needle should immediately flush the area with:
    a. alcohol
    b. hydrogen peroxide
    c. betadine
    d. bleach
    e. water

123. Which immunization must be available free to all health care employees?
    a. Hepatitis A
    b. Hepatitis C
    c. Hepatitis B
    d. HIV
    e. TB

124. Use of alcohol-based hand rub is acceptable in which of the following situations?
    a. Before and after eating
    b. Before and after using the rest room
    c. After contact with body excretions
    d. After decontamination of a work area
    e. Following processing of microbiologic specimens

125. Which of the following is NOT an OSHA requirement for housekeeping in a medical setting?

   a. Routine decontamination of reusable containers

   b. Double-bagged soiled linens

   c. Biohazard waste collected in impermeable red containers

   d. Sharps containers stored in an upright condition

   e. Alcohol-based hand rub available at all times

126. Materials Safety Data Sheet (MSDS):

   a. is used for training programs only

   b. commends manufacturers

   c. must be assembled and maintained

   d. indicates when not to use PPE

   e. briefly explains the level of risk for each product

127. When performing CPR on an infant or child, circulation is checked by assessing pulse at which pulse point?

   a. Carotid

   b. Axial

   c. Femoral

   d. Brachial

   e. Dorsal pedis

128. The method used to clear an airway obstruction in an unconscious adult is:

   a. finger sweep

   b. back blows

   c. chest thrust

   d. two rescue breaths

   e. CPR

129. A burn that has penetrated to the bone would be considered:

   a. superficial

   b. partial thickness

   c. 100%

   d. full thickness

   e. 75%

130. Which of the following is NOT a step in controlling bleeding from an open wound on the arm?

   a. Applying direct pressure

   b. Elevating the arm

   c. Wrapping the wound tightly

   d. Applying pressure to the appropriate artery

   e. Disinfecting the area

131. Appropriate first aid for a patient with a case of acute frostbite would include:

   a. immersing the area in warm water

   b. warming the area by creating friction

   c. immediately raising the patient's core body temperature

   d. applying heavy moisturizing cream to the area

   e. immediately debriding necrotic tissues

132. Appropriate treatment for an acute sprain or strain would include all BUT which of the following?
    a. Ice
    b. Rest
    c. Compression
    d. Range of motion
    e. Elevation

133. A medication that is to be taken twice a day would be indicated as:
    a. qd
    b. tid
    c. qid
    d. bid
    e. od

134. Which type of manual identifies the specific methods for performing tasks?
    a. Policy
    b. Training
    c. Procedures
    d. Personnel
    e. Benefits

135. What is the primary purpose of managed care plans?
    a. To allow patients to manage their own care
    b. To control patients' access to providers
    c. To encourage patients to explore alternative medicine treatments
    d. To provide acute care only
    e. To provide comprehensive health care at a reasonable cost

136. How are claims managed when both parents are covered by health insurance?
    a. The father's plan is always primary.
    b. Claims for the family are paid according to the birthday rule.
    c. The mother's plan is always primary.
    d. Double benefits are paid for the children.
    e. The duplication of benefits rule is put into effect.

137. Why are accurate medical records legally important?
    a. Because they are needed to provide referrals
    b. Because they assist in controlling health care costs
    c. Because they aid in billing
    d. Because they are written documentation used to prove patient care
    e. Because they are essential to quality patient care

138. Meaningful use of health information technology is a term for:
    a. rules and regulations
    b. reimbursement purposes
    c. family coordination
    d. reasonable and customary fees
    e. eligible patients

139. Which type of check is used most often for writing payroll checks?

   a. Voucher check

   b. Traveler's check

   c. Certified check

   d. Cashier's check

   e. Money order

140. What is the role of a computer firewall?

   a. A computer firewall limits potential damage from viruses.

   b. A computer firewall protects the computer in the event of a fire.

   c. A computer firewall does not allow outside computers access to your computer.

   d. A computer firewall allows outside access to an office computer but not to databases.

   e. A computer firewall prevents employees from surfing the Internet for personal reasons.

141. How should a letter that requires a written receipt be mailed?

   a. Registered mail

   b. Priority mail

   c. Third-class mail

   d. Certified mail

   e. First-class mail

142. Which of the following are used in conjunction with CPT codes?

   a. V codes

   b. Preventive care codes

   c. Injury codes

   d. Modifiers

   e. E codes

143. What must happen when more than one policy pays on a claim?

   a. Coinsurance

   b. Coordination of benefits

   c. Co-pay

   d. Deductible

   e. Exclusions

144. When alphabetizing and assigning units for filing order, titles are considered:

   a. as part of the last name

   b. as the first indexing unit

   c. as the third indexing unit

   d. as part of the patient's surname

   e. as a separate unit at the end

145. A person who is injured on the job may be covered by:

   a. workers' compensation

   b. CHAMPUS

   c. Medicaid

   d. disability insurance

   e. HCFA

146. Which of the following is an advantage of accepting credit cards in an ambulatory care setting?
    a. Maintaining patient confidentiality is not a problem.
    b. There are no fees to be paid by the practice.
    c. The money is available to the practice within 1 day.
    d. The money is usually available to the practice within 10 days.
    e. Accepting credit cards eliminates having to file insurance claims.

147. What is the key to having an effective scheduling system?
    a. Accommodating patient preferences
    b. Customizing the system to the type of practice
    c. Tailoring the system to provider preferences
    d. Accommodating the requirements of the insurance carriers
    e. Effectively monitoring the use of time versus the dollars produced

148. Which scheduling system assigns two patients to the same time?
    a. Clustering
    b. Stream
    c. Modified wave
    d. Double booking
    e. Open hours

149. Which program provides health care coverage for low-income individuals?
    a. CHAMPUS
    b. Workers' compensation
    c. Medicare
    d. CHAMPVA
    e. Medicaid

150. Which of the following is a critical issue regarding the use of a fax machine in a medical office?
    a. The speed at which the machine works
    b. The time required to train personnel
    c. Compromised confidentiality due to access by unauthorized personnel
    d. The clarity of the documents received
    e. The volume of documents the machine can handle

151. Which of the following is used when there is not enough information to find a more specific code?
    a. NEC
    b. NOS
    c. CC
    d. V codes
    e. E codes

152. Which of the following tells the computer hardware what to do?
    a. Application software
    b. The motherboard
    c. The modem
    d. System software
    e. Servers

153. Which of the following conditions is most frequently related to the repetitive use of a computer?
    a. Eyestrain
    b. Fatigue
    c. Carpal tunnel syndrome
    d. Lower back pain
    e. Tension headaches

154. When seeking employment, a person who has job experience should use:
    a. a targeted résumé
    b. a functional résumé
    c. a complete résumé
    d. an information mapping résumé
    e. a chronological résumé

155. Which type of résumé highlights one's special qualities?
    a. Targeted
    b. Functional
    c. Chronologic
    d. Concise
    e. Career-oriented

156. Which statement is accurate regarding a cover letter?
    a. The cover letter may be addressed "To whom it may concern."
    b. The purpose of the cover letter is to ask for an interview.
    c. The cover letter includes résumé information.
    d. The cover letter should be bulleted.
    e. The cover letter should include a list of references.

157. Which of the following tasks is NOT assigned to the human resources manager?
    a. Creating office manuals
    b. Hiring and firing personnel
    c. Interpreting legal regulations
    d. Providing employee training
    e. Performing employee evaluations

158. Tiffany wants a well-paying position as a medical assistant. Which statement is accurate regarding her search?
    a. Every CMA (AAMA) is guaranteed a well-paying position.
    b. Using an employment agency is her most effective tool in finding a well-paying position.
    c. Networking is her most effective tool in finding a well-paying position.
    d. Running down all leads is her most effective tool in finding a well-paying position.
    e. Cold calling to offices that are not advertising will produce excellent leads.

159. Which federal law requires employers to verify the right of employees to work in the United States?
    a. Immigration Reform Act
    b. Equal Pay Act
    c. Civil Rights Act
    d. Fair Labor Standards Act
    e. Americans with Disabilities Act

160. Which of these interviewing tips is accurate?
    a. Think carefully before answering questions.
    b. Do not ask questions, as you may appear confused.
    c. Answer questions "off the cuff" so your responses do not seem rehearsed.
    d. Place your personal belongings—coat, purse, and so on—on the interviewer's desk.
    e. Give lengthy answers to all questions, even when you are not sure of the answer.

161. Which of the following statements about completing an employment application form is accurate?
    a. Write "See résumé" rather than repeating information.
    b. Using either a pen or pencil is acceptable.
    c. Try to complete the application without referring to your résumé.
    d. Complete the application quickly to demonstrate how well you work.
    e. Following instructions is very important.

162. Which of the following is the best networking resource for recruiting new personnel?
    a. Newspapers
    b. Family and friends
    c. Current employees
    d. Patients
    e. AAMA's national office

163. Which of the following is NOT vital résumé information?
    a. Home address
    b. Current telephone number
    c. Education
    d. Date of birth
    e. Work experience

164. Which payroll forms must be submitted to the Social Security Administration each year?
    a. W-4
    b. W-2
    c. W-6
    d. 1099
    e. 941

165. A policy manual should include all of the following EXCEPT:
    a. employment practices
    b. insurance billing techniques
    c. wage and salary scales
    d. evaluation schedules
    e. continuing education policies

166. In order to track inventory in an office, the most appropriate type of software to use would be:
    a. word processing
    b. billing
    c. contact management
    d. spreadsheet
    e. EMR

167. When taking a telephone message, everything BUT the following should be included:
    a. full name of person leaving message
    b. reason for the call
    c. time and date of call
    d. expected action
    e. diagnosis of the patient the message is about

168. An office operating on a wave schedule will:
    a. have groups of patients arriving at relatively the same time throughout the day
    b. schedule two patients for the same appointment time
    c. schedule patients in specific time increments (e.g., every 15 minutes)
    d. allow for walk-in patients at any time
    e. provide "catch up" time for the provider

169. When scheduling an outpatient procedure, each of the following should be completed EXCEPT:
    a. obtaining necessary preauthorizations
    b. making arrangements with the facility
    c. notifying the patient of the arrangements
    d. determining and scheduling preprocedure testing
    e. precertifying the admission

170. A block letter style includes:
    a. centered paragraphs with all other components at the left margin
    b. all components starting at the left margin
    c. centered address and signature lines with paragraphs starting at the left margin
    d. centered address, signature line, and first paragraph
    e. all components centered

171. Source-oriented medical records are organized by the:
    a. cause of a patient's medical diagnosis
    b. location of a patient's medical record
    c. nature of a patient's complaint
    d. treatment methods being used
    e. professionals who have documented in the record

172. Each of the following is objective information EXCEPT:
    a. laboratory data
    b. diagnosis
    c. prescribed treatment
    d. patient's complaint
    e. examination findings

173. Color coding medical records assists with each of the following EXCEPT:
    a. increasing efficiency with filing
    b. increasing the ability to identify filing errors
    c. identifying a patient's diagnosis
    d. identifying patients who are due for a physical during a specific month
    e. removing inactive files

174. Tickler files are helpful in:
    a. sending billing notices
    b. scheduling the provider's time
    c. providing reminders for routine medical appointments
    d. submitting insurance claims
    e. processing payroll

175. Providers' fees are generally set by each of the following descriptors EXCEPT:
    a. reasonable
    b. insurance
    c. customary
    d. usual
    e. geographic region

176. Accounts receivable refers to:
    a. money collected by a practice during a day
    b. accounts turned over to a debt collection agency
    c. money owed by the practice
    d. money owed to a practice
    e. petty cash expenditures

177. Manually posting charges usually involves each of the following EXCEPT:
    a. day sheet
    b. ledger card
    c. account summary
    d. encounter form
    e. HCFA 1500

178. The Truth in Lending Act requires:
    a. lower interest rates for medical services
    b. an increased amount of time for repayment of medical loans
    c. use of an independent billing service
    d. accurate information regarding finance charges
    e. routine billing statements

179. Calls made to a patient's home in order to collect money owed to a practice are regulated by:
    a. the Truth in Lending Act
    b. CLIA
    c. the Fair Debt Collection Act
    d. OSHA
    e. the AMA

180. Once an account has been submitted to a collection agency, the medical assistant should:
    a. discontinue sending statements to the patient
    b. continue to send routine billing statements to the patient
    c. send copies of billing statements to emergency contacts listed in the patient's chart
    d. file for legal action in small claims court
    e. telephone the patient in order to attempt to collect the debt

181. Best practices with manual bookkeeping involve all of the following EXCEPT:

    a. proficiency with 10-key typing

    b. using consistent methods

    c. writing with red ink

    d. writing numbers clearly

    e. double checking all math

182. In managing practice finances, an adjustment would be used for:

    a. recording payment

    b. recording charges

    c. indicating past due accounts

    d. indicating discounts or write-offs

    e. indicating accounts turned over to collections

183. When preparing a check to a supplier, the medical assistant should:

    a. verify the expense has been approved

    b. endorse with "for deposit only"

    c. reconcile the bank statement

    d. record the payment on the correct ledger card

    e. file a I-9 tax form

184. If an office determines it will accept personal checks as payment, it is important to:

    a. clearly post the policy

    b. implement use of a restrictive endorsement

    c. follow Truth in Lending guidelines

    d. verify policies with the practice's bank

    e. follow Fair Debt Collection Act guidelines

185. Mrs. Jones's insurance requires that she pay for $400 of medical expenses before she is eligible for insurance payment for medical services. The $400 would be referred to as:

    a. a co-payment

    b. coinsurance

    c. a deductible

    d. a premium

    e. an exclusion

186. Mr. Johnson's insurance company has stated that it will not pay for treatment of his asthma because he was known to have the disease prior to the time when his policy was purchased. His asthma would be considered a(n):

    a. exclusion

    b. preexisting condition

    c. concurrent condition

    d. secondary diagnosis

    e. subjective condition

187. The type of Medicare coverage that provides benefits for inpatient medical care is:

    a. Medicare B

    b. Medicare D

    c. Medicare E

    d. Medicare A

    e. Medicare F

188. Most managed care organizations provide a capitated payment for services. This means that:

    a. a maximum payment for services is set

    b. patients must pay excess charges out of their own pocket

    c. they will not pay for services covered by another company

    d. the government sets the maximum allowed charge for a service

    e. patients' premiums will never change

189. RBRVS payment structures are based on all EXCEPT which of the following?

    a. Level of work

    b. Malpractice expenses

    c. Regional charges

    d. Diagnosis of patient

    e. Experience of the provider

190. E codes in the ICD book are used to identify:

    a. wellness-related procedures

    b. cardiovascular diseases

    c. morphology

    d. neurologic diseases

    e. accidents

191. V codes in the ICD book are used to identify:

    a. accidents

    b. cardiovascular disease

    c. wellness-related procedures

    d. morphology

    e. neurologic diseases

192. Which of the following would be considered a commercial form of health insurance?

    a. Medicare

    b. Medicaid

    c. CHAMPUS

    d. Blue Cross/Blue Shield

    e. Workers' compensation

193. Patient Sally Kane arrives at your office as a new patient. While copying her insurance card you notice that she will need to pay 20 percent of the cost of the visit. That percentage is referred to as:

    a. co-payment

    b. coinsurance

    c. deductible

    d. premium

    e. exclusion

194. In order to accurately locate an ICD code, which section of the book would you use first?

    a. Volume II

    b. Volume I

    c. Volume III

    d. Volume IV

    e. Appendix

195. Which of the following is NOT a section in the CPT book?

    a. Anesthesia

    b. Surgery

    c. Pathology and Laboratory

    d. Rehabilitation

    e. Medicine

196. Deliberately billing a service at a higher level than what was completed would be considered:

    a. downcoding

    b. bundling

    c. unbundling

    d. upcoding

    e. proper procedure

197. A business letter sent from an office would be processed through which class of mail?

    a. Second class

    b. Third class

    c. First class

    d. Fourth class

    e. Priority

198. Hospital inpatient payments are based on:

    a. APG

    b. DRG

    c. usual fees

    d. reasonable fees

    e. customary fees

199. Electronic charts corrections are made by:

    a. hitting the delete key

    b. hitting the backspace key

    c. using the word processing strike-through feature

    d. using the word processing tracking device

    e. hitting a different color font

200. Dr. Abernathy provides you with the accompanying growth chart and asks you to explain it to the child's mother, who is concerned that the child is not as tall as other children his age. You would explain to the mother that:

    a. the child is actually slightly above average on the growth chart

    b. the child is actually slightly below average on the growth chart

    c. the child is actually well above average on the growth chart

    d. the child is actually well below average on the growth chart

    e. the child is of average height on the growth chart

CDC Growth Charts: United States

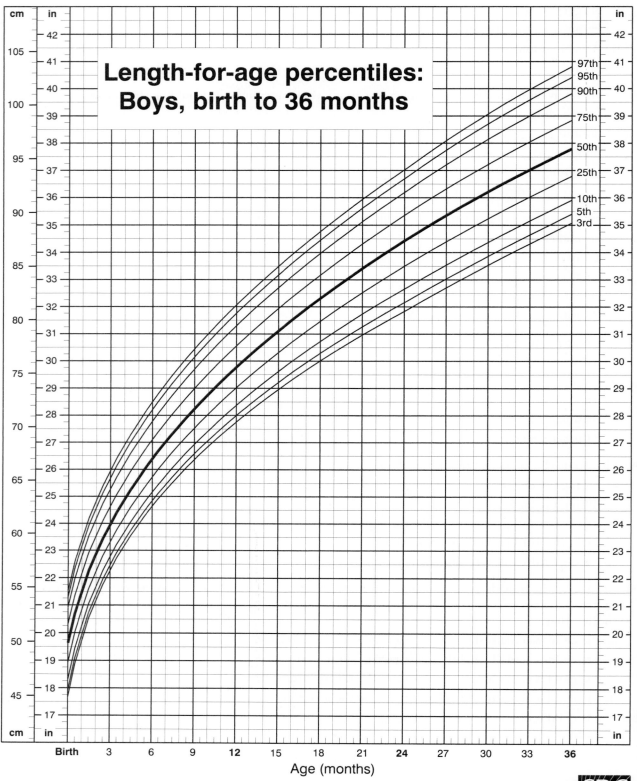

Length-for-age percentiles:
Boys, birth to 36 months

Age (months)

Published May 30, 2000.
SOURCE: Developed by the National Center for Health Statistics in collaboration with
the National Center for Chronic Disease Prevention and Health Promotion (2000).

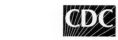

SAFER · HEALTHIER · PEOPLE™

Courtesy of the Centers for Disease Control and Prevention